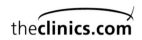

RADIOLOGIC CLINICS
of North America

Multidetector CT of the Abdomen

JOHN R. HAAGA, MD
DEAN A. NAKAMOTO, MD
Guest Editors

November 2005 • Volume 43 • Number 6

SAUNDERS

An Imprint of Elsevier, Inc.
PHILADELPHIA   LONDON   TORONTO   MONTREAL   SYDNEY   TOKYO

W.B. SAUNDERS COMPANY
A Division of Elsevier Inc.

1600 John F. Kennedy Boulevard • Suite 1800 • Philadelphia, Pennsylvania 19103-2899

http://www.theclinics.com

RADIOLOGIC CLINICS OF NORTH AMERICA	**Volume 43, Number 6**
November 2005	**ISSN 0033-8389**
Editor: Barton Dudlick	**ISBN 1-4160-2763-7**

Reprints: For copies of 100 or more, of articles in this publication, please contact the Commercial Reprints Department, Elsevier Inc., 360 Park Avenue South, New York, New York 10010-1710. Tel.: (+1) 212-633-3813; Fax: (+1) 212-462-1935; E-mail: reprints@elsevier.com.

The ideas and opinions expressed in *Radiologic Clinics of North America* do not necessarily reflect those of the Publisher. The Publisher does not assume any responsibility for any injury and/or damage to persons or property arising out of or related to any use of the material contained in this periodical. The reader is advised to check the appropriate medical literature and the product information currently provided by the manufacturer of each drug to be administered to verify the dosage, the method and duration of administration, or contraindications. It is the responsibility of the treating physician or other health care professional, relying on independent experience and knowledge of the patient, to determine drug dosages and the best treatment for the patient. Mention of any product in this issue should not be construed as endorsement by the contributors, editors, or the Publisher of the product or manufacturers' claims.

Radiologic Clinics of North America   (ISSN 0033-8389) is published bimonthly by W.B. Saunders Company. Corporate and editorial offices: 1600 John F. Kennedy Boulevard, Suite 1800, Philadelphia, Pennsylvania 19103-2899. Accounting and circulation offices: 6277 Sea Harbor Drive, Orlando, FL 32887-4800. Periodicals postage paid at Orlando, FL 32862, and additional mailing offices. Subscription prices are USD 235 per year for US individuals, USD 350 per year for US institutions, USD 115 per year for US students and residents, USD 275 per year for Canadian individuals, USD 430 per year for Canadian institutions, USD 320 per year for international individuals, USD 430 per year for international institutions and USD 155 per year for Canadian and foreign students/residents. To receive student and resident rate, orders must be accompanied by name of affiliated institution, date of term, and the *signature* of program/residency coordinator on institution letterhead. Orders will be billed at individual rate until proof of status is received. Foreign air speed delivery is included in all *Clinics* subscription prices. All prices are subject to change without notice. POSTMASTER: Send address changes to *Radiologic Clinics of North America,* W.B. Saunders Company, Periodicals Fulfillment, Orlando, FL 32887-4800. **Customer Service: 1-800-654-2452 (US). From outside of the US, call (+1) 407-345-4000.**

Radiologic Clinics of North America also is published in Greek by Paschalidis Medical Publications, Athens, Greece.

Radiologic Clinics of North America is covered in *Index Medicus, EMBASE/Excerpta Medica, Current Contents/Life Sciences, Current Contents/Clinical Medicine, RSNA Index to Imaging Literature, BIOSIS, Science Citation Index,* and *ISI/BIOMED.*

Printed in the United States of America.

GOAL STATEMENT

The goal of the *Radiologic Clinics of North America* is to keep practicing radiologists and radiology residents up to date with current clinical practice in radiology by providing timely articles reviewing the state of the art in-patient care.

ACCREDITATION

The *Radiologic Clinics of North America* is planned and implemented in accordance with the Essential Areas and Policies of the Accreditation Council for Continuing Medical Education (ACCME) through the joint sponsorship of the University of Virginia School of Medicine and Elsevier. The University of Virginia School of Medicine is accredited by the ACCME to provide continuing medical education for physicians.

The University of Virginia School of Medicine designates this educational activity for a maximum of 90 category 1 credits per year, 15 category 1 credits per issue, toward the AMA Physician's Recognition Award. Each physician should claim only those credits that he/she actually spent in the activity.

The American Medical Association has determined that physicians not licensed in the US who participate in this CME activity are eligible for AMA PRA category 1 credit.

AMA PRA category 1 credit can be earned by reading the text material, taking the examination online at http://www.theclinics.com/home/cme, and completing the evaluation. After taking the test, your will be required to review any and all incorrect answers. Following completion of the test and the evaluation, your credit will be awarded and you may print your certificate.

FACULTY DISCLOSURE/CONFLICT OF INTEREST

The University of Virginia School of Medicine, as an ACCME accredited provider, endorses and strives to comply with the Accreditation Council for Continuing Medical Education (ACCME) Standards of Commercial Support, Commonwealth of Virginia statutes, University of Virginia policies and procedures, and associated federal and private regulations and guidelines on the need for disclosure and monitoring of proprietary and financial interests that may affect the scientific integrity and balance of content delivered in continuing medical education activities under our auspices.

The University of Virginia School of Medicine requires that all CME activities accredited through this institution be developed independently and be scientifically rigorous, balanced and objective in the presentation/discussion of its content, theories and practices.

All authors/editors participating in an accredited CME activity are expected to disclose to the readers relevant financial relationships with commercial entities occurring within the past 12 months (such as grants or research support, employee, consultant, stock holder, member of speakers bureau, etc.). The University of Virginia School of Medicine will employ appropriate mechanisms to resolve potential conflicts of interest to maintain the standards of fair and balanced education to the reader. Questions about specific strategies can be directed to the Office of Continuing Medical Education, University of Virginia School of Medicine, Charlottesville, Virginia.

The authors/editors listed below have identified no financial or professional relationships for themselves or their spouse/partner:
Shweta Bhatt, MD; Vikram S. Dogra, MD; Barton Dudlick; John R. Haaga, MD; Ihab R. Kamel, MD, PhD; Preet S. Kang, MD; Eleni Liapi, MD; Lisa A. Miller, MD; Raj Mohan Paspulati, MD; Michael A. Patak, MD; J. Thomas Payne, PhD; Tatiana C. Rocha, MD; Pablo R. Ros, MD, MPH; Deborah J. Rubens, MD; Geoffrey D. Rubin, MD; and, Kristina A. Siddall, MD.

The authors/editors listed below have identified financial or professional relationships for themselves or their spouse/partner:
Matthew A. Barish, MD is a consultant and patent holder for Barco, Inc., and is on the speakers' bureau for EZ-EM, Inc. (virtual colonoscopy).
Elliot K. Fishman, MD is a consultant for Siemens Medical Solutions and GE Healthcare, and additionally the co-founder of Hip Graphics, Inc.
Koenraad J. Mortele, MD is a consultant for EZ-EM, Inc.

The authors listed below have not provided disclosures for themselves or their spouse/partner:
Jeffrey C. Hellinger, MD; Mark D. Hiatt, MD; Ercan Kocakoc, MD; Dean A. Nakamoto, MD; K. Shanmuganathan, MD; James W. Spain, MD, PhD; and, Dominik Fleischmann, MD.

Disclosure of Discussion of Non-FDA Approved Uses for Pharmaceutical and/or Medical Devices:
The University of Virginia School of Medicine, as an ACCME provider, requires that all authors identify and disclose any "off label" uses for pharmaceutical and medical device products. The University of Virginia School of Medicine recommends that each physician fully review all the available data on new products or procedures prior to clinical use.

TO ENROLL

To enroll in the Radiologic Clinics of North America Continuing Medical Education program, call customer service at 1-800-654-2452 or sign up online at http://www.theclinics.com/home/cme. The CME program is available to subscribers for an additional annual fee USD 205.

FORTHCOMING ISSUES

RECENT ISSUES

THE CLINICS ARE NOW AVAILABLE ONLINE!

Access your subscription at:
http://www.theclinics.com

GUEST EDITORS

JOHN R. HAAGA, MD, Professor, Department of Radiology, University Hospitals of Cleveland, Cleveland, Ohio

DEAN A. NAKAMOTO, MD, Assistant Professor, Department of Radiology, University Hospitals of Cleveland, Cleveland, Ohio

CONTRIBUTORS

MATTHEW A. BARISH, MD, Assistant Professor (Radiology), Department of Radiology; and Director, 3D & Image Processing Center, Brigham and Women's Hospital, Harvard Medical School, Boston, Massachusetts

SHWETA BHATT, MD, Fellow, Department of Imaging Sciences, University of Rochester School of Medicine and Dentistry, Rochester, New York

VIKRAM S. DOGRA, MD, Professor (Radiology) and Associate Chair (Education and Research), Department of Imaging Sciences, University of Rochester School of Medicine and Dentistry, Rochester, New York

ELLIOT K. FISHMAN, MD, Professor, Russell H. Morgan Department of Radiology and Radiological Sciences, Johns Hopkins Hospital, Baltimore, Maryland

DOMINIK FLEISCHMANN, MD, Assistant Professor, Division of Cardiovascular Imaging, Department of Radiology, Stanford University Medical Center, Stanford, California

JEFFREY C. HELLINGER, MD, Clinical Instructor, Division of Cardiovascular Imaging, Department of Radiology, Stanford University Medical Center, Stanford, California

MARK D. HIATT, MD, Cardiovascular Imaging Fellow, Division of Cardiovascular Imaging, Department of Radiology, Stanford University Medical Center, Stanford, California

IHAB R. KAMEL, MD, PhD, Associate Professor, Russell H. Morgan Department of Radiology and Radiological Sciences, Johns Hopkins Hospital, Baltimore, Maryland

PREET S. KANG, MD, Assistant Professor (Radiology), Case Western Reserve University; and Staff Radiologist, Department of Radiology, University Hospitals of Cleveland and Veterans Affairs Medical Center, Cleveland, Ohio

ERCAN KOCAKOC, MD, Associate Professor, Department of Radiology, Faculty of Medicine, Firat University, Elazig, Turkey

ELENI LIAPI, MD, Post-Doctoral Fellow, Russell H. Morgan Department of Radiology and Radiological Sciences, Johns Hopkins Hospital, Baltimore, Maryland

LISA A. MILLER, MD, Assistant Professor (Trauma Radiology), Department of Radiology, University of Maryland Medical Center, Baltimore, Maryland

KOENRAAD J. MORTELE, MD, Associate Director, Division of Abdominal Imaging and Intervention; Director, Abdominal and Pelvic MRI; Director, Continuing Medical Education, Department of Radiology, Brigham and Women's Hospital; and Assistant Professor (Radiology), Harvard Medical School, Boston, Massachusetts

v

RAJ MOHAN PASPULATI, MD, Assistant Professor, Department of Radiology, University Hospitals of Cleveland, Case Western Reserve University, Cleveland, Ohio

MICHAEL A. PATAK, MD, Research Fellow, Department of Radiology, Brigham and Women's Hospital, Harvard Medical School, Boston, Massachusetts

J. THOMAS PAYNE, PhD, Director, Radiation Safety, Abbott Northwestern Hospital, Minneapolis, Minnesota

TATIANA C. ROCHA, MD, Research Fellow, Department of Radiology, 3D & Image Processing Center, Brigham and Women's Hospital, Harvard Medical School, Boston, Massachusetts

PABLO R. ROS, MD, MPH, Executive Vice Chair and Associate Radiologist-in-Chief, Department of Radiology, Brigham and Women's Hospital; and Professor (Radiology), Harvard Medical School, Boston, Massachusetts

DEBORAH J. RUBENS, MD, Professor and Associate Chair, Department of Imaging Sciences, University of Rochester Medical Center, Rochester, New York

GEOFFREY D. RUBIN, MD, Associate Professor and Chief, Division of Cardiovascular Imaging, Department of Radiology, Stanford University Medical Center, Stanford, California

K. SHANMUGANATHAN, MD, Professor (Trauma Radiology), Department of Radiology, University of Maryland Medical Center, Baltimore, Maryland

KRISTINA A. SIDDALL, MD, Department of Imaging Sciences, University of Rochester Medical Center, Rochester, New York

JAMES W. SPAIN, MD, PhD, Assistant Professor (Radiology), Case Western Reserve University; and Staff Radiologist, Department of Radiology, University Hospitals of Cleveland and Veterans Affairs Medical Center, Cleveland, Ohio

CONTENTS

Image quality is proportional to radiation dose. Improvements in image quality come at a cost of increased radiation dose. CT scanners are more robust today than even 5 years ago. X-ray tubes are capable of producing high levels of almost continuous radiation for rapid CT volume acquisitions and angiographic studies. All parameters of modern CT scanners provide rapid subsecond, large-volume CT acquisitions. How high we go needs to be tempered by how high we should go regarding radiation dose from CT examinations. Radiologists, referring physicians, medical physicists, CT technologists, CT equipment manufacturers, and regulators need to evaluate the appropriateness of radiation dose for different CT studies.

Multidetector CT angiography (MDCTA) is redefining traditional imaging strategies of the vascular structures of the abdomen. Angiographic depiction of normal and variant anatomy is becoming the standard for evaluation and has a significant impact in transplant and oncologic surgery. MDCTA is increasingly being used for assessing diseases affecting the vasculature of the abdominal organs, including the abdominal aorta for treatment planning and post therapy follow-up.

CT commonly is indicated for the evaluation of suspected hepatic and biliary pathology. The recent introduction of multidetector CT (MDCT) provides unique capabilities that are valuable especially in hepatic volume acquisitions, combining short scan times, narrow collimation, and the ability to obtain multiphase data. These features result in improved lesion detection and characterization. Concomitant advances in computer software programs have made three-dimensional applications practical for a range of hepatic image analyses and displays. This article discusses the specific areas of hepatic and biliary pathology where MDCT has a significant diagnostic impact.

ELSEVIER
SAUNDERS

Radiol Clin N Am 43 (2005) xi

RADIOLOGIC
CLINICS
of North America

Preface

Multidetector CT of the Abdomen

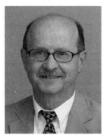 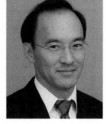

John R. Haaga, MD   Dean A. Nakamoto, MD
Guest Editors

Revolutions and evolutions in scientific endeavors have occurred throughout medical history, but the greatest number and most notable in radiology have occurred in the past 30 years with the advent of new electronics, computers, detectors, and contrast agents. When crystal technology and radiographic tube design were primitive, there were theoretical questions posed about the feasibility of real time or fluoroscopic CT. The conclusion in the early years was that it was impossible to have sufficient photon production and unlikely that crystals could scintillate/reduce afterglow enough to achieve such speed.

And now the multidetector CT (MDCT) revolution has begun! Current MDCT scanners have crystal detectors that are 99% efficient and have favorable afterglow properties such that thousands of slices with superior spatial resolution can be achieved. Acquisition, display, and processing of three-dimensional datasets are routine with separation of different vascular phases during contrast administration. It is ironic that earlier technologies such as DSA were once promoted as a replacement for CT, because the MDCT scanners can now totally replace catheter angiography for evaluation of the vasculature for many parts of the body, including the lungs and heart. This is the subject of this issue of the *Radiologic Clinics of North America*.

We are proud to have assembled a group of talented, innovative, well-recognized authors to con-

tribute to this work. Each author has extensive experience in their areas of expertise and provides valuable insights and paradigms for the diagnosis of intra-abdominal pathology. Rationale use of this new technology is important in view of the need for responsible radiologists to tailor the examinations to minimize potential radiation dose to individual patients.

While the past 30 years of CT have been exciting, we anticipate even more exciting developments in the future. It is our belief that functional MDCT will provide molecular information by the use of various vasoactive drugs that modulate blood flow to tumors and normal tissues. Rapid volume scanning may also promote evolution of robotic interventions and treatments.

John R. Haaga, MD
Department of Radiology
University Hospitals of Cleveland
11100 Euclid Avenue
Cleveland, OH 44106, USA
E-mail address: haaga@uhrad.com

Dean A. Nakamoto, MD
Department of Radiology
University Hospitals of Cleveland
11100 Euclid Avenue
Cleveland, OH 44106, USA

0033-8389/05/$ – see front matter © 2005 Elsevier Inc. All rights reserved.
doi:10.1016/j.rcl.2005.09.003

radiologic.theclinics.com

**ELSEVIER
SAUNDERS**

Radiol Clin N Am 43 (2005) 953 – 962

**RADIOLOGIC
CLINICS**
of North America

CT Radiation Dose and Image Quality

J. Thomas Payne, PhD*

Radiation Safety, Abbott Northwestern Hospital, Minneapolis, MN, USA

CT scanning burst on the diagnostic imaging scene in 1973, sprinted for almost a decade, and then settled into comfortable midlife. But the quiet life did not last long. Technologic advances thrust CT scanning back to center stage. High-frequency generators with ever-higher power ratings and specially designed CT x-ray tubes with ever-higher heat storage permitted the advent of faster subsecond scans. These advances along with the development of slip ring electrical energy transfer allowed for continuous gantry rotation and the birth of spiral or helical scanning [1]. If that were not enough, multirow detector arrays were developed to increase the area of coverage during one gantry rotation. This facilitates volume CT scanning of whole organs in a single breath-hold. Improvements in software have led to real-time 3-D displays of volume-rendered data, as used in virtual CT colonoscopy, CT angiography, CT coronary calcium scoring, and other useful applications [2].

These technologic advances have expanded the role of CT in diagnostic imaging greatly. The annual number of CT studies in the United States more than tripled from 3.6 million in 1980 to 13.3 million in 1990 and then more than doubled to 33 million in 1998 [3]. By 2001, CT scanning comprised more than 13% of all radiology procedures. Unfortunately, the collective radiation dose from CT procedures increased even faster than the increase in the number of studies. The National Radiological Protection Board in the United Kingdom indicated that in 1989, CT studies comprised only 2% of all imaging studies but contributed to 20% of the total patient dose. Subsequent study analysis showed that CT contribution to overall patient dose has risen to 40% [4]. In a 2000 report of the United Nations Scientific Committee on the Effects of Atomic Radiation, the frequency of CT examinations for all imaging procedures was approximately 5%, but the CT radiation dose was approximately 34% of the total imaging dose and was the largest single sector of radiation dose [5]. In the United States, CT contribution to overall patient dose in some departments may be as high as 67% [4]. The rising total patient radiation dose from CT primarily is the result of its increased use and increased number of images per examination. In the early days, a CT study consisted of 20~50 images. Today, it is not unusual to have CT studies with 200–1000 images or more. Initially, CT was used almost exclusively to rule out malignant disease or replace procedures of even graver danger (*Does anyone remember the air contrast pneumoencephalogram?*) and radiation dose was not an issue in most of these cases. Today, with the capability of performing rapid multiphase contrast enhanced studies, screening studies, and increased use, the collective CT radiation patient dose is adding up.

What is lacking is good radiation dose management in CT imaging [6]. Since their inception, CT studies have been performed with standard one-size-fits-all technique protocols [7]. A series of journal articles in 2001 concerning the risk of radiation-induced fatal cancer in pediatric patients, and the fact that pediatric patients were being imaged with adult CT protocols, caught media attention and caused considerable public and professional outcry [8–11]. This had the positive effect of focusing attention on better CT radiation dose use and implementation of as-low-as-reasonably-achievable (ALARA) concepts into CT technique protocols. Appropriateness criteria now are recommended in the selection of CT imaging

---
* Radiation Safety (Internal 17611), Abbott Northwestern Hospital, 800 East 28th Street, Minneapolis, MN 55407.

E-mail address: thomas.payne@allina.com

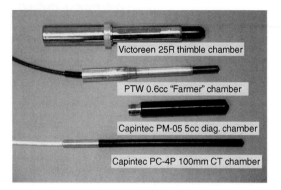

Fig. 1. Radiation ionization chambers.

examinations. The ALARA concept is evoked for CT radiation dose management. Questions are being asked: What is an appropriate amount of radiation for CT procedures? How can the radiation needed for CT scanning be optimized? Answering these questions requires a basic understanding of CT radiation dose and the factors that determine the amount of radiation used in CT scanning.

CT radiation dose

What is radiation dose? How is it measured? What terminology has been developed specifically to characterize CT radiation dose?

Radiation dose is a measure of the amount of energy imparted by ionizing radiation to a small mass of material. The unit of absorbed dose in the International System of Units (SI) is the gray (Gy), which is the deposition of 1 joule of energy by ionizing radiation into 1 kg of material. Some of us (including the author) were around before the formal establishment of the Gy and learned a different unit, the radiation absorbed dose (rad). 1 rad = 100 erg/gram. The conversion between the rad and Gy is 1 Gy = 100 rad. Currently in radiation therapy, a substitute term for the rad, centigray (cGy), often is used to specify radiation dose. Even though it is easy to specify rad, it is not easy to measure it directly. The most common way to measure radiation is to use a thimble-sized ionization chamber and measure the ionization or exposure produced by ionizing radiation. This is not a direct measure of dose but a measure of the ionization exposure in a small air cavity produced by the radiation. Early commercial versions of an ionization chamber were made by the Victoreen Company (Cardinal Health, Cleveland, Ohio) and called Victoreen R chambers. Today, similar chambers are made by several manufactures in different sizes and shapes. These chambers typically are cylindric in shape, a few centimeters in length, and a few millimeters in diameter (Fig. 1). The chamber is placed in a radiation field and it collects the ionization or electronic discharge produced inside of its specifically designed active volume. The chamber contains regular air and the unit of measure is called the air kerma unit (the old unit was the roentgen [R]). Air kerma stands for kinetic energy released in material [12]. The air kerma value then is multiplied by appropriate conversion factors to obtain absorbed dose.

With CT scanners, there are several problems with measuring and specifying radiation dose. First, the radiation beam for early CT scanners was a thin-sectioned fan beam, typically, only approximately 10- to 13-mm thick at isocenter. This beam is thinner

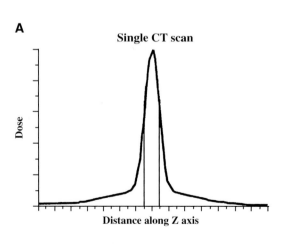

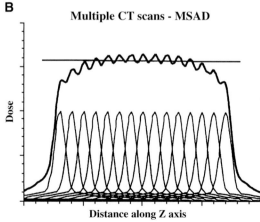

Fig. 2. (*A*) Single CT slice dose profile. (*B*) Multiple scan average dose profile.

than the length of a typical ionization chamber and the thimble chamber; therefore, it undermeasures the amount of radiation exposure produced per unit volume. Second, the CT scanning process is a step-and-scan process, wherein patients are moved past the CT beam to acquire volume acquisition data over a considerable length of patient anatomy (typically 20–60 cm or more). A single scan produces what is called a single scan dose profile, which has a bell-shaped distribution with radiation dose tails (penumbra) that extend several centimeters on either side of the central portion of the beam (Fig. 2A). When a sequence of CT scans is performed, as is done in all CT patient studies, the penumbra regions of each CT beam add to one another to produce a resultant dose distribution that has peak radiation dose values considerably larger than for a single scan. This resultant dose distribution is known as the multiple scan average dose (MSAD) (see Fig. 2B). Depending on the scan-to-scan interval and extent of the penumbra region, the MSAD is 20%–50% greater than the peak single scan dose. The MSAD can be measured using a special dosimeter made from finely spaced thermoluminescent dosimeter (TLD) chips, but it is not practical to do this in the field on a routine basis [13–16].

CT dose index

Instead of measuring the MSAD for a CT acquisition of multiple CT slices, a method was developed using the principles of calculus to measure the radiation dose distribution from only one CT slice and then to calculate the dose for multiple slices. This is called the CT dose index (CTDI), described in a paper by Shope and colleagues [17]. The CTDI value is the integral of the radiation dose distribution profile in the z-axis (along the axis of the patient table) of a single CT slice (Eq. 1)

$$\text{CTDI} = 1/T \int_{-\infty}^{\infty} D(z)dz \tag{1}$$

where T is slice thickness and $D(z)$ is dose as a function of position along the z-axis. Shope and colleagues [17] show that the CTDI can be used to determine MSAD, where MSAD is $T/I \times$ CTDI and single CT scans are spaced at any interval (I).

Because of the practical difficulty of measuring the dose over an infinite distance, the Food and Drug Administration (FDA) Center for Devices and Radiological Health formally decided to measure the dose

over a distance of 7 CT slices on either side of center (±7 T). The FDA CTDI (CTDI$_{\text{FDA}}$) currently is defined in FDA code regulations (Eq. 2) [18]

$$\text{CTDI}_{\text{FDA}} = 1/nT \int_{-7T}^{7T} D(z)dz \tag{2}$$

where n is the number of slices per scan, T slice thickness, and $D(z)$ dose as a function of position along z-axis.

To measure the CTDI$_{\text{FDA}}$, a special pencil ionization chamber is used. To meet the requirement of ±7 T (14 CT slices), it only need be longer than 14 T (in theory, different sized chambers can be used as long as they are greater than 14 times the slice thickness). Two phantoms of different sizes are designated for used with the pencil ionization chamber. The phantoms are cylindric plastic polymethylmethacrylate (PMMA) blocks with diameters of 16 cm and 32 cm and length of 14 cm or longer. Holes of 1 cm in diameter are drilled in the centers and 1 cm from the outer edge at locations of 12:00, 3:00, 6:00, and 9:00 (Fig. 3A and B). Dose for CTDI$_{\text{FDA}}$ is specified as the absorbed dose to the phantom material, which is PMMA. This requires a correction factor of 7.8 mGy/R (f-factor of 0.78) for PMMA.

To allow for a constant length pencil ionization chamber and eliminate the ±7 T requirement, the International Electrotechnical Commission defined a new CT dose descriptor, CTDI$_{100}$, in 1999 [19]. For CTDI$_{100}$, the dose is measured with a fixed-length 10-cm pencil ionization chamber (referred to as a CT dose chamber). Measurements still are made using the PMMA cylindric (16- and 32-cm diameter) phantoms; however, the dose is specified in air rather than PMMA. Thus, the conversion factor is 8.7 mGy/R (f-factor of 0.87), which is 11% higher than the CTDI$_{\text{FDA}}$ value for the same CT technique factors. CTDI$_{100}$ is expressed in Eq. 3.

$$\text{CTDI}_{100} = 1/nT \int_{-50mm}^{+50mm} D(z)dz \tag{3}$$

Another CT dose descriptor was defined by the International Electrotechnical Commission , which better reflects the average absorbed dose over the axial x-y scan plane of the PMMA CT phantoms [20]. Because radiation dose decreases with increasing depth, the dose is higher at the surface of an object than at the center. Because most of the dose is peripheral (near the surface), a 2/3 peripheral to 1/3 central weighting was selected. The term used for

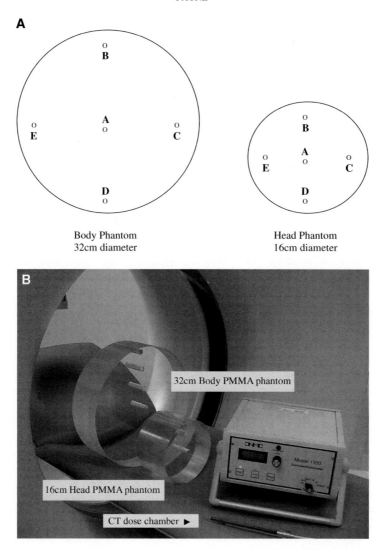

Fig. 3. (*A*) Diagram of CTDI phantoms with measurement locations. (*B*) CTDI phantoms with electrometer and CT dose chamber.

this CT dose descriptor is $CTDI_W$ (*W* represents weighted). $CTDI_W$ provides a weighted average dose to more nearly represent the average dose distribution from the periphery to the center within the same scan plane. $CTDI_W$ is determined by Eq. 4:

$$CTDI_W = (2/3)CTDI_{100} \text{ (periphery of phantom)}$$
$$+ (1/3)CTDI_{100} \text{ (center of phantom)} \tag{4}$$

The $CTDI_W$ dose adequately reflects the weighted average dose for within a single scan plane but does not take into account the dose along the z-axis (multiple slices or spiral slices) in clinical CT volume scanning. For clinical scanning of patient volume, the average dose also depends on the table feed between axial scans or table feed per rotation in spiral scanning. Thus, a patient volume dose descriptor, or $CTDI_{Vol}$, is used to provide a weighted dose value over the x, y, and z directions or total CT volume scanned. $CTDI_{Vol}$ is determined by $CTDI_{Vol} = CTDI_W/pitch$ or $CTDI_{Vol} = CTDI_W/(N \cdot T/I)$, where pitch is table travel in one full rotation/total collimated beam width, *n* is number of slices per scan, and *T* is slice thickness.

Initially, the basic dose descriptor of CT radiation dose was described and is the MSAD. The Interna-

Table 1
CT radiation dose descriptors

CT dose descriptor	How determined	Units	Dose conversion factor	Year introduced
MSAD	Measured by TLD	rad	Not specified	1978
CTDI$_{FDA}$	CT dose chamber in 16- or 32-cm–diameter plastic blocks	MGy:PMMA	7.8 mGy/R (f-factor of 0.78)	1981
CTDI$_{100}$	CT dose chamber in 16- or 32-cm–diameter plastic blocks	MGy:air	8.7 mGy/R (f-factor of 0.87)	1999
CTDI$_W$	CT dose chamber in 16- or 32-cm–diameter plastic blocks	MGy:air	8.7 mGy/R (f-factor of 0.87)	2002
CTDI$_{Vol}$	CT dose chamber in 16- or 32-cm–diameter plastic blocks	MGy:air	8.7 mGy/R (f-factor of 0.87)	2002

tional Electrotechnical Commission [20] shows that CTDI$_{Vol}$ is equivalent to MSAD:

$$CTDI_{Vol} = (N \cdot T/I) \times CTDI_W$$

and

$$MSAD = (N \cdot T/I) \times CTDI$$

therefore

$$MSAD = CTDI_{Vol}$$

This brings us full circle. CTDI$_{Vol}$ is the preferred CT radiation dose descriptor. In Europe, the Interna-

tional Electrotechnical Commission recommends that all CT scanners calculate and display, on the operator console, the CTDI$_{Vol}$ value for each selected CT scan protocol. The unit of CTDI$_{Vol}$ is mGy. Because 1 Gy = 100 rad, 1 mGy = (1/1000) × 100 rad or 1 mGy = 10 rad and 1 rad = 0.1 mGy. For those who work with the rad as a reference dose unit, simply take the value of CTDI$_{Vol}$ in mGy, for example 47 mGy, and divide it by 10 to get the dose in rad (eg, 47mGy = 4.7 rad). The author finds this helpful, because his radiation dose knowledge base is in units of rad rather than mGy. Table 1 lists these CT radiation dose descriptors.

Currently the FDA does not require CT manufacturers to calculate and display CTDI$_{Vol}$ dose values

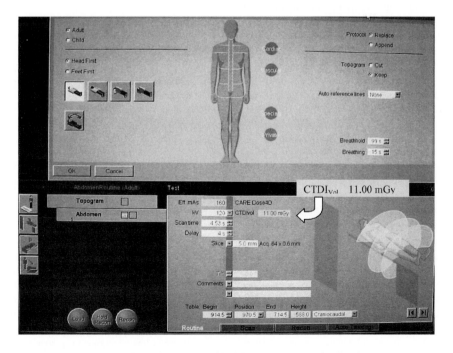

Fig. 4. CT monitor screen with abdomen CTDI$_{Vol}$ value listed.

on the CT operator's console. Virtually all current CT scanners have this capability, however, and $CTDI_{Vol}$ usually is displayed whenever a patient protocol is selected (Fig. 4). This is the only radiation dose descriptor that is readily available for any type of CT patient scan. It can and should be used to evaluate the radiation dose for a particular CT examination. The $CTDI_{Vol}$ radiation dose descriptor is meant to be an index of radiation dose and is not an accurate measure of real patient dose. The $CTDI_{Vol}$ value is determined with an air dose conversion factor of 8.7 mGy/R, where real tissue has a conversion factor of 9.4 mGy/R (8% higher). Furthermore, the dose is measured in either a 16-cm diameter plastic cylinder for head studies or a 32-cm diameter plastic cylinder for body studies. Thus, for pediatric patients who have small heads or small bodies, the actual CT dose may be higher by as much as 3–6 times [21]. $CTDI_{Vol}$ is not perfect as an evaluation of patient dose, but it is available at the moment. $CTDI_{Vol}$ is useful as an approximate value of patient dose—so let's use it.

Effective dose

$CTDI_{Vol}$ does provide a reasonable estimate of radiation dose but it does not provide information on radiation risk. For this purpose the concept of effective dose was introduced by the International Commission on Radiological Protection (ICRP) to provide a risk-based dose from the nonhomogeneous irradiation of human beings [22]. In the context of CT examinations, the effective dose is a weighted sum of the dose to the various organs and tissues from the CT study to a limited patient volume, where the weighting factor is the radiation detriment of a given organ as a fraction of the total radiation detriment. A good reference paper on effective dose is by McCollough and Schueler [23].

Although it is possible to determine effective dose by measurements in a whole body phantom (Alderson phantom), it generally is calculated by Monte Carlo simulation [24]. The calculation of effective dose by Monte Carlo simulation entails the mathematic modeling of the radiation beam and the patient. The calculation needs to take into account such factors as x-ray beam propagation, x-ray beam quality, gantry motion, scan volume, the organs included in the scan volume, and the organs affected by scattered radiation. For each organ, the radiation dose that it receives from a CT scan has to be calculated and then multiplied by its particular weighted radiation risk factor. Then, the weighted organ dose values are

Table 2
Typical effective dose values for various radiation imaging examinations

Examination	Effective dose (mSv)
CT head	1–2
CT chest	5–7
CT abdomen and pelvis	8–11
CT colon cancer screening	6–11
CT coronary calcium scoring (retro)	2–4
CT coronary artery angiogram (retro)	9–12
Conventional coronary angiogram	3–10
Posteroanterior and lateral chest radiograph	0.04–0.06
Average background in US	3.6

summed to get the effective dose. The concept of effective dose allows for a comparison of radiation dose risk from different radiograph and CT examinations. The units of effective dose are sieverts (Sv) or, more commonly, millisieverts (mSv). The older unit, which has been replaced by the Sv, is the roentgen equivalent man (rem);1 Sv = 100 rem. Effective dose organ risk weighting factors are published by the ICRP. Because of its conceptual nature, several methods exist to calculate effective dose. The results generally are in good agreement [22]. A reasonable approximation of CT effective dose can be obtained from Eq. 5:

$$E = k \times DLP \qquad (5)$$

where E is effective dose, k is a conversion unit (mSv/mGy $\times$ cm^{-1}), and DLP is dose length product (CT dose $\times$ CT scan length in units of mGy $\cdot$ cm).

Typical effective dose values for various radiation imaging examinations are listed in Table 2 from data provided by Morin and colleagues [24] and McNitt-Gray [15].

How can CT radiation dose be managed?

Appropriate CT scan protocols

How are the current CT scan protocols in a department established? Almost invariably they are supplied by the CT manufacturer and then modified by an applications specialist and a lead CT operator at the time of CT installation. Periodic software updates generally are supplied by the manufacturer and CT protocol modification often is made at this time. How many times has someone in a department sat down and reviewed all of the CT protocols with the lead

CT technologist? Is it ever done in consultation with a qualified medical physicist who is knowledgeable in CT dose? Now might be a good time to go through all of the patient protocols and evaluate the appropriateness of radiation dose indicated by the CTDI$_{Vol}$ values for the various CT examinations. There are limited guidelines for acceptable dose values, but some do exist. The European Commission has published reference dose levels for several CT studies [15]. CTDI$_{Vol}$ reference dose levels are shown in Table 3. European Commission reference dose levels for brain, abdomen, and pediatric abdomen have been adopted by the American College of Radiology (ACR) in their CT accreditation program. Dose values higher than reference dose levels should be questioned and evaluated. A premise that still exists in many CT protocols is that one size fits all. For too many years a single CT protocol has been used for patients of all shapes and sizes. A single CT protocol may be acceptable for head scans, where various adult head heads are not dramatically different in size, but it is certainly no longer acceptable for body imaging. In no other area of x-ray imaging is a single manual technique used for all studies. Patient size–adjusted technique protocols need to be established and used.

CT parameters that affect dose

The parameters for operator-controlled CT parameters that affect radiation dose are as follows: x-ray tube current (mA), scan time/rotation (sec), x-ray tube voltage (kVp), volume of patient scanned, pitch factor in spiral scanning, and beam collimation (number of multislices used with multirow detector systems). These operator-controlled CT parameters

should be evaluated with regard to the quality of the study and the amount of radiation required. For body and extremity studies, patient size–based CT protocols should be established by modifying the mA, scan time, pitch factor, and kVp. Collectively, radiologists need to move toward optimization of CT procedures to provide the necessary information to make an accurate interpretation with a minimum amount of radiation dose. Over the past 3 decades of CT development, the technologic drive has been toward what is achievable. Now it is time to raise the bar and implement the principle of ALARA in CT parameter selection.

Progress is being made. CT vendors and the radiologic physics community are working to develop radiation dose reduction methods and automatic exposure control processes [25–28]. Currently, x-ray beam modulation (adjustment of the x-ray current during a scan) based on patient size and beam transmission is implemented by the CT vendors. Commercial versions of this mA modulation are called CAREdose 4D (Siemens, Malvern, Pennsylvania), SmartScan (General Electric, Milwaukee, Wisconsin), and SUREExposure (Toshiba, New York, New York).

A more prominent display of radiation dose with each CT image and a list of CT radiation dose in other text locations might help radiologists, CT operators, and referring physicians to become more aware of high-dose procedures. In addition to displaying dose, it is important to link the dose data to each patient procedure. The radiation dose information should be included in the Digital Imaging and Communications in Medicine (DICOM) information of a patient's study for future analysis.

Radiologists, technologists, and medical physicists should review current CT scan protocols and evaluate where the tube current (mA) might be reduced. CT technologists should be encouraged to become more involved in assisting with the optimization of CT protocols. Review all spiral scan acquisitions and seriously question those protocols where a pitch factor is less than 1.0. For body imaging, select a pitch factor greater than 1.0 (preferably 1.5). Always limit the scan volume to the area needed for the CT examination by using the digital localization information to set scan boundaries. Wherever possible, shield critical organs, such as the thyroid, breast, lens of eye, and gonads, particularly in children or young adults. This can result in as much as a 30%–60% reduction in dose to these organs. As radiologists, ensure that patients are not irradiated unjustifiably. CT scanning in pregnancy is not a de facto contraindication, particularly in emergency situations. CT examinations of the pelvis of pregnant

Table 3
CTDI$_{Vol}$ reference dose levels

| CT examination | Reference dose levels CTDI$_{Vol}$ (mGy) | | |
	European Commission	ACR	CRCPD
Brain	60	60	50.3
Chest	30	—	—
Abdomen	35	35	—
Pelvis	35	—	—
Osseous pelvis	25	—	—
Face and sinuses	35	—	—
Vertebral trauma	70	—	—
HRCT lung	35	—	—
Liver and spleen	35	—	—
Pediatric	25	25	—

Data from Refs. [15,34,35].

women should be evaluated carefully, however. As CT scanning becomes more prevalent, a record of previous patient CT examinations is important to avoid unnecessarily repeating a CT study within a short time interval. Finally, a record of patient dose and technique factors should be made a part of the permanent record and provided in radiologists' reports. Furthermore, a periodic review on at least an annual basis should be made by every facility that uses CT as an ongoing part of the quality assurance program. This review should analyze the types of CT studies, number of CT studies, and the radiation dose of these CT studies. This allows evaluation the CT trends from year to year.

Image quality versus dose

What is meant by image quality? For CT scanning, image quality refers to how faithfully actual physical structures with different linear attenuation values can be seen in a reconstructed CT image. The fidelity of the CT imaging process determines image quality. Because CT scanning involves numeric sampling (eg, measuring x-ray transmission through an object), a CT image is subject to sampling statistics. The statistic uncertainty of the final CT image greatly affects the observer's perception of the overall image quality. The primary factors affecting image quality are measuring errors, positioning errors, and discontinuity errors [29]. A general expression for image quality is described by Stapleton [30]:

$$\text{image quality} \sim \text{sharpness}^2 \times \text{contrast}^2 / \text{noise power}$$

There is no exact mathematic relationship between image quality and radiation dose. Image quality is influenced by dose, however. Currently, there is considerable emphasis on dose reduction but few people are interested in a reduction of image quality; therein lies the rub. To understand this relationship further, image quality as it relates to dose is discussed.

Image sharpness

Image sharpness depends on good spatial resolution. Extensive work has been conducted over the past 50 years to measure and quantify spatial resolution. The main methods of quantifying resolution include the point-spread function (PSF), the line-spread function (LSF), and the modulation transfer function (MTF) [29]. The PSF describes the unsharpness of a point when it is spread out or blurred by the imaging process. The LSF describes the unsharpness of a line or slit object when it is spread out or blurred by the imaging process. The MTF is derived from either the PSF or the LSF through Fourier transformation. The MTF is a measure of the resolution capabilities of an imaging system that is obtained by breaking down an object into its frequency components [31]. The MTF value generally varies from 1.0 to 0 when going from lower frequency structures to higher frequency structures. An MTF of 1 suggests that the imaging system has recorded the object faithfully, whereas an MTF of 0 indicates that there is no transfer of the object to the image. A nonmathematic method of spatial resolution evaluation (referred to as high-contrast spatial resolution) involves the imaging of line pair bar patterns. In the ACR CT performance evaluation phantom, the bar pattern spatial frequencies vary from 4 to 12 line pairs per centimeter [32]. To increase image sharpness requires finer spatial object sampling. This requires higher radiation dose. In the development of CT scanning, spatial resolution improved quickly in the beginning but pretty much leveled off. There has not been routine introduction of 1024 × 1024 or higher matrix images or CT spatial resolution approaching that of conventional x-ray imaging of 100 line pairs per centimeter.

Image contrast

Image contrast in CT is the ability to differentiate small changes in tissue contrast (small changes in linear x-ray attenuation between different tissues). This is the main imaging advantage of CT over conventional radiographs. CT machines can differentiate tissue attenuation differences of less than 0.5%, whereas x-ray imaging is hard pressed to get below 2%–3%. CT contrast detectability depends on the statistical fluctuations in the measurement of voxel (volume element) values. This often is referred to as quantum mottle or image noise. One way to characterize the statistical fluctuations in voxel values is to compute the SD of voxels in a uniform water phantom scan. To differentiate tissues with low contrast, good sampling statistics are needed, which require higher radiation dose. Image noise is inversely proportional to the square root of dose: noise $\alpha \ 1/\sqrt{}$ dose. Thus, to reduce the noise by half requires at least a fourfold increase in radiation dose. Because of reasonable limits to radiation dose, CT images almost always are noise limited.

The CT parameters of slice thickness, mA, and pitch all are related directly to dose. Thus, decreasing any of these parameters requires an increase in radiation dose to maintain image noise. One of the primary reasons for an increase in CT dose is the desire to have thin slices for good volume-rendered 3-D images with isotropic voxels. In the ACR phantom, there is a section containing low-contrast cylindric objects of decreasing diameter (6-mm diameter pins down to 2-mm diameter pins) to evaluate low-contrast detectability. The contrast of these objects is approximately 5 Hounsfield units or approximately 0.5%.

Noise also is affected by patient size. An increase in patient thickness increases the noise and requires an increase in dose to maintain a desired noise level. Alternatively, a decrease in patient thickness permits a decrease in dose (eg, the opportunity to reduce dose in pediatric or small patients). The ImPACT group in the United Kingdom illustrates these relationships on their Web site [33].

Summary

Image quality is proportional to radiation dose. Improvements in image quality come only at a cost of increased radiation dose. This is a continuing challenge in CT imaging. Because of technologic improvements, CT scanners are more robust today than they were even 5 years ago. The x-ray tubes are capable of producing high levels of almost continuous radiation for rapid CT volume acquisitions and angiographic studies. All parameters of modern CT scanners have been technologically turbo-charged to provide rapid subsecond, large-volume CT acquisitions. The only restraint is a human one. How high we go needs to be tempered by how high we should go with regard to radiation dose from CT examinations. We are at another crossroads. Radiologists, referring physicians, medical physicists, CT technologists, CT equipment manufacturers, and regulators collectively need to evaluate the appropriateness of the radiation dose for different CT studies and get the word out to all facilities. Techniques from appropriateness criteria and evidenced-based medicine should be used to guide in selection and use of optimized CT studies. Patients deserve no less.

References

[1] Kalender W, Seissler W, Klotz E, et al. Spiral volumetric CT with single-breath-hold technique, continuous transport and scanner rotation. Radiology 1990;176:181–3.

[2] McCollough C, Zink F. Performance evaluation of a multi-slice CT system. Med Phys 1999;26:2223–30.

[3] Nickoloff E, Alderson P. Radiation exposures to patients from CT: reality, public perception and policy. AJR Am J Roentgenol 2001;177:285–7.

[4] Golding S, Shrimpton P. Radiation dose in CT: are we meeting the challenge. BJR 2002;75:1–4.

[5] United Nations Scientific Committee on the Effects of Atomic Radiation 2000. Report to the General Assembly with scientific annexes, vol. 1, sources, annex D. In: Medical radiation exposures. New York: United Nations Publications; 2001.

[6] Haaga J. Radiation dose management: weighing risk versus benefit. AJR Am J Roentgenol 2001;177: 289–91.

[7] Haaga JR, Miraldi F, MacIntyre W, et al. Effect of MAS variation upon CT image quality. Radiology 1991;138:449–54.

[8] Rogers L. Dose reduction in CT: how low can we go? AJR Am J Roentgenol 2002;179:299.

[9] Brenner D, Elliston C, Hall E, et al. Estimated risks of radiation-induced fatal cancer form pediatric CT. AJR Am J Roentgenol 2001;176:289–96.

[10] Paterson A, Frush D, Donnelly L. Helical CT of the body: are settings adjusted for pediatric patients? AJR Am J Roentgenol 2001;176:297–301.

[11] Donnelly L, Emery K, Brody A, et al. Minimizing radiation dose for pediatric body applications of single-detector helical CT: strategies at a large children's hospital. AJR Am J Roentgenol 2001;176:303–6.

[12] International Commission on Radiation Units and Measurements. ICRU report 10a. Oxford (UK): Oxford University Press; 1962.

[13] McCullough E, Payne JT. Patient dose in computed tomography. Radiology 1978;129:457–63.

[14] McCullough E, Payne JT. Radiation dose. In: Seeram E, editor. Computed tomography technology. Philadelphia: WB Saunders; 1982. p. 139–51.

[15] McNitt-Gray M. Radiation issues in computed tomography screening. Semin Roentgenol 2003;38: 87–99.

[16] Rothenberg L, Pentlow K. CT dosimetry and radiation safety. RSNA categorical course in diagnostic radiology physics: CT and US cross-sectional imaging 2000; 171–88.

[17] Shope T, Gagne R, Johnson G. A method for describing the doses delivered by transmission x-ray computed tomography. Med Phys 1981;8:488–95.

[18] US Food and Drug Administration. Centers for devices and radiological health. [Title 21; Chapter I; Part 1020; Sec. 1020.33]. Available at: http://www.accessdata.fda.gov/scripts/cdrh/cfdocs/cfCFR/CFRSearch.cfm?fr=1020.33. Accessed April 1, 2005.

[19] European Commission. European Guidelines on Quality Criteria for Computed Tomography. Report EUR 16262. Brussels (Belgium): European Commission; 1999.

[20] International Electrotechnical Commission. Medical electrical equipment: particular requirements for safety of x-ray equipment for computed tomography (part 2–44). IEC publication no. 60601-2-44. Ge-

neva (Switzerland): International Electrotechnical Commission; 2002.

[21] Nickoloff E, Dutta A, Lu Z. Influence of Phantom diameter, kVp an dscan mode upon computed tomography dose index. Med Phys 2003;30:395–403.

[22] International Commission on Radiological Protection. ICRP publication 26. Oxford (UK): International Commission on Radiological Protection; 1977.

[23] McCollough C, Schueler B. Calculation of effective dose. Med Phys 2000;27:828–37.

[24] Morin R, Gerber T, McCollough C. Radiation dose in computed tomography of the heart. Circulation 2003; 107:917–22.

[25] Cohnen M, Fischer H, Hamacher J, et al. CT of the head by use of reduced current and kilovoltage: relationship between image quality and dose reduction. AJNR Am J Neuroradiol 2000;21:1654–60.

[26] Tack D, Maertelaer D, Gevenois P. Dose reduction in multidetector CT using attentuation-based online tube current modulation. AJR Am J Roengenol 2003;181: 331–4.

[27] Gies M, Kalender W, Wolf H, et al. Dose reduction in CT by anatomically adapted tube current modulation. I. Simulation studies. Med Phys 1999;26: 2235–47.

[28] Kalender W, Wolf H, Suess C. Dose reduction in CT by anatomically adapted tube current modulation. II. Phantom measurements. Med Phys 1999;26:2248–53.

[29] Boyd D. Image quality. In: Seeram E, editor. Computed tomography technology. Philadelphia: WB Saunders; 1982. p. 123–38.

[30] Stapleton R. Image quality in x-ray systems. X-ray Focus 1976;14:46–55.

[31] Hay G. X-ray imaging. J Physiol [E] 1978;11:377–86.

[32] McCollough C, Bruesewitz M, McNitt-Gray M, et al. The phantom portion of the American College of Radiology Computed Tomography accreditation program: practical tips, artifact examples and pitfalls to avoid. Med Phys 2004;31:2423–42.

[33] impactscan.org. RSNA 2003 presentations. Available at: http://www.impactscan.org/rsna2003presentations. htm. Accessed April 1, 2005.

[34] American College of Radiology. Phantom testing criteria. Available at: http://www.acr.org/s_acr/bin.asp? CID=596&DID=15333&DOC=FILE.DOC. Accessed April 1, 2005.

[35] Conference of Radiation Control Program Directors, Inc. 25 years of NEXT Trifold. Available at: http://www.crcpd.org/computedtomography(ct).asp. Accessed April 1, 2005.

ELSEVIER
SAUNDERS

Radiol Clin N Am 43 (2005) 963 – 976

RADIOLOGIC
CLINICS
of North America

Multidetector CT Angiography of the Abdomen

Preet S. Kang, MD[a,b,*], James W. Spain, MD, PhD[a,b]

[a]Case Western Reserve University, Cleveland, OH, USA
[b]Department of Radiology, University Hospitals of Cleveland and Veterans Affairs Medical Center, Cleveland, OH, USA

Multidetector CT angiography (MDCTA) is redefining body imaging owing to exceptional quality scanning and reconstruction capabilities. An undeniable paradigm shift is occurring from axial imaging to volumetric imaging. MDCTA allows one to scan larger volumes in less time using advancements in software. There is improved spatial and temporal resolution. In addition, the faster scanning makes it possible to image different vascular phases using the same contrast bolus, impacting the number of scans that can be done. Newer types of studies can be included in the armamentarium of CT imaging. The volume data can be reconstructed and rotated in different planes for optimal representation of anatomy and abnormalities. This capability allows for the assessment of complex findings and easier communication to referring clinicians. Many catheter-based diagnostic angiographic studies are being replaced by MDCTA. The acquisition of large data sets requires better software and robust workstations for handling the images, including archiving and retrieving the scans. Hard copy review of these studies is no longer feasible. Overall, MDCTA provides an exciting opportunity for a dramatic improvement in diagnostic acumen; however, it also poses challenges with respect to manipulation and review of the large volumes of data [1–5].

Technical considerations

There are several vendors of MDCTA devices, each with various iterations, the details of which are beyond the scope of this article. Four-row detector CT scanners, which were amazing a few years ago, have been replaced by 16-row detector equipment. Currently, 64-row detector CT scanners are becoming a significant and growing segment of the market [5]. Despite multiple detectors, there still remains a single x-ray point source, which emits in a fan shape; therefore, the relatively simple filtered back projection mathematical data reconstruction has been replaced by a more complex spiral cone beam reconstruction. Fortunately, concurrent advances in software and hardware technology have facilitated this radiologic advance. Each vendor has also developed unique features designed to provide optimal imaging. Regardless of the scanner model, one must use scan parameters that result in isotropic voxel acquisition, which produces a volume data set. Simply put, the computer reconstruction produces a numeric attenuation value for a tissue volume that is a regular cube.

Optimal vascular imaging requires a reliable intravenous access capable of injecting iodinated contrast bolus at the rate of 3 to 5 mL per second. A saline bolus chase is optional but can help keep the bolus tight and reduce the volume of contrast required. The timing of scan initiation can be estimated based on different organs or can be tailored to each patient using contrast bolus detection technology offered by various manufacturers. The latter is becoming more desirable with tight bolus administration and critical timing requirements to obtain a particular vascular phase.

* Corresponding author. Department of Radiology, University Hospitals of Cleveland and Veterans Affairs Medical Center, 11100 Euclid Avenue, Cleveland, OH 44106.
    E-mail address: kang@uhrad.com (P.S. Kang).

Post scan processing is critical for rapid and accurate diagnosis. When evaluated by a well-trained radiologist, the 500 to 1000 axial images can often be entirely diagnostic; however, the point of post processing is to reduce dramatically the time required to come to that diagnosis. Ten years ago, three-dimensional reconstructions were usually "cute toys" whose primary import was to wow clinicians. Today, reconstructions can make subtle axial findings clearly diagnostic in other planes or in three-dimensional reconstruction. Given the number of slices acquired in a typical study, the radiologist needs this advantage to remain efficient [6,7].

The simplest processing is multiplanar reconstruction (MPR), which takes the volume acquisition and displays it in a coronal or sagittal projection rather than axial projection. With a volume acquisition, there is no loss of resolution. This acquisition can be refined further to curved MPR, allowing for display of blood vessels and other tortuous structures. This method is suitable for assessing luminal narrowing, especially in calcified vessels, and involvement of blood vessels by malignancy [1,2,5,8].

Maximum intensity projection (MIP) is a technique that produces a planar image from a volume of data. Consider a ray passing through a data volume in a selected projection (any projection can be used, which is a considerable strength of this technique). The maximum attenuation along the path of that ray is represented on the two-dimensional surface, and an image of the high attenuation structures is obtained. On a CT scan, bones will have a prominent role in the image. Vascular contrast enhancement would be another high attenuation structure on CT angiography. Techniques are available to sculpt away the bones, but these are relatively time intensive. Lately, a sliding thin slab MIP has been gaining favor. This technique involves evaluating a thin (user-defined thickness) slab of tissue volume in any tissue plane [9]. The slab can be moved easily through the tissue, resulting in the targeted evaluation of critical structures. This technique is probably the best available for evaluating small arteries [1,2,5,7,9].

The volume rendering technique is a computer reconstruction of the volume with an attenuation threshold for display. Typically, there is a gradient using a color scale for attenuation display, allowing easy differentiation of structures with differing attenuations. This gradient can be user defined and can be a source of considerable artifact if poorly conceived. Specifically, small arteries can disappear, and severe stenosis can appear to be occlusion. MPR or curved planar reconstructions are better for intra-luminal assessment (Fig. 1). Again, skeletal elements are prominently displayed on the initial rendering. Sculpting techniques are available to eliminate the undesirable structures from the final picture. Once the image has been cleaned up, it can be rotated in real time to best display the critical finding. This ability to find rapidly and intuitively the best projection to view

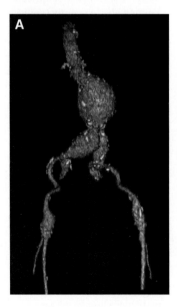
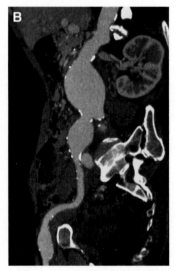

Fig. 1. Multiple aneurysms. (*A*) Three-dimensional volume rendered image gives a global view of the aneurysmal disease affecting the abdominal aorta, bilateral common and internal iliac, and femoral arteries. (*B*) Curved planar reconstruction of the aorta and the right iliac arteries is suitable for assessment of luminal patency and endovascular treatment planning.

the abnormality is the most important feature of the volume rendering technique [1,2,5]. The ability to interrogate critically any subtle abnormality is extremely important. Unfortunately, manipulation of this data is best performed by the interpreting radiologist, which places an additional burden while already struggling with hundreds or thousands of axial images. The importance of an easy to use advanced workstation that is user friendly cannot be overemphasized [7]. After the data have been manipulated, critical images demonstrating the finding can be easily stored on picture archiving and communication systems (PACS) or printed. In some cases, a series of images can be made into a movie, which gives referring clinicians a better understanding of the three-dimensional ramifications of the findings.

Clinical applications

MDCTA of the abdomen includes the abdominal aorta and visceral organs for anatomic vascular assessment and the diagnosis of abnormalities affecting the vascular system [10]. Increasingly, it is being used for preoperative planning for endovascular therapies, oncologic treatment, transplant surgery, and multisystem trauma. Most of these studies are replacing conventional catheter angiography. There are increasing reports of the use of MDCTA in planning various laparoscopic procedures, such as living donor nephrectomy, gastrectomy, and splenectomy [11–13].

MDCTA is a quick and accurate imaging modality for assessing patients who have multisystem trauma [14]. Head-to-pelvis imaging can be performed at the same setting following a single intravenous contrast bolus in trauma cases. A recent review concluded that MDCT was a powerful modality primarily because of its exquisite spatial resolution, coverage speed, and diagnostic multiplanar and volume rendering reconstructions allowing for vascular, solid organ, and skeletal assessment [15]. MDCT comprises the essential criteria necessary for a fast and global evaluation of traumatic injury.

Pediatric applications are being reported, with the best use of the technology being determined as experience is increasing. Chan and Rubin [16] concluded that advances in MDCT technology have contributed substantially to diagnosis, treatment planning, and follow-up in pediatric vascular disease.

Abdominal aorta

Imaging of the abdominal aorta is commonly performed for atherosclerotic disease such as aneurysms, stenotic or occlusive vessels, ulceration, plaques, and dissection. Other indications include pseudoaneurysms, arteriovenous fistulas, arteritis, and aortoduodenal fistulas (Fig. 2). Frauenfelder and coworkers [17] reported a rapid diagnosis using MDCTA for nontraumatic emergent abdominal vascular conditions, decreasing delay by avoiding the transfer of patients for catheter angiography. Ruptured or leaking abdominal aortic aneurysms can be imaged and MPR used for defining the anatomy and possible site of leakage (Fig. 3). MDCTA may be the modality of choice for complete evaluation of the entire aorta for dissection, especially in the acute setting [18]. The evaluation of aortic dissection starts above the aortic arch and extends to the pelvis. Assessment of true and false lumens can be performed, as well as determin-

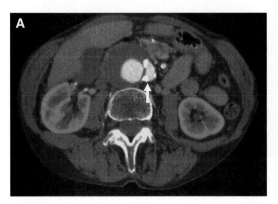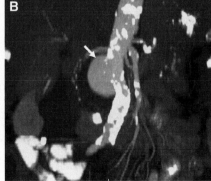

Fig. 2. Aortic aneurysm. (*A*) Axial image through an abdominal aortic aneurysm (*arrow*) has a double lumen appearance suggesting the presence of a dissection. (*B*) Thin slab MIP clarifies that the aneurysm (*arrow*) is saccular rather than fusiform, and the inferior extension of the sac mimics a false appearance of dissection.

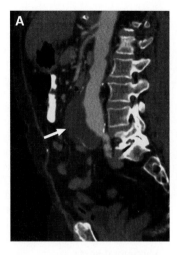
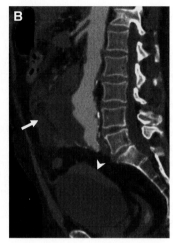

Fig. 3. Ruptured abdominal aortic aneurysm. (*A*) Sagittal MPR in a patient with pain and suspected abdominal aortic aneurysm rupture shows a large aneurysm with intramural thrombus (*arrow*). (*B*) Same patient after 2 days and worsening abdominal pain shows ruptured aneurysm (*arrow*) with intraperitoneal blood above the urinary bladder (*arrowhead*).

ing the patency of mesenteric and renal arteries. The extension of dissection into the iliac artery can be visualized [17,18]. As an alternative modality, MR imaging is radiation free, has an advantage in its ability to diagnose aortic regurgitation, and may be preferable for monitoring chronic aortic dissection.

Rydberg and coworkers [19,20] and Diehm and coworkers [21] have suggested that MDCTA is the imaging modality of choice for the preoperative and postoperative assessment of abdominal aortic aneurysms with endovascular aneurysm repair. Diehm and colleagues concluded that MDCTA had the potential

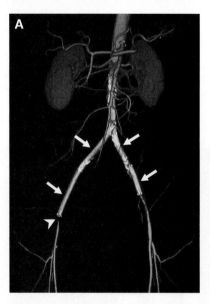
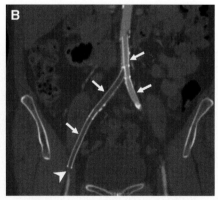

Fig. 4. CT angiography to evaluate right leg ischemic symptoms in a patient following endovascular intervention performed at an outside hospital. (*A*) Three-dimensional volume rendered image shows the extent of the vascular repair performed with multiple covered stents in the iliac arteries (*arrows*) and occlusion of the right common femoral artery (*arrowhead*). (*B*) Oblique MPR clearly demonstrates the occlusion of the right-sided covered stents, most likely owing to overextension of the left-sided common iliac covered stent into the aorta. MPR image shows the advantage over volume rendering for luminal imaging.

to replace digital subtraction angiography (DSA) as an imaging method before endovascular aneurysm repair. MDCTA is suitable owing to its ability to assess true aneurysm size, intramural thrombus, aortic rupture or contained rupture, inflammatory aneurysm, and co-existing disease, which may influence management. Following open repair of abdominal aortic aneurysm, imaging is infrequently used for assessing recurrence or other complications such as iliac limb thrombosis (Fig. 4). A reimplanted inferior mesenteric artery or bypass renal artery graft can be imaged. In a study evaluating the abdominal aorta and its branches, Stueckle and coworkers [22] reported that MDCTA seemed to be similar to conventional DSA for abdominal vessels if multiplanar projections were used. MDCTA helps to differentiate infrarenal abdominal aortic aneurysms reliably from juxtarenal or suprarenal aortic aneurysms. The selection of patients for endovascular treatment of abdominal aortic aneurysms is currently performed using CT parameters.

Planning for endovascular treatment

The length and diameter of the aneurysm neck in relation to the lower-most renal artery are measured to determine the feasibility and selection of the endograft. A small accessory renal artery may be sacrificed during the endograft placement. Measurements of the neck length, angulation, diameter, calcification, and intramural thrombus determine the adequacy of the proximal seal of the endograft. An assessment of the iliac and femoral arteries is performed to determine the patency, tortuosity, and calcification for delivery of endograft components. Most commonly bifurcated aortoiliac modular devices and, occasionally, uni-iliac devices are used, the dimensions of which are determined based on CT scan measurements [19,20].

Determination of the need for pre-endograft coiling of internal iliacs can be performed if the aneurysm extends into the common iliacs, and there is a need to extend the iliac component of the endograft into the external iliac artery to achieve a distal seal (Fig. 5). MPR including curved planes, volume rendering, and MIP reconstruction methods are useful for displaying different aspects of vascular structures. The curved MPR is useful for assessing luminal narrowing owing to stenosis, thrombus, or plaques, whereas MIP images show the distribution of calcium. The volume rendered images are useful for overall display of the aneurysm and its extent. Co-existing renal artery stenosis can be visualized by MDCTA and can be treated before endograft placement.

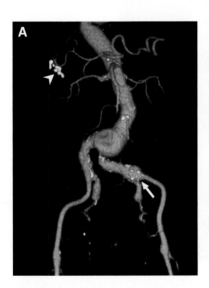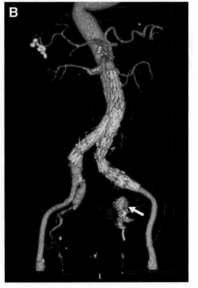

Fig. 5. Pre- and postendovascular aortobi-iliac endograft. (*A*) Three-dimensional volume rendered image shows morphology of the aortic and left common iliac artery aneurysm with involvement of the left internal iliac artery (*arrow*), necessitating its embolization before endovascular graft placement. Gallstones are evident (*arrowhead*). (*B*) Following successful endovascular treatment, a three-dimensional volume rendered image shows the aorto bi-iliac endograft extending into the left external iliac artery and the embolization coils (*arrow*) in the left internal iliac artery.

A post endovascular evaluation is useful for detecting endoleakage or other complications such as graft migration, iliac limb thrombosis, kinking or angulation of the endograft component, or groin access complications. The patency of lumbar arteries and the inferior mesenteric artery can be demonstrated, which are the main causes of type II endoleakage. The post endovascular repair follow-up CT scan should include delayed scans at 2 to 3 minutes to detect slow endoleakage (Fig. 6).

Kidney

MDCTA is an excellent modality for imaging the renal arteries and veins. Tunaci and Yekeler [23] reported that the superior application techniques of MDCT rendered it one of the most distinguished modalities in the detection of congenital anomalies, tumors, transplants, trauma, and arterial disease (Fig. 7). An aberrant renal arterial branch or accessory artery or vein may be responsible for uretero-

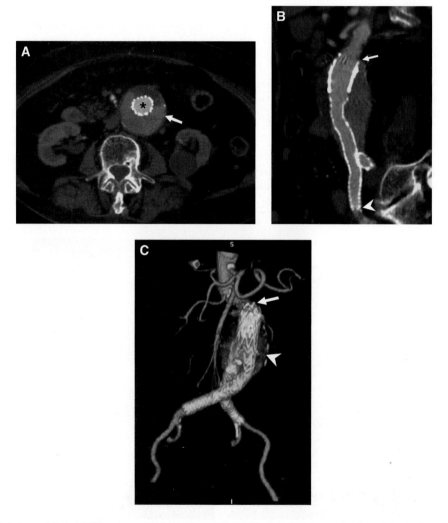

Fig. 6. Endoleakage. (*A*) Axial CT angiography image in a patient with endovascular repair of an abdominal aortic aneurysm shows contrast within the endograft (*) as well as within the dependent portion of the aneurysm sac (*arrow*), diagnostic of endoleakage. (*B*) Curved planar reconstruction in a sagittal oblique plane shows the low position of the proximal endograft attachment and the site of type 1 endoleakage (*arrow*). The distal iliac landing site is sealed (*arrowhead*). (*C*) Three-dimensional volume rendered image shows the tortuous neck of the abdominal aortic aneurysm (*arrow*) and endoleakage, resulting in opacification of the aneurysm sac (*arrowhead*).

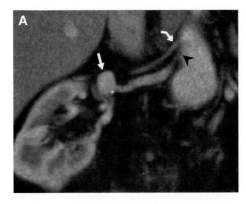 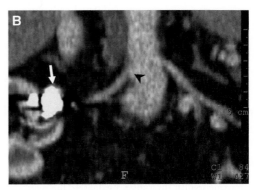

Fig. 7. Renal artery stenosis and aneurysm in a patient with hypertension. (*A*) Oblique MPR shows osteal stenosis (*arrowhead*) and an aneurysm (*arrow*) of the main right renal artery. An accessory renal artery is also seen (*curved arrow*). (*B*) Oblique MPR shows a patent main right renal artery following angioplasty of the ostium (*arrowhead*) and platinum coils (*arrow*) within the embolized aneurysm sac. Note the beam hardening artifacts from the coils.

pelvic junction obstruction [24]. Fleishmann [25] reported that renal CT angiography was an accurate and reliable test for visualizing vascular anatomy and renal artery stenosis and a viable alternative to MR angiography in the assessment of patients with renovascular hypertension and potential living related renal donors. Renal artery stenosis owing to aortic plaque involving the orifice or atherosclerotic narrowing of the main renal artery and the presence of calcified plaque can be detected. Post stent placement MDCTA helps visualize the patency of the stent and renal artery. Raza and coworkers [26] suggested that MDCTA might be a useful noninvasive screen for

renal artery stent restenosis. Arteriovenous malformations, fistulas, and aneurysms can be detected and management decided based on the imaging. Angiomyolipoma can be diagnosed and exquisitely depicted on MDCTA. The feeding arterial branches can be delineated and treatment planning performed based on the findings. The presence of multiple angiomyolipomas in patients who have tuberous sclerosis makes percutaneous catheter embolization a better option to preserve renal tissue (Fig. 8).

Renal tumor imaging and staging can be performed based on information from MDCT and CT angiography and can be used to plan surgery. Renal

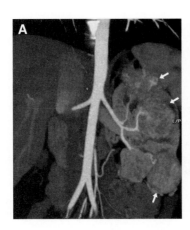 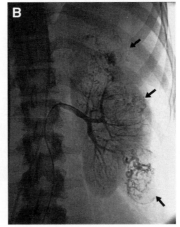

Fig. 8. Angiomyolipoma. (*A*) Thin slab coronal oblique MIP in a pediatric patient demonstrates multiple renal angiomyolipomas (*arrows*) and prominent vascularity in the left upper and lower pole lesions. (*B*) Pre-embolization selective left renal angiogram demonstrates strong correlation with the CT angiography images showing multiple angiomyolipomas (*arrows*).

vein or vena caval invasion can be determined. The display of arterial and venous anatomy is helpful in planning surgical procedures, especially the presence of variant anatomy [23].

Transplant imaging

CT angiography of renal arteries and veins can be performed for pretransplant donor imaging of kidneys. Kim and coworkers reported that for CT angiographic evaluation of living related donors, sliding thin slab reconstruction was superior to thick slab reconstruction [9]. In a study evaluating the renal venous system in potential laparoscopic renal donors, Kawamoto and coworkers [27] reported that late arterial phase images obtained 25 seconds after the start of contrast injection could reveal adequate renal vein anatomy, suggesting that venous phase imaging was not necessary. The prehilar branching pattern of the renal artery and the presence of a precaval accessory renal artery are significant findings in urologic surgery, particularly for laparoscopic living donor nephrectomy (Fig. 9) [28].

Pretransplant imaging of the recipient arterial system, particularly the common and external iliac arteries, can be helpful in older patients. Evaluation of calcification, atherosclerotic plaques, or stenotic disease can be done and the site for a kidney transplant determined. Sebastia and coworkers [29] reported normal findings and early and late complications on helical CT following a kidney transplant.

Vascular complications include arterial stenosis, thrombosis, arteriovenous fistulas, aneurysms, and pseudoaneurysms, which can be visualized with MDCTA, although ultrasound with Doppler is the initial modality of choice (Fig. 10). Proximal native iliac arterial stenosis can also be imaged. These posttransplant complications are amenable to percutaneous intervention in the form of angioplasty and stenting for stenosis or embolization of arteriovenous fistulas, all of which can be planned using MDCTA.

Mesenteric vasculature and visceral organs

Mesenteric vasculature

Iannaccone and coworkers [30] reported that multislice CT angiography was a valuable tool to visualize the mesenteric vessels with excellent detail. MDCTA can be a part of the evaluation for acute or chronic mesenteric ischemia as reported by Cademartiri and coworkers [31] in a study of patients with abdominal angina. Imaging of the mesenteric vessels can be performed to look for mesenteric artery stenosis or occlusion and thromboembolic disease in the arterial and venous system. The acquisition is performed in the arterial and portal venous phases using water for oral contrast with intravenous iodine contrast. MPR including curved reformats is optimal for the diagnosis of celiac or mesenteric arterial narrowing. The portal and mesenteric venous system can

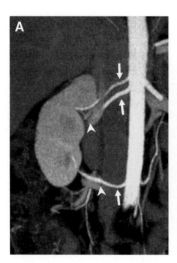
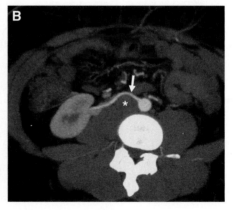

Fig. 9. Kidney donor. (*A*) Thin slab coronal oblique MIP shows three right renal arteries (*arrows*) and two renal veins (*arrowheads*). (*B*) Thin slab axial MIP shows that the lowermost right accessory renal artery (*arrow*) is precaval. The asterisk denotes the inferior vena cava.

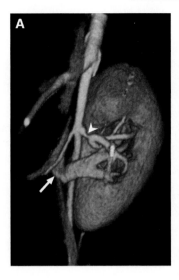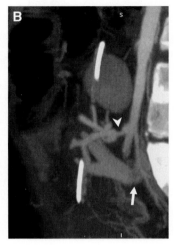

Fig. 10. Pediatric renal transplant artery stenosis. (*A*) Three-dimensional volume rendered image in a pediatric patient with a kidney transplant shows moderate stenosis in the proximal transplant renal artery (*arrowhead*) that was difficult to assess on axial images. A patent transplant renal vein anastomosis is also seen (*arrow*). (*B*) The findings are confirmed with a thin slab oblique MIP.

similarly be imaged [30,31]. The presence of collateral circulation can also be visualized, as well as any radiologic evidence of ischemic bowel injury.

All forms of mesenteric, celiac, or splenic vascular lesions, such as aneurysms, arteriovenous malformations, or fistulas, and traumatic or postinflammatory pseudoaneurysms can be imaged adequately with MDCTA (Fig. 11). A preoperative assessment for laparoscopic splenectomy can also be performed on MDCT including splenic vascular anatomy [13].

Pancreas

Arterial, parenchymal, and portal venous phase imaging provides complete pancreatic evaluation [32]. A precontrast scan may be performed to look for calcifications or stones. Staging for pancreatic malignancy based on vascular encasement, such as of the celiac axis, portal vein, superior mesenteric vein, and splenic vein, can be performed best using curved MRP. The decision as to the respectability of a

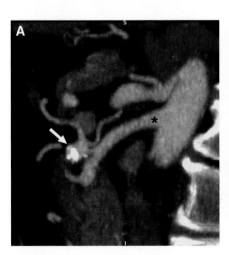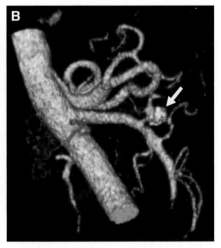

Fig. 11. Superior mesenteric artery branch aneurysm. (*A*) Thin slab oblique sagittal MIP shows a partially calcified aneurysm (*arrow*) arising from the inferior pancreaticoduodenal branch of the superior mesenteric artery (*). (*B*) Three-dimensional volume rendered image showing the same aneurysm (*arrow*) from a right lateral oblique projection.

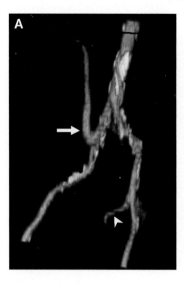

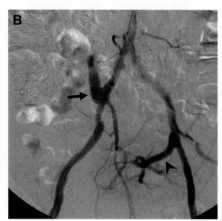

Fig. 12. Simultaneous pancreas and kidney transplant in a diabetic patient with end-stage renal disease. (*A*) Three-dimensional volume rendered image shows a patent pancreatic arterial conduit (*arrow*) and patent left iliac kidney transplant (*arrowhead*). (*B*) Corresponding pelvic arteriogram.

carcinoma in the pancreas can be made based on the extent of tumor spread and vascular involvement as reported by Brugel and coworkers [8].

Imaging of a pancreas transplant for evaluation of the arterial supply via a venous graft or synthetic conduit can be performed by MDCTA (Fig. 12).

Pancreatic graft thrombosis after transplantation is the main nonimmunologic cause for graft failure and usually results in pancreatectomy [33]. The thrombosed arterial supply can be displayed exquisitely with curved planar reconstruction, which helps in treatment planning (Fig. 13). Portal vein thrombosis

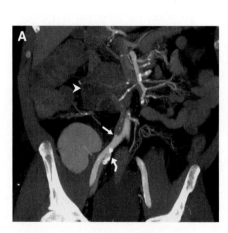

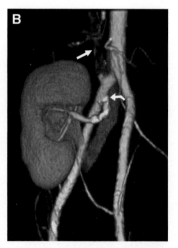

Fig. 13. Thrombosed pancreatic transplant arterial conduit. (*A*) Curved planar reconstruction in a patient with a failing pancreatic transplant who also has a simultaneous kidney transplant. The transplant pancreas (*arrowhead*) is swollen and does not show enhancement. The arterial conduit (*arrow*) is thrombosed. The patent kidney transplant is evident in the right iliac fossa (*curved arrow*). (*B*) Three-dimensional volume rendered image shows the patent right iliac kidney transplant (*curved arrow*); however, it is limited for assessment of the thrombosed pancreatic arterial conduit (*arrow*).

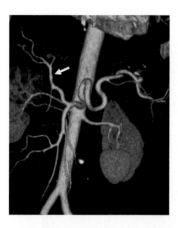

Fig. 14. Replaced hepatic artery. Three-dimensional volume rendered representation of the mesenteric arteries shows a replaced right hepatic artery (*arrow*) arising from the superior mesenteric artery.

owing to bland thrombus or tumor thrombus can be imaged, as well as arterial and venous complications of pancreatitis.

Liver

MDCTA can provide an exquisite display of vascular anatomy in the liver. The major role of CT is for characterizing liver masses, tumor staging, and treatment planning. Atasoy and Akyar [34] have reported that MIP and volume rendering methods can demonstrate the three-dimensional anatomy of the hepatic arteries and portal and hepatic veins successfully, providing useful information before hepatic resection or intra-arterial chemotherapy. MDCTA is a noninvasive method for preoperative planning for hepatectomy for limited metastatic disease and transcatheter tumor chemo-embolization in patients with colorectal metastasis to the liver as reported by Sahani and coworkers [35]. Variations of hepatic arterial distribution are important when placing a chemotherapy infusion pump and in transcatheter chemo-embolization. The presence of a replaced right hepatic artery from the superior mesenteric artery would exclude a patient from chemoinfusion pump placement (Fig. 14). MDCT is helpful in the pretransplant evaluation of a living donor to assess the vascular supply, including anomalies, and to calculate liver volume [36]. Another report by Sahani and coworkers concluded that MDCTA and MR angiography are complementary modalities that permit comprehensive accurate preoperative delineation of hepatic vascular anatomy and evaluation of parenchyma in patients undergoing liver surgery,

obviating multiple invasive studies including catheter angiography [37]. Vascular anomalies can be imaged and treatment planned. Post transplant vascular complications such as portal vein stenosis, hepatic artery stenosis, or thrombosis can be imaged and therapy planned [38]. Portosystemic venous collaterals resulting from hepatic or extrahepatic portal hypertension can be imaged with MDCTA. Kamel and coworkers [39] reported the utility of MDCTA in delineating collateral pathways in extrahepatic portal hypertension before surgery to avoid possible bleeding complications.

Venous multidetector CT angiography in the abdomen

Imaging of the pelvic and ovarian veins can be performed as part of the evaluation of pelvic congestion syndrome. The large ovarian veins and the presence of reflux are indications of incompetent venous valves, which are mostly seen in multiparous women. Nevertheless, Hiromura and coworkers [40] reported the MDCTA findings of contrast reflux into the left ovarian vein in asymptomatic women, with an increasing grade of reflux with opacification of the parauterine and uterine veins. In men, the presence of large gonadal veins is associated with infertility, which also can be imaged with MDCTA. Volume

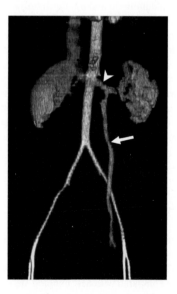

Fig. 15. Left ovarian vein. Three-dimensional volume rendered image shows a dilated left ovarian vein (*arrow*) opacified by contrast reflux from the left renal vein (*arrowhead*) in the early phase imaging of CT angiography. The pelvic varices were seen better on the axial images.

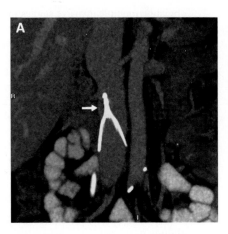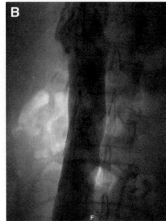

Fig. 16. Inferior vena cava filter. A patient with a history of lower extremity deep venous thrombosis underwent placement of a retrievable vena cava filter for prophylaxis during cessation of anticoagulation for pelvic surgery. (*A*) Oblique coronal MPR image following pelvic surgery shows the position of the vena cava filter (*arrow*) without any trapped clots. (*B*) Corresponding venogram of the inferior vena cava at the time of filter retrieval a few days later shows similar findings. The filter was successfully retrieved.

rendering or MIP methods can be used for display of the gonadal venous anatomy and reflux (Fig. 15).

The inferior vena cava can be imaged to detect the presence of thrombus or anomalies such as a duplicate inferior vena cava or retroaortic renal veins. CT angiography for iliofemoral deep venous thrombosis can be performed for diagnostic purposes and for treatment planning including thrombolysis or stent placement. In 56 patients with acute iliofemoral deep vein thrombosis evaluated with spiral CT venography, Chung and coworkers [41] found an underlying anatomic abnormality in a majority of the cases.

Follow-up imaging after placement of a retrievable inferior vena cava filter can be performed with imaging in the venous phase at 2 to 3 minutes after injection of contrast. The lack of any trapped thrombus with the filter makes it safe for retrieval if the patient has no further indication for the filtration (Fig. 16).

Summary

Advances in MDCT have significantly improved CT angiography applications in the entire vascular system. The wider availability and lower cost of a CT scan when compared with MR imaging are reasons for its status and preference for vascular imaging. Willmann and coworkers [42] found no statistical difference between three-dimensional MR angiography and MDCTA in the detection of hemodynamically significant arterial stenosis of the aortoiliac and renal

arteries. The review of CT angiography data using post processing techniques requires knowledge of the strength and weakness of the display methods for optimal diagnosis and treatment planning. CT angiography requires the use of three-dimensional reconstruction software not only for extracting vascular information but also for creating three-dimensional images to communicate optimally with referring physicians. MR angiography saves time owing to the ease of post processing data and the lack of overlying bone artifacts; however, it is not suitable for the assessment of vascular calcification. Although the time needed to perform three-dimensional reconstructions and image analysis is significantly longer with CT angiography, it has better patient acceptance when compared with MR angiography. Limitations exist in patients with a history of iodine contrast reaction, which has become rare with the use of low or nonionic contrast media. MR imaging is free from radiation exposure and may be the preferred imaging modality in conditions requiring long-term assessment. Poor kidney function is a relative contraindication. In patients with mild renal dysfunction, adequate hydration and the use of less contrast, supplemented with a saline bolus, may permit adequate scanning.

MDCTA has multifaceted applications in the abdomen with its ability to image the various vascular territories. With the advent of minimally invasive, laparoscopic, and endovascular therapies, the need for accurate and minimally invasive imaging is increasing, with MDCTA at the center of this evolution. While MDCT technology, imaging protocols, and interpretation techniques are continuing to overcome challenges, MDCTA provides the most comprehensive noninvasive modality for accurate vascular diagnosis and treatment planning in the abdomen.

References

[1] Wintersperger BJ, Nikolaou K, Becker CR. Multidetector-row CT angiography of the aorta and visceral arteries. Semin Ultrasound CT MR 2004;25(1):25–40.

[2] Napoli A, Fleischmann D, Chan FP, et al. Computed tomography angiography: state-of-the-art imaging using multidetector-row technology. J Comput Assist Tomogr 2004;28(Suppl 1):S32–45.

[3] Brink JA. Spiral CT angiography of the abdomen and pelvis: interventional applications. Abdom Imaging 1997;22(4):365–72.

[4] Fishman EK, Lawler LP. CT angiography: principles, techniques and study optimization using 16-slice multidetector CT with isotropic datasets and 3D volume visualization. Crit Rev Comput Tomogr 2004; 45(5–6):355–88.

[5] Duddalwar VA. Multislice CT angiography: a practical guide to CT angiography in vascular imaging and intervention. Br J Radiol 2004;77(Spec No 1):S27–38.

[6] Kalra MK, Maher MM, D'Souza R, et al. Multidetector computed tomography technology: current status and emerging developments. J Comput Assist Tomogr 2004;28(Suppl 1):S2–6.

[7] Maher MM, Kalra MK, Sahani DV, et al. Techniques, clinical applications and limitations of 3D reconstruction in CT of the abdomen. Korean J Radiol 2004; 5(1):55–67.

[8] Brugel M, Rummeny EJ, Dobritz M. Vascular invasion in pancreatic cancer: value of multislice helical CT. Abdom Imaging 2004;29(2):239–45.

[9] Kim JK, Kim JH, Bae SJ, et al. CT angiography for evaluation of living renal donors: comparison of four reconstruction methods. AJR Am J Roentgenol 2004; 183(2):471–7.

[10] Guven K, Acunas B. Multidetector computed tomography angiography of the abdomen. Eur J Radiol 2004; 52(1):44–55.

[11] El Fettouh HA, Herts BR, Nimeh T, et al. Prospective comparison of 3-dimensional volume rendered computerized tomography and conventional renal arteriography for surgical planning in patients undergoing laparoscopic donor nephrectomy. J Urol 2003;170(1): 57–60.

[12] Matsuki M, Kani H, Tatsugami F, et al. Preoperative assessment of vascular anatomy around the stomach by 3D imaging using MDCT before laparoscopy-assisted gastrectomy. AJR Am J Roentgenol 2004; 183(1):145–51.

[13] Napoli A, Catalano C, Silecchia G, et al. Laparoscopic splenectomy: multi-detector row CT for preoperative evaluation. Radiology 2004;232(2):361–7.

[14] Shanmuganathan K. Multi-detector row CT imaging of blunt abdominal trauma. Semin Ultrasound CT MR 2004;25(2):180–204.

[15] Mullinix AJ, Foley WD. Multidetector computed tomography and blunt thoracoabdominal trauma. J Comput Assist Tomogr 2004;28(Suppl 1):S20–7.

[16] Chan FP, Rubin GD. MDCT angiography of pediatric vascular diseases of the abdomen, pelvis, and extremities. Pediatr Radiol 2005;35(1):40–53.

[17] Frauenfelder T, Wildermuth S, Marincek B, et al. Nontraumatic emergent abdominal vascular conditions: advantages of multi-detector row CT and three-dimensional imaging. Radiographics 2004;24(2): 481–96.

[18] Willoteaux S, Lions C, Gaxotte V, et al. Imaging of aortic dissection by helical computed tomography (CT). Eur Radiol 2004;14(11):1999–2008.

[19] Rydberg J, Kopecky KK, Lalka SG, et al. Stent grafting of abdominal aortic aneurysms: pre-and postoperative evaluation with multislice helical CT. J Comput Assist Tomogr 2001;25(4):580–6.

[20] Rydberg J, Kopecky KK, Johnson MS, et al. Endovascular repair of abdominal aortic aneurysms: assessment with multislice CT. AJR Am J Roentgenol 2001; 177(3):607–14.

[21] Diehm N, Herrmann P, Dinkel HP. Multidetector CT angiography versus digital subtraction angiography for aortoiliac length measurements prior to endovascular AAA repair. J Endovasc Ther 2004;11(5):527–34.

[22] Stueckle CA, Haegele KF, Jendreck M, et al. Multislice computed tomography angiography of the abdominal arteries: comparison between computed tomography angiography and digital subtraction angiography findings in 52 cases. Australas Radiol 2004;48(2):142–7.

[23] Tunaci A, Yekeler E. Multidetector row CT of the kidneys. Eur J Radiol 2004;52(1):56–66.

[24] Herts BR. Helical CT and CT angiography for the identification of crossing vessels at the ureteropelvic junction. Urol Clin North Am 1998;25(2):259–69.

[25] Fleischmann D. MDCT of renal and mesenteric vessels. Eur Radiol 2003;13(Suppl 5):M94–101.

[26] Raza SA, Chughtai AR, Wahba M, et al. Multislice CT angiography in renal artery stent evaluation: prospective comparison with intra-arterial digital subtraction angiography. Cardiovasc Intervent Radiol 2004;27(1): 9–15.

[27] Kawamoto S, Lawler LP, Fishman EK. Evaluation of the renal venous system on late arterial and venous phase images with MDCT angiography in potential living laparoscopic renal donors. AJR Am J Roentgenol 2005;184(2):539–45.

[28] Yeh BM, Coakley FV, Meng MV, et al. Precaval right renal arteries: prevalence and morphologic associations at spiral CT. Radiology 2004;230(2):429–33.

[29] Sebastia C, Quiroga S, Boye R, et al. Helical CT in renal transplantation: normal findings and early and late complications. Radiographics 2001;21(5): 1103–17.

[30] Iannaccone R, Laghi A, Passariello R. Multislice CT angiography of mesenteric vessels. Abdom Imaging 2004;29(2):146–52.

[31] Cademartiri F, Raaijmakers RH, Kuiper JW, et al. Multi-detector row CT angiography in patients with abdominal angina. Radiographics 2004;24(4):969–84.

[32] Tunaci M. Multidetector row CT of the pancreas. Eur J Radiol 2004;52(1):18–30.

[33] Gilabert R, Fernandez-Cruz L, Real MI, et al. Treatment and outcome of pancreatic venous graft thrombosis after kidney–pancreas transplantation. Br J Surg 2002;89(3):355–60.

[34] Atasoy C, Akyar S. Multidetector CT: contributions in liver imaging. Eur J Radiol 2004;52(1):2–17.

[35] Sahani DV, Krishnamurthy SK, Kalva S, et al. Multi-detector-row computed tomography angiography for planning intra-arterial chemotherapy pump placement in patients with colorectal metastases to the liver. J Comput Assist Tomogr 2004;28(4):478–84.

[36] Coskun M, Kayahan EM, Ozbek O, et al. Imaging of hepatic arterial anatomy for depicting vascular variations in living related liver transplant donor candidates with multidetector computed tomography: comparison with conventional angiography. Transplant Proc 2005;37(2):1070–3.

[37] Sahani D, Mehta A, Blake M, et al. Preoperative hepatic vascular evaluation with CT and MR angiography: implications for surgery. Radiographics 2004; 24(5):1367–80.

[38] Katyal S, Oliver 3rd JH, Buck DG, et al. Detection of vascular complications after liver transplantation: early experience in multislice CT angiography with volume rendering. AJR Am J Roentgenol 2000;175(6): 1735–9.

[39] Kamel IR, Lawler LP, Corl FM, et al. Patterns of collateral pathways in extrahepatic portal hypertension as demonstrated by multidetector row computed tomography and advanced image processing. J Comput Assist Tomogr 2004;28(4):469–77.

[40] Hiromura T, Nishioka T, Nishioka S, et al. Reflux in the left ovarian vein: analysis of MDCT findings in asymptomatic women. AJR Am J Roentgenol 2004; 183(5):1411–5.

[41] Chung JW, Yoon CJ, Jung SI, et al. Acute iliofemoral deep vein thrombosis: evaluation of underlying anatomic abnormalities by spiral CT venography. J Vasc Interv Radiol 2004;15(3):249–56.

[42] Willmann JK, Wildermuth S, Pfammatter T, et al. Aortoiliac and renal arteries: prospective intraindividual comparison of contrast-enhanced three-dimensional MR angiography and multi-detector row CT angiography. Radiology 2003;226(3):798–811.

ELSEVIER
SAUNDERS

Radiol Clin N Am 43 (2005) 977–997

RADIOLOGIC
CLINICS
of North America

Liver and Biliary System: Evaluation by Multidetector CT

Ihab R. Kamel, MD, PhD*, Eleni Liapi, MD, Elliot K. Fishman, MD

Russell H. Morgan Department of Radiology and Radiological Sciences, Johns Hopkins Hospital, Baltimore, MD, USA

CT commonly is indicated for the evaluation of suspected hepatic and biliary pathology. The recent introduction of multidetector CT (MDCT) provides unique capabilities that are valuable especially in hepatic volume acquisitions, combining short scan times, narrow collimation, and the ability to obtain multiphase data. These features result in improved lesion detection and characterization [1–3]. Concomitant advances in computer software programs have made three-dimensional (3-D) applications practical for a range of hepatic image analyses and displays. This article discusses the specific areas of hepatic and biliary pathology where MDCT has a significant diagnostic impact.

Imaging and image processing techniques

The main objective in scanning the liver using MDCT is to obtain timed hepatic arterial phase (HAP) and portal venous phase (PVP) accurately, each in a single breath-hold. For scanning the liver using a 16-detector CT, a detector collimation of 0.75 mm and table speed of 12 mm provide adequate coverage in a single breath-hold of 20 to 25 seconds. Image reconstruction of 0.75 mm can be performed in such cases. A 64-detector CT allows thinner (0.6-mm) collimation and smaller (0.5-mm) reconstruction interval. This results in true isotropic volumetric datasets and superior 3-D image reconstruction and volume-rendering (VR) technique. Contrast enhancement typically is achieved using 120 to 150 mL (2 mL/kg) of nonionic contrast media injected intravenously,

with a power injector, at a rate of 3 mL per second. Scan delay is 20 to 25 seconds and 60 to 65 seconds for HAP and PVP, respectively. Positive oral contrast is not administered in such cases because it may degrade image reconstruction. In these cases, 750 to 1000 mL of water is recommended as a negative contrast agent.

The indication for the study determines whether or not single-, dual-, or triple-phase scanning is performed. Routine imaging of the liver is performed in the PVP. Dual-phase scanning in the HAP and PVP generally is indicated in patients who have cirrhosis and hypervascular metastases. Recently, triple-phase scanning in the arterial phase, portal vein inflow phase, and PVP has been suggested [1,2,4–6]. The first two phases typically are acquired in a single breath-hold. The first phase depicts small branches of the hepatic arteries and the second phase is best for depicting hypervascular metastases. The third acquisition is in the PVP and is best for hypovascular metastases. Because of concerns about radiation dose, however, the authors do not perform triple-phase scanning routinely.

Noncontrast CT is unnecessary except for the detection of fat, as in fatty infiltration or adenoma; calcification, such as in mucinous metastases; or hemorrhage. Delayed CT images of the liver may be obtained 10 to 15 minutes after the initiation of contrast injection and are useful for specific indications. Tumors with a large component of fibrosis demonstrate prolonged hyperdense enhancement of the stroma. This feature is characteristic of cholangiocarcinoma [7]. Delayed images also can be obtained in cases of hepatic masses believed possibly to represent cavernous hemangioma, where progressive centripetal enhancement of the hemangioma is one of its characteristic features [8,9].

At the authors' institution, all CT imaging data, in the original resolution of 512 × 512, are sent from the

* Corresponding author. Russell H. Morgan Department of Radiology and Radiological Sciences, Johns Hopkins University Hospital, 600 North Wolfe Street, Baltimore, MD 21287.

E-mail address: ikamel@jhmi.edu (I.R. Kamel).

doi:10.1016/j.rcl.2005.07.003

scanner to a freestanding workstation for postprocessing (Leonardo with In Space software, Siemens
Medical Solutions, Malvern, Pennsylvania). Multiplanar VR allows the best approach to visualizing the
liver compared with other rendering algorithms, such
as multiplanar reconstruction (MPR) and maximum
intensity projection (MIP). VR uses all the attenuation information in any given slab of tissue and
real time adjustments can be performed to accentuate
the hepatic vasculature and parenchyma. Histograms
of the relative density values are manipulated through
trapezoid control of variables, such as width, level,
opacity, and brightness. This function assigns opacity
and color to each voxel and can be adjusted to alter
the final display. Interactive application of different
orientations and cut planes enhance the visualization
of the hepatic arterial and venous anatomy and allows
accurate scrutiny of the liver parenchyma. These
techniques provide robust evaluation of the hepatic
parenchyma and use the full potential of the acquired
thin-slice acquisition without the need for additional
phases or digital image subtraction.

Multidetector CT of hepatic vascular anatomy

Hepatic arterial anatomy and pathology

The complex arterial anatomy of the liver can be
delineated easily by MDCT with advanced image

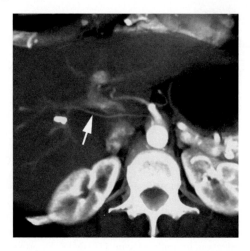

Fig. 2. Small right hepatic artery (*arrow*) arising directly
from the aorta, as seen on axial oblique MIP image.
Small vessels are difficult to visualize in the axial plane
but can be delineated clearly along their entire course on
3-D image processing.

processing. The high incidence of normal vascular
variants, reported in 45% of patients, reinforces the
need for accurate vascular imaging before surgery or
vascular intervention [10–12] (Figs. 1–3). Providing the surgeon with intra- and extrahepatic vascular
road maps may be essential to the technical success
before liver transplantation and may decrease the rate
of vascular complications. Mapping of the hepatic

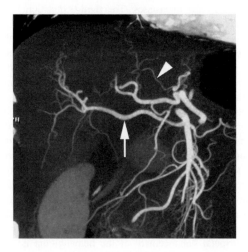

Fig. 1. Replaced right hepatic artery (*arrow*) arising from
the superior mesenteric artery, and accessory left hepatic artery (*arrowhead*) arising from the left gastric, as seen on MIP
image of the HAP. Notice exquisite details of the vascular
anatomy. The coronal plane provides more intuitive delineation of the vascular anatomy compared with the axial plane.

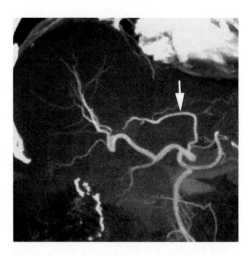

Fig. 3. Replaced left hepatic artery (*arrow*) arising from the
left gastric artery. Preoperative knowledge of this vascular
variant in important before intra-arterial chemotherapy
infusion pump to ensure adequate positioning of the pump
catheter within the desired artery.

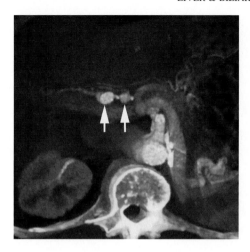

Fig. 4. Incidental hepatic artery aneurysms. Axial oblique MIP image demonstrates two saccular aneurysms (*arrows*) and clearly delineates their communication with the hepatic artery. These could be mistaken for hypervascular masses in the axial plane.

arteries before intra-arterial chemotherapy infusion pump is valuable in delineating the relationship of tumor to adjacent vessels and ensures adequate positioning of the pump catheter within the desired artery. It identifies accessory or replaced vessels that may be sacrificed for the success of the procedure [13].

In addition to the delineation of normal arterial anatomy and vascular variants, MDCT can be used to diagnose a variety of arterial pathologies, including aneurysm and pseudoaneurysm of the hepatic artery and hepatic infarctions.

Hepatic artery aneurysm and pseudoaneurysm

The hepatic artery is the fourth most common abdominal artery to develop aneurysm, after the infrarenal aorta, iliac arteries, and splenic artery. The most common cause is atherosclerosis, followed by medial degeneration, vasculitis, and mycotic infection [14]. Pseudoaneurysm of the hepatic artery also is reported after trauma and after liver transplantation [15]. On axial arterial phase CT, aneurysms and pseudoaneurysms appear as well defined, focal enhancing lesions that may simulate hypervascular tumors [16]. They enhance with attenuation similar to that of the hepatic arteries in the arterial phase and PVP. Although aneurysms and pseudoaneurysms usually are detected on the axial images, MDCT with image processing easily delineates the size and extent of the aneurysm and establishes communication with the hepatic ar-

tery (Fig. 4). Confident diagnosis can be made in the majority of these cases.

Hepatic infarctions

Hepatic infarction may be the result of hypercoagulable states, neoplasm, trauma, and transcatheter arterial embolization, particularly in patients who have vascular disease [17,18]. Most reported cases are the result of hepatobiliary surgery [19,20]. Hepatic infarction can be segmental, lobar, or diffuse. Segmental or lobar infarction is described classically as a peripheral well-defined, wedge-shaped hypodense lesion with no mass effect or capsular bulge (Fig. 5). It also may contain gas. Infarctions also may be rounded, oval, or irregular lesions paralleling the bile ducts [19]. Caudate lobe involvement typically is rare. Diffuse infarction that leads to necrosis and abscess formation is rare and could complicate chemoembolization if performed on patients who have portal vein thrombosis or occlusion [19].

After liver transplantation, MDCT with MIP and VR can document vascular patency accurately and noninvasively. It also is valuable in detecting complication. The clinical presentation of hepatic arterial complications is variable, ranging from mild elevation in hepatic enzymes to fulminant hepatic failure. Imaging, therefore, is critical in early diagnosis of suspected arterial complications. In a study of 35 patients who have suspected vascular and biliary com-

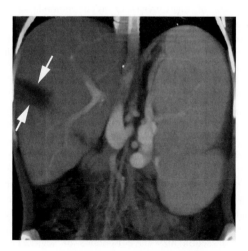

Fig. 5. Hepatic infarction after liver transplantation. Coronal VR image demonstrates peripheral low-density region in the right lobe of the liver. The sharp borders (*arrows*) in this coronal VR image reflect the vascular etiology of the lesion. Notice massive splenomegaly and retroperitoneal collaterals resulting from portal hypertension.

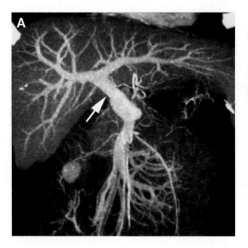
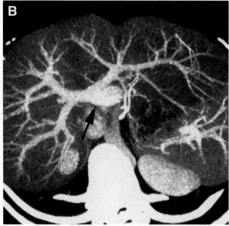

Fig. 6. Normal portal venous anatomy. Coronal (*A*) and axial (*B*) MIP images in the PVP demonstrate excellent delineation of the main portal vein (*arrow*) and its branches.

plications after orthotopic liver transplantation, MDCT detected 10 hepatic artery stenoses, six hepatic artery thromboses, and two hepatic artery pseudoaneurysms [21]. Hepatic artery thrombosis is associated with other complications, including graft ischemia, bile duct necrosis, bilomas, and abscesses. Stenosis of the hepatic artery generally occurs at the site of anastomosis within 3 months after transplantation. Blood flow should be re-established by balloon angioplasty or revascularization surgery. Extrahepatic pseudoaneurysms usually develop at the site of anastomosis or as a complication to angioplasty. When ruptured, these can lead to massive intraperitoneal hemorrhage. Treatment includes surgical resection, embolization, or exclusion with stent placement [22].

Portal venous anatomy and pathology

MDCT easily can delineate portal venous anatomy (Fig. 6) and accurately identify normal venous variants. Variations in portal venous anatomy are common and may complicate hepatic resection and transplantation [11,23]. The anterior branch of the right portal vein rarely may originate from the left portal vein. In these cases, patients who undergo left lobe resection may have ischemia of segments V and VIII, normally supplied by the anterior branch of the anterior right portal vein. In 20% of cases, a single right portal vein truck is absent, resulting in a portal trifurcation branching (Fig. 7). When a right hepatectomy is performed in living donor transplantation, this results in more than one portal vein anastomosis

in the recipient, with an increased risk of postoperative portal vein thrombosis [11].

In addition to the delineation of portal venous anatomy, MDCT can be used to delineate the site, extent, sequela, and possible cause of portal vein thrombosis (Fig. 8). Portal vein thrombosis can occur in cirrhosis, infection, trauma, hypercoagulable states, extrinsic tumor compression, or direct invasion. The presence of arterial phase enhancement of the thrombus and expansion of the portal vein suggests tumor thrombus, and these findings help distinguish tumor thrombus from bland thrombus [24]. Pro-

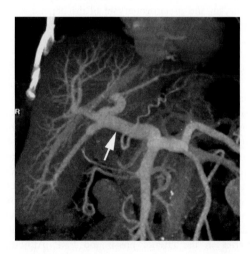

Fig. 7. Trifurcation of the main portal vein. MIP image of the portal venous system shows trifurcation of the main portal vein (*arrow*) into anterior, posterior, and left branches. No right portal vein trunk is seen.

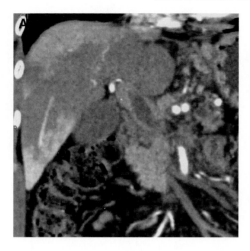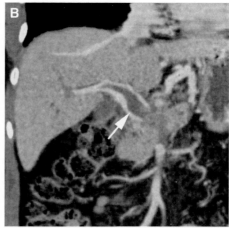

Fig. 8. Nonocclusive PV thrombosis resulting from pancreatic adenocarcinoma. (*A*) Coronal reconstruction in the arterial phase shows large perfusion change in both lobes of the liver. (*B*) Coronal reconstruction in the PVP shows a nonocclusive clot in the main PV (*arrow*).

longed thrombosis results in cavernous transformation of the main portal vein, and the appearance of dilated periportal collaterals (Fig. 9). Alternatively, recanalization of thrombosed portal vein may occur.

Portal vein thrombosis no longer is considered an absolute contraindication to liver transplantation. Several surgical techniques are available for the management of such cases. Acute portal vein thrombosis is treated by manual thrombectomy at the time of surgery. If chronic portal vein thrombosis is present, the donor portal vein is anastomosed to the spleno-mesenteric confluence. Diffuse chronic thrombo-

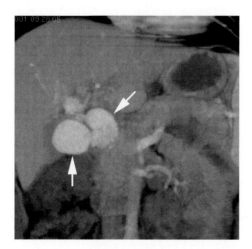

Fig. 9. Cavernous transformation of the main portal vein in a patient who had portal hypertension. Coronal VR image reveals large periportal varix (*arrows*).

sis of the portal vein and the superior mesenteric vein remains a contraindication to liver transplantation [24].

After liver transplantation, MDCT can delineate accurately the site of extrahepatic portal vein anastomosis and any possible stenosis, narrowing, or thrombosis. Portal vein thrombosis or stenosis is reported in 1% to 3% of cases of orthotopic liver transplantation and results from vascular malalignment, difference in caliber of anastomosed vessels, previous portal vein thrombosis or calcification, or hypercoagulable states [22]. MDCT can demonstrate filling defects within the portal vein or focal narrowing at the site of anastomosis. Treatment includes transluminal angioplasty, surgical thrombectomy, placement of a venous graft, or retransplantation.

Hepatic venous anatomy and pathology

MDCT easily can delineate hepatic venous anatomy and accurately identify normal venous variants (Figs. 10–12). Hepatic vein mapping is important before liver resection or transplantation, as the course of the middle hepatic vein determines the plane for formal right or left hepatectomy and allows preoperative prediction of the postoperative liver volume [11,12]. This plane may not be avascular, and in the majority of patients one or more large veins may be transected during surgery [25]. In potential living donors, this plane determines the size of the graft, which is essential to maintain liver function in the recipient. Important venous variants also include

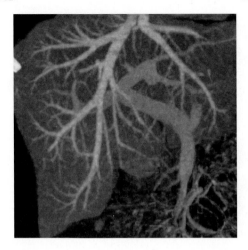

Fig. 10. Normal hepatic venous anatomy. MIP image in the coronal plane allows for adequate visualization of the hepatic veins along their entire course.

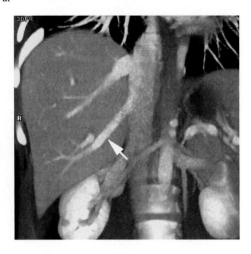

Fig. 12. Accessory inferior right hepatic vein (*arrow*) as seen on coronal VR image. This vein should be preserved during living donor transplantation to reduce the risk of graft malfunction.

accessory inferior hepatic veins (see Fig. 12), and these should be preserved in case of living donors to reduce the risk of graft malfunction [11].

In addition to the delineation of hepatic venous anatomy, MDCT can be used to detect hepatic vein or IVC thrombosis in patients who have Budd-Chiari syndrome (Fig. 13) [26]. Narrowing or nonvisualization of the hepatic veins or inferior vena cava (IVC) also may occur in such cases. Secondary changes include the development of intraparenchymal collaterals and dilatation of the azygos vein. The syndrome

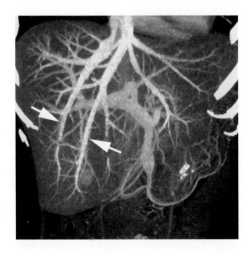

Fig. 11. Two large right hepatic veins (*arrows*) draining the right lobe of the liver as seen on MIP projection image. Preoperative venous mapping can delineate this incidental variant accurately.

most commonly is idiopathic. Other causes are hematologic and myeloproliferative diseases, hypercoagulable states, tumors, and infections. Parenchymal liver changes also can be observed resulting from venous obstruction. In an acute stage, the hepatic segments that are drained by the obstructed vein appear swollen because of stagnant venous flow. Wedge-shaped increased enhancement in the arterial phase can be seen, similar to portal vein thrombosis, but with the vertex of the wedge-shaped areas pointing to the IVC rather than the hepatic hilum [27]. Heterogeneous enhancement persists in the PVP [28] and becomes homogenous on delayed scans [29]. Compensatory hypertrophy of the caudate lobe may occur as a result of a separate unaffected venous drainage directly into the IVC. Fibrosis and segmental volume loss may occur if the disease becomes chronic. Benign regenerative nodules also may occur. Caution must be used when making the diagnosis of Budd-Chiari syndrome on MDCT, because nonopacification of the hepatic veins occurs if scanning is performed in the arterial phase, or in patients who have heart failure or poor cardiac output.

Multidetector CT of hypervascular liver masses

Multidetector CT of hemangioma

The classic features on CT that distinguish hemangioma from other hepatic tumors include attenua-

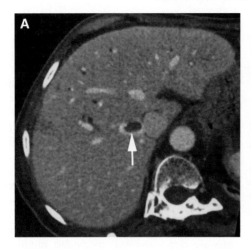
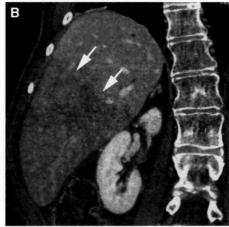

Fig. 13. Hepatic vein thrombosis resulting in perfusion change in the right lobe. (*A*) Nonocclusive filling defect in the right hepatic vein (*arrow*). (*B*) Coronal reconstruction shows well-delineated (*arrows*) hypoperfusion in the right lobe.

tion similar to that of the blood vessels on unenhanced CT and peripheral nodular enhancement, with a centripetal filling on portal venous and delayed images (Fig. 14). The attenuation of the enhancing areas is identical to that of the aorta on the HAP images and to the blood pool in later phases. The speed of contrast enhancement of hemangioma is related not to the size of the tumor but to the size of the vascular spaces. Several studies suggest the slow fill-in within large vascular spaces and fast fill-in in small vascular spaces and large interstitium [30–32]. Delayed enhancement of hemangioma likely is related to lower retention of contrast material in larger intravascular spaces, resulting from slow flow, puddling, and partial thrombosis.

Although most hemangiomas have typical enhancement on CT, some may have atypical enhancement. Complete hyalinization may result in unenhancement of hemangioma, even on delayed images, as a result of obliteration of the vascular spaces. Hemangioma may have arterioportal shunt, even though this feature is of malignant tumors, in particular hepatocellular carcinoma (HCC). This results in peritumoral enhancement, which is wedge-shaped, or irregular enhancement and opacification of vascular structures adjacent to the tumor, as seen during the early phase

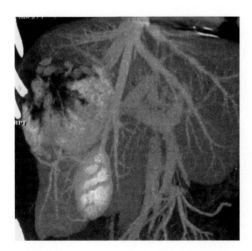
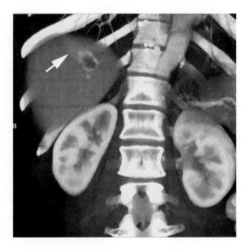

Fig. 14. Classic liver hemangioma. Notice peripheral nodular enhancement with centripetal flame-shaped filling in the PVP.

Fig. 15. Classic hemangioma in the dome of the liver. Notice wedge-shaped peritumoral enhancement (*arrow*) resulting from arterioportal shunting.

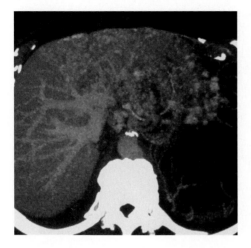

Fig. 16. Giant hemangiomas replacing the entire left lobe. Notice peripheral puddling of contrast in the PVP.

of dynamic enhancement (Fig. 15) [8]. Intratumoral structural variations may result in centrifugal enhancement from the center to the periphery [33]. It is likely that apparent central enhancement of hemangioma in the axial plane may be the result of a peripheral nodular enhancement from the superior or inferior aspects of the lesion. This can be detected easily with MDCT and VR.

Small hemangioma may be hypoattenuating and may be difficult to diagnose. MDCT occasionally may help in identifying tiny enhancing dots in a hemangioma, also known as bright dot sign [34]. These dots do not progress to the classic peripheral

nodular enhancing because of slow flow and slow fill-in pattern resulting from relatively large vascular spaces. Small hemangiomas also may have rapid enhancement resulting from the small vascular spaces and large interstitium [32]. These may be difficult to differentiate from hypervascular metastases. The presence of transient peritumoral enhancement favors hemangioma [8]. Giant hemangioma is significantly less common than the classic type. It is defined as lesions that are greater than 4 cm in diameter, although some investigators define giant hemangioma as lesions greater than 6 cm in diameter [35]. Giant hemangiomas can reach a massive size, replacing an entire lobe (Fig. 16) or most of the hepatic parenchyma. Patients who have giant hemangioma may develop abdominal discomfort resulting from liver enlargement and capsular distension.

Multidetector CT of focal nodular hyperplasia

The characteristics of focal nodular hyperplasia (FNH) on helical CT are reported in the literature [36,37]. The lesion typically has a smooth surface with ill-defined margin unless a pseudocapsule is present, is homogeneously hyperattenuating in the HAP, and is attenuating to the surrounding liver parenchyma on unenhanced phase, PVP, and delayed phase. A fibrous central scar had been reported in 35% of lesions 3 cm or smaller and in 65% of lesions greater than 3 cm. When present, a central scar is hypoattenuating to the surrounding lesion on HAP and PVP and typically demonstrates enhancement on

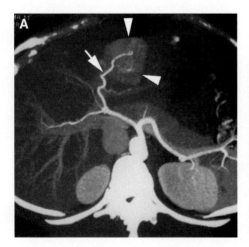
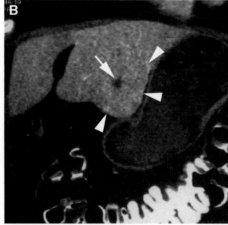

Fig. 17. Focal nodular hyperplasia. (*A*) Axial MIP image in the arterial phase shows the left hepatic artery (*arrow*) supplying the center of the lesion. Notice reticular pattern of enhancement and peripheral septations (*arrowheads*). (*B*) Coronal VR image in the PVP shows central scar (*arrow*) and pseudocapsule (*arrowheads*).

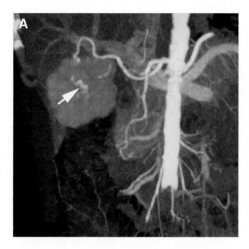 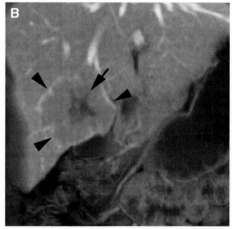

Fig. 18. Focal nodular hyperplasia. (*A*) Coronal MIP image in the arterial phase shows large branches from the right hepatic artery supplying the lesion. Notice central artery within the scar (*arrow*). (*B*) Coronal VR image in the same plane shows lobular tumor with typical reticular pattern of enhancement, central scar (*arrow*), pseudocapsule (*arrowheads*), and draining middle hepatic vein.

delayed (5- to 10–minute) images. Although some of these features can be delineated in the axial plane, they may be detected more readily with image processing (Figs. 17 and 18). One or more enlarged feeding arteries may be identified, depending on the size of the lesion. Feeding arteries may be peripheral, septal, or central in location within the lesion. The entire course of feeding arteries can be delineated easily using sliding MIP images of the arterial phase acquisition. The feeding artery usually divides into small penetrating branches, resulting in a reticular or net-like pattern. No neovascularity in the form of short serpiginous vessels with abrupt angulation, serrated appearance, and variable diameter is seen, because these findings usually represent malignant vessels. Lesions typically are ill defined, with no peritumoral enhancement, as is reported in hemangioma, HCC, and metastases [38–40].

Several small anomalous sinusoids and draining veins may be identified surrounding FNH, and they become more confluent toward a hepatic vein (Fig. 19). Larger tumors may have several draining

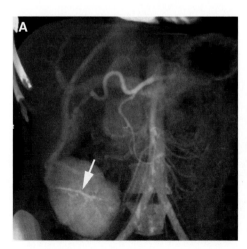 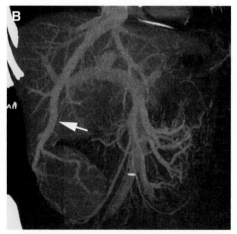

Fig. 19. Predominantly exophytic focal nodular hyperplasia. (*A*) Coronal VR image in the arterial phase shows large branch from the right hepatic artery (*arrow*) supplying the center of the lesion. Notice typical reticular pattern of enhancement. (*B*) Coronal MIP image in the PVP shows several large veins draining into the middle hepatic vein (*arrow*).

veins and may result in displacement of major hepatic and portal venous branches because of mass effect. Portal venous drainage is unusual in FNH [41] and is seen more commonly in patients who have HCC resulting from significant arteriovenous shunting. Hepatic venous drainage is demonstrated best on MIP images of the PVP, as the entire vessel course can be delineated [40]. On VR images, lesions show fine homogeneous granularity or tumor blush resulting from accumulation of contrast material in tumor interstitium, often with a linear lucency resulting from a central scar.

If present, a pseudocapsule may appear as a thin hypodense rim in the arterial phase that becomes hyperdense in the PVP. This is pronounced particularly in larger lesions and may be the result of dilated surrounding vessels orsinusoids or because of compressed liver parenchyma [36,40–42]. A pseudocapsule is seen best on VR images of the PVP acquisition (see Figs. 17B and 18B).

A scar is a region of low attenuation in or near the center of the lesion and is seen best on VR image of the PVP, because VR enhances the difference in attenuation between the central scar and the surrounding tumor (see Figs. 17B and 18B). A scar may extend through thin septations toward the surface of the lesion. A feeding artery penetrating into a central scar can be identified easily on MIP images of the arterial phase (see Fig. 18A). Linear septations may be seen radiating from the central scar peripherally to the surface of the lesion. They may result in surface lobularity of the lesion. Similar to a central scar, septations are seen best on VR images of the PVP [40].

Multidetector CT of hypervascular metastases

Metastases account for the majority of liver masses that are detected by imaging. The most common metastatic tumors to the liver are colon, breast, lung, pancreas, melanoma, and sarcoma [43]. Metastatic disease in the liver usually appears as multiple, focal, and discrete lesions. MDCT appearances of hepatic metastases depend on the vascularity of the lesions compared with normal surrounding liver parenchyma. Hypovascular lesions, such as metastases of colorectal adenocarcinoma, have lower attenuation compared with normal liver and are detected best on PVP images [44]. Larger lesions may have irregular margins, and may have central low attenuation because of necrosis or cystic degeneration. Hypervascular metastases, including islet cell tumors, melanoma, sarcoma, renal cell carcinoma, and certain subtypes of breast and lung carcinoma, enhance more rapidly than normal liver and are detected best on HAP images. The addition of arterial phase acquisitions in the evaluation of hypervascular metastases is reported to demonstrate 8% more lesions compared with PVP images only [45]. Another study shows increased conspicuity of hypervascular lesions smaller than 1.5 cm using dual-phase imaging [46]. MDCT with VR may improve lesion detection. It can demonstrate pooling of contrast material that may occur during the arterial phase,

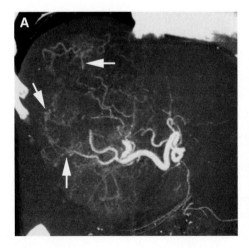
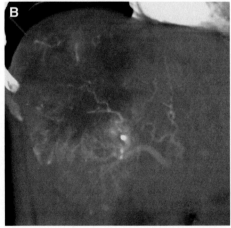

Fig. 20. Carcinoid metastases. (*A*) Coronal MIP image reveals neovascularity in the form of short serpiginous vessels with abrupt angulation, serrated appearance, and variable diameter (*arrows*). These are features of malignancy. (*B*) Coronal VR image reveals tumor stain.

resulting in tumor blush. Neovascularity in the form of short serpiginous vessels with abrupt angulation, serrated appearance, and variable diameter may be seen. These are features of malignancy and may help in lesion characterization (Fig. 20).

Multiplanar VR and MIP techniques allow for the evaluation of feeding vessels and vascular variants, with an accuracy that could surpass digital angiography [11,12,47]. Vascular delineation also results in accurate segmental localization that is essential before hepatic resection. Demonstration of lesion proximity to major vein helps to predict response to radiofrequency ablation. Lesions treated with radiofrequency are more likely to recur if they are in close proximity to major veins, as blood flow in these vessels causes heat dispersion [48,49].

Multidetector CT of vascular shunts

MDCT with advanced image processing is useful in delineating uncommon hypervascular liver lesions that may simulate tumors on arterial phase imaging. Many of these lesions can be recognized by their characteristic appearance on MDCT. Familiarity with the appearance of these lesions may reduce the need for additional imaging, follow-up, or histologic correlation.

Arterioportal shunt

Communications exist between a hepatic arterial branch and the portal veins at the level of the main

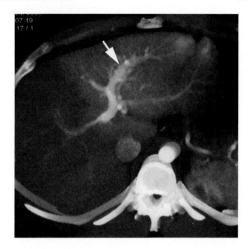

Fig. 22. Postbiopsy arterioportal fistula. Axial VR image in the arterial phase reveals early enhancement and distention of the left portal vein (*arrow*). Notice increased perfusion of the left hepatic lobe.

vessels, sinusoids, and peribiliary venules [16]. These may result in transient hepatic attenuation differences, commonly seen in cirrhotic liver in response to compromise to the portal venous flow [50]. These also are seen in a large variety of liver disorders, including in patients who have HCC or metastatic liver disease, and may precede the appearance of obvious hepatic neoplasm [51]. In these cases, the hepatic parenchyma should be scrutinized carefully for possible neoplasm.

After trauma or interventional procedures, such as hepatic biopsy and percutaneous biliary or abscess drainage, CT may demonstrate wedge-shaped transient subsegmental enhancement at the site of needle entry (Fig. 21) [52]. Occasionally, arterioportal fistula may occur (Fig. 22) and may result in rapid development of portal hypertension and high output cardiac failure. Passage of contrast material from high-pressure arterial branch into a low-pressure portal branch leads to early enhancement of focal area of the liver before the adjacent parenchyma. At MDCT, these may be detected easily. Early enhancement of the peripheral portal vein may occur during the HAP and before enhancement of the main portal vein. The abnormally enhancing vein often is distended because of high systemic pressure that is transmitted by the hepatic artery. An enlarged feeding hepatic artery also may be seen proximal to the shunt. Arterioportal shunting also can be seen in cases of arteriovenous malformation of the liver. At MDCT, these may have a beaded or grape-like appearance,

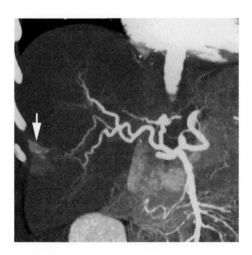

Fig. 21. Postbiopsy transient perfusion change. Coronal MIP images in the arterial phase reveal wedge-shaped transient subsegmental enhancement (*arrow*) at site of needle biopsy.

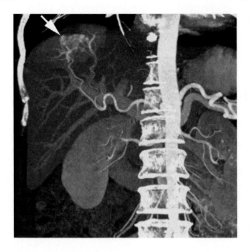

Fig. 23. Spontaneous arteriovenous malformation. Coronal MIP image reveals grape-like hypervascular lesions in dome of liver (*arrow*), with surrounding increased perfusion.

with surrounding heterogeneous mottled capillary blush (Fig. 23).

Intrahepatic portosystemic venous shunt

Intrahepatic portosystemic venous shunt is a high-flow shunt between the portal vein and the hepatic veins, resulting in compromise of the portal venous supply to the liver parenchyma. Congenital shunt may be the result of persistent communication between the omphalomesenteric venous system and the inferior vena cava. This shunt is considered a portosystemic collateral vessel because it occurs usually in association with portal hypertension and hepatic encephalopathy [53]. Acquired shunts may occur in patients who have cirrhosis or after biopsy. There usually is concomitant increase in hepatic arterial flow to the affected segment of the liver to compensate for the decreased hepatic perfusion. At MDCT with image processing, communication between a portal vein branch and a hepatic vein branch can be established with early and asymmetric enhancement of the involved hepatic vein (Fig. 24).

Anomalous paraumbilical venous drainage

The falciform ligament is the remnant of the ventral mesentery and contains the round ligament, which is the obliterated umbilical vein, and persistent paraumbilical vein draining the ventral surface of the diaphragm and the epigastric abdominal wall. These vessels act as portosystemic collaterals in case of portal hypertension, resulting in the recanalyzed umbilical vein (Fig. 25). They may communicate inferiorly with the inferior epigastric vein, resulting in caput medusae (Fig. 26). These vessels commonly communicate with the inferior vein of Sappey, resulting in hypoperfusion adjacent to the falciform ligament seen in the PVP. In addition, these vessels communicate with the superior vein of Sappey, which receives systemic blood flow from the diaphragm and chest wall. In cases of superior vena cava obstruction, increased flow through these collaterals can cause early hepatic enhancement adjacent to the falciform ligament in segment IVa (Fig. 27). MDCT with advanced image processing can delineate easily the vascular communication between the region of he-

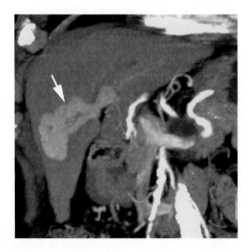

Fig. 24. Spontaneous venous malformation. Coronal MIP image shows tubular venous malformation (*arrow*) arising from the right portal vein.

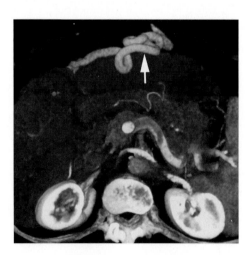

Fig. 25. Portal hypertension in a cirrhotic patient. VR axial image reveals a large recanalyzed umbilical vein (*arrow*) along the surface of the liver.

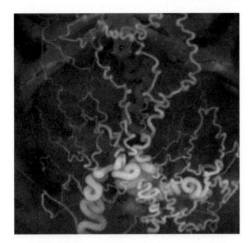

Fig. 26. Large dilated venous collaterals radiating from the umbilicus and forming caput medusae. Detailed knowledge of these collaterals is important to avoid inadvertent interruption and uncontrollable bleeding during surgical and nonsurgical interventions.

patic hyperenhancement and the systemic venous channels along the chest wall (Fig. 28).

Multidetector CT of hepatic cirrhosis and hepatocellular carcinoma

Cirrhosis is the end result of hepatic injury and may be the result of chronic infection by hepatitis viruses, especially hepatitis C. Up to 50% of patients who have hepatitis C eventually may develop cirrhosis [54]. Other causes include alcoholic liver disease,

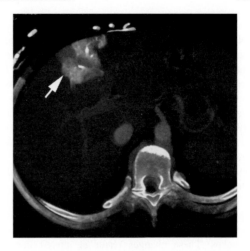

Fig. 28. Early hepatic enhancement adjacent to the falciform ligament (*arrow*) in a patient who had superior vena cava obstruction. Notice collaterals along the anterior chest wall.

primary biliary cirrhosis, primary sclerosing cholangitis, congestive heart failure (cardiac cirrhosis), and hemochromatosis.

In early cirrhosis, the liver may appear normal in up to 25% of cases [55,56]. With progression of the disease, nodularity of the liver surface and generalized heterogeneity of the hepatic parenchyma can be seen (Fig. 29). Parenchymal nodules can be micro, macro, or mixed. Micronodular cirrhosis is characterized by regenerative nodules of relatively uniform small size. This pattern is seen in chronic alcoholic

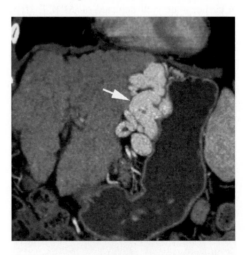

Fig. 29. Cirrhosis and portal hypertension. Coronal reconstruction image reveals nodular contour and heterogeneous enhancement of the liver compatible with cirrhosis. There is hypertrophy of the caudate and lateral segment of the left lobe. Notice retroperitoneal collaterals (*arrow*) medial to the stomach.

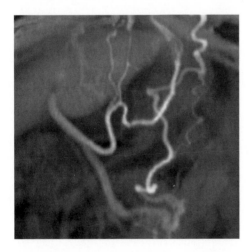

Fig. 27. Superior vena cava obstruction. Coronal VR image reveals collaterals along the surface of the liver and anterior abdominal wall.

cirrhosis, hepatitis C, and biliary cirrhosis. In macro-nodular cirrhosis, the parenchymal nodules are larger, coarser, and more variable in size. The most common cause of macronodular cirrhosis is chronic hepatitis B. Nodular lesions commonly found in cirrhotic livers include regenerative nodules, which may progress to dysplastic nodules, and HCC. Ferumoxide-enhanced MR, combined with MDCT findings, may help in the differentiation of different nodules found in patients who have cirrhosis [57,58]. HCC also is shown to develop independent of regenerative or dysplastic nodules [59].

In advanced cirrhosis, periportal fibrosis and regenerative nodules cause extrinsic compression and tapering of the intrahepatic portal and venous branches. These changes result in altered hepatic perfusion, trans-sinusoidal arterioportal anastomoses, and portal hypertension [16,60,61]. The portal vein may become narrowed, and slow or retrograde flow may result in portal vein thrombosis and calcification (Figs. 8 and 30) [62]. Preoperative knowledge of these findings is important because proper surgical planning (typically thrombectomy for nonocclusive thrombus or bypass venous graft in occlusive thrombus) reduces the risk of rethrombosis. Compensatory hypertrophy of the hepatic artery often occurs in advanced cirrhosis [63]. It becomes enlarged and beaded or tortuous (Fig. 31) and it may be the major vascular supply to the hepatic parenchyma if portal vein thrombosis is present.

The patterns of altered blood flow that result from cirrhosis are well depicted on MDCT. Hepatic

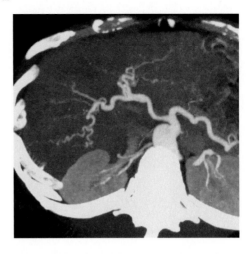

Fig. 31. Hepatic arterial changes in cirrhosis. Axial MIP reveals arterial enlargement and tortuosity.

enhancement is characteristically heterogeneous because of regenerating nodules, periportal fibrosis, and microcirculatory shunts that form between the portal venous and hepatic venous systems [64–66]. Collateral vessels and varices secondary to portal hypertension appear as brightly enhancing structures on the PVP of MDCT. These commonly are seen in the distal esophagus, gastrohepatic ligament, and splenic hilum (Figs. 29 and 32). Additionally, the paraumbilical vein may be recanalyzed (Fig. 25). Esophageal varices are the most clinically important collaterals to demonstrate by MDCT and are present

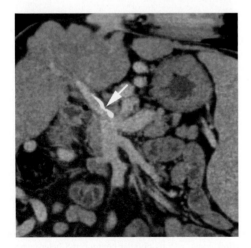

Fig. 30. Portal vein calcification in a patient who had cirrhosis and portal hypertension. Coronal reconstruction image shows linear calcification (*arrow*) along the portal vein.

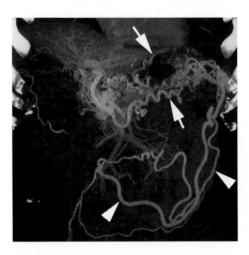

Fig. 32. Cirrhosis and portal hypertension. Coronal MIP image reveals a small liver, extensive gastric (*arrows*), and gastroepiploic (*arrowheads*) collaterals.

in 65% of patients who have advanced cirrhosis being the cause of massive hematemesis and death in approximately half these patients. MPR with MDCT demonstrate these vascular channels in relationship to the liver and major vessels.

Hepatocellular carcinoma in cirrhotic livers

HCC may present as solitary mass, a dominant mass with surrounding satellite lesions, a multifocal mass, or a diffusely infiltrating neoplasm. Small (less than 3 cm) HCCs usually show diffuse homogenous enhancement in the arterial phase, with rapid washout in the PVP (Fig. 33) [4]. This is because of the increase in arterial blood flow and the development of tumor vessels. Therefore, dual-phase CT in the HAP and PVP is necessary in evaluating the cirrhotic liver for HCC. Demonstration of a hypervascular mass on the HAP phase of a dual-phase CT scan is highly suggestive of HCC. Many investigators have shown that the HAP demonstrates significantly more HCC lesions than PVP or unenhanced images [67–69]. Lesion conspicuity is increased in the HAP because most HCC are hypervascular and because the cirrhotic liver receives less portal venous inflow as a result of portal hypertension. The addition of arterial phase imaging to unenhanced and PVP imaging depicts up to 30% more tumor nodules and, in approximately 10% of patients who have HCC, it may be the only method to show the tumor mass

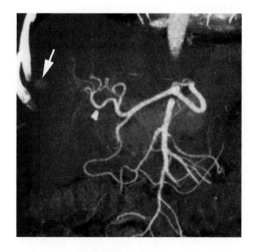

Fig. 33. HCC in a patient who had hepatitis C. Coronal MIP image in the HAP reveals a subtle hypervascular mass (*arrow*). Proper technique and diligent evaluation of the liver parenchyma are necessary to identify this tumor, which becomes isodense to the liver parenchyma in the PVP.

[69,70]. Large tumors have heterogeneous or mosaic pattern of enhancement in the HAP. CT images during the PVP are useful in the detection of less vascularized tumors, such as early or well-differentiated HCC. CT also may demonstrate a capsule or an enhancing septation. Occasionally, it may be difficult to differentiate abnormal liver parenchyma of cirrhosis from diffuse or multifocal HCC. Focal contour abnormality, vascular invasion or thrombosis, and mass effect on the hepatic vasculature are clues to the diagnosis of an underlying tumor. Large necrotic tumors may bleed, and subcapsular tumors may present with signs and symptoms of hemoperitoneum.

MDCT with VR allows for the detection of subtle lesions that may be difficult to visualize on axial images, particularly in cirrhotic livers with heterogeneous parenchyma. It also may demonstrate vascular encasement or invasion, which are reliable signs of malignancy. The encased artery appears serrated or serpiginous and may progress to complete occlusion. HCC frequently is associated with venous invasion and thrombosis of the portal or hepatic veins. Venous invasion is characteristic of HCC and is rare in other neoplasms and metastases. The HAP images are useful in differentiating portal tumor thrombus from portal bland thrombus, because the tumor thrombus enhances in the arterial phase. Prolonged portal venous thrombosis and occlusion may result in the development of small venous collaterals around the portal vein, also known as cavernous transformation. Occasionally, lymphadenopathy may be present (Fig. 34).

The sensitivity of MDCT in detecting HCC in patients who have cirrhosis recently was reported by Murakami and colleagues [71]. Using MDCT and multiphase scanning that included two sets of arterial phase images, overall reported sensitivity was 86%. Double arterial phase imaging showed greater sensitivity and specificity than either phase alone in the detection of HCC. The study concludes that fast imaging of the liver using MDCT provides a diagnostic advantage over single-slice helical CT.

Hepatocellular carcinoma in noncirrhotic livers

Although in Asia HCC occurs almost exclusively in patients who have chronic liver damage from hepatitis [72], in North America it is estimated that 22% to 40% of patients develop HCC without cirrhosis or known risk factors [73,74]. HCC occurring in the noncirrhotic liver has several distinguishing features compared with HCC occurring in patients who have cirrhosis [73,75]. Noncirrhotic patients are younger and more likely to present

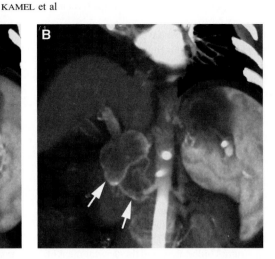

Fig. 34. HCC in a patient who had cirrhosis. (*A*) Coronal VR image in the arterial phase reveals a heterogeneously enhancing hypervascular mass (*arrow*) in the dome of the liver. (*B*) Coronal VR image in a slightly posterior plane reveals enlarged rim enhancing porta hepatic lymph nodes (*arrows*), with central necrosis.

with symptoms, to have a single or dominant mass, and to survive after liver resection [76]. They also have a better prognosis, with a median survival of 2.7 years and with 25% of patients surviving for at least 5 years [75]. HCCs are predominantly moderately to well differentiated. Serum tumor markers, such as α-fetoprotein or des-γ-carboxyprothrombin usually are elevated in these patients.

The radiologic appearance of HCC in the noncirrhotic liver recently has been described [74]. The tumors are significantly larger in noncirrhotic than in cirrhotic patients, predominantly solitary or dominant with satellite lesions, and often are partially encapsulated, with areas of necrosis and hemorrhage (Fig. 35). Obstruction or invasion of portal or hepatic veins is present in 38% of patients and bile duct invasion in 44%. Tumors are predominantly in the right hepatic lobe, without central scar or calcification, and with little or no evidence of fibrosis. Upper abdominal lymphadenopathy is uncommon and may be the result of reactive hyperplasia rather than lymphatic metastases.

Multidetector CT of biliary disease

Detailed knowledge of biliary tract morphology is essential for diagnostic assessment of patients who have suspected biliary disease, preoperative evaluation of potential living liver donors, hepatic and biliary surgical candidates, and postoperative noninvasive follow-up for patients after transplantation or laparoscopic biliary procedures [77–80]. Endoscopic retrograde cholangiopancreatography is an accurate but invasive technique of evaluating the biliary system and has a 1.4% to 5% rate of major complications [81,82]. Percutaneous transhepatic cholangiography allows direct visualization under positive pressure of the biliary tree but also is associated with many complications [83]. Magnetic resonance cholangiopancreatography (MRCP) is an excellent means by which the level and cause of biliary obstruction can be determined but has disadvantages in terms of time and cost and contraindications, such as the presence of certain cardiac pacemakers, cerebral aneurysm clips, or claustrophobia [84].

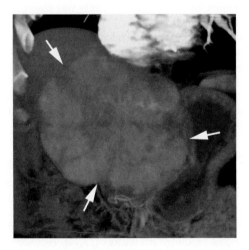

Fig. 35. HCC in a noncirrhotic patient. Coronal VR image reveals a large mass in the left lobe of the liver (*arrows*). Notice tumor stain and short serpiginous vessels with variable diameter typically seen in malignancy.

CT cholangiography was described first in 1982 by Greenberg and colleagues, who demonstrated satisfactory opacification of the distal common bile duct by using an oral hepatotropic contrast agent [85]. Before the era of MDCT, visualization of the biliary tree was achieved using conventional or spiral CT scanners, with or without the administration of oral or intravenous biliary excreted contrast material [86–89]. CT cholangiography also is used for biliary assessment before cholecystectomy, identification of choledocholithiasis, detection of anatomic biliary variants, diagnosis of biliary strictures, and evaluation of biliary complications after liver transplantation [87,90,91]. High-resolution images, detailed imaging of the periampullary area, functional information showing free passage of contrast medium into the duodenum, and delineation of segmental duct obstruction are some of the advantageous features of CT cholangiography over MRCP [92]. The use of IV cholangiographic agents, however, is reported to produce minor and major allergic reactions and hepatic and renal toxicity [88]. Earlier studies also report a long postprocessing time; however, continuous hardware and software evolution have facilitated postimaging reformatting [93].

The introduction of MDCT has enhanced imaging quality of the biliary tree [79,94,95]. The use of advanced image processing, including MIP, MPR, and VR, may demonstrate superior 3-D visualization of vascular structures and the biliary tree with or without the administration of biliary contrast media

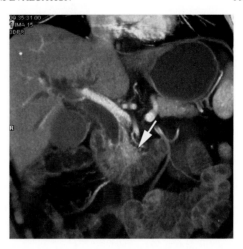

Fig. 37. Mass in the head of pancreas in a patient presenting with obstructive jaundice. Coronal VR image shows dilated intrahepatic and common duct and abrupt transition at the level of the pancreas resulting from an enhancing mass (*arrow*). Mass also involves the duodenum.

[77,79,94,95]. The resulting images are comparable to conventional cholangiographic series even without the use of biliary contrast agents [95], especially when minimum intensity (MinIP) images are used. MDCT cholangiography studies with VR or MinIP are shown to delineate the site and cause of biliary obstruction effectively without the additional administration of a cholangiographic contrast agent (Figs. 36 and 37) [77,95,96]. Coronal oblique reformatted and thin-slab MinIP images can show stones in the common bile duct (Figs. 38 and 39), whereas

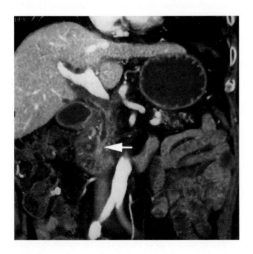

Fig. 36. Infiltrating adenocarcinoma of the distal common bile duct. Coronal VR image reveals wall thickening, enhancement and ill-defined soft tissue mass along the common duct (*arrow*) consistent with cholangiocarcinoma. Calcification and tiny pseudocyst in the pancreatic head resulting from chronic pancreatitis.

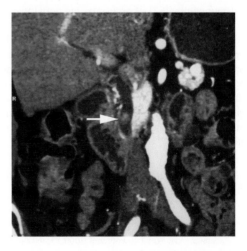

Fig. 38. Distal common duct stone in a patient who had right upper quadrant pain. Coronal reconstruction image demonstrates a filling defect (*arrow*) in the distal common duct.

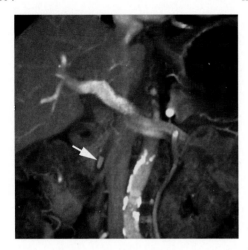

Fig. 39. Status post open cholecystectomy for gallbladder cancer. Coronal VR image shows surgical clip in distal common duct (*arrow*), believed to represent a stone on axial images.

oblique plane images in the plane along the course of the intrahepatic duct may depict intrahepatic duct stones. A recent study comparing the effectiveness of MDCT cholangiography without biliary contrast media to MRCP confirms the high diagnostic quality of the former [97].

MDCT cholangiography with additional use of intravenous cholangiographic contrast media reveals satisfactory visualization of second-order biliary branches in living liver donor candidates [98]. A prior study shows that MDCT cholangiography enables significantly better visualization of second-order bile ducts than conventional or excretory MR cholangiography [92]. If necessary, the portal venous system easily may be assessed concurrently, so as to depict aberrant vascular or biliary anatomy preoperatively [99]. A potential application of MDCT data is the fusion of the generated vascular and biliary images using advanced postprocessing software tools [100]. This multiphase fusion imaging of the liver may aid surgeons in exploring their field beforehand, thus minimizing operation time and related complications [100].

References

[1] Foley WD, Mallisee TA, Hohenwalter MD, et al. Multiphase hepatic CT with a multirow detector CT scanner. AJR Am J Roentgenol 2000;175:679–85.

[2] Ji H, McTavish JD, Mortele KJ, et al. Hepatic imaging with multidetector CT. Radiographics 2001; 21 Spec No:S71–80.

[3] Hu H, He HD, Foley WD, et al. Four multidetector-row helical CT: image quality and volume coverage speed. Radiology 2000;215:55–62.

[4] Mitsuzaki K, Yamashita Y, Ogata I, et al. Multiple-phase helical CT of the liver for detecting small hepatomas in patients with liver cirrhosis: contrast-injection protocol and optimal timing. AJR Am J Roentgenol 1996;167:753–7.

[5] Murakami T, Kim T, Takahashi S, et al. Hepatocellular carcinoma: multidetector row helical CT. Abdom Imaging 2002;27:139–46.

[6] Paulson EK, McDermott VG, Keogan MT, et al. Carcinoid metastases to the liver: role of triple-phase helical CT. Radiology 1998;206:143–50.

[7] Lacomis JM, Baron RL, Oliver 3rd JH, et al. Cholangiocarcinoma: delayed CT contrast enhancement patterns. Radiology 1997;203:98–104.

[8] Kim T, Federle MP, Baron RL, et al. Discrimination of small hepatic hemangiomas from hypervascular malignant tumors smaller than 3 cm with three-phase helical CT. Radiology 2001;219:699–706.

[9] Leslie DF, Johnson CD, Johnson CM, et al. Distinction between cavernous hemangiomas of the liver and hepatic metastases on CT: value of contrast enhancement patterns. AJR Am J Roentgenol 1995;164: 625–9.

[10] Erbay N, Raptopoulos V, Pomfret EA, et al. Living donor liver transplantation in adults: vascular variants important in surgical planning for donors and recipients. AJR Am J Roentgenol 2003;181: 109–14.

[11] Kamel IR, Kruskal JB, Pomfret EA, et al. Impact of multidetector CT on donor selection and surgical planning before living adult right lobe liver transplantation. AJR Am J Roentgenol 2001;176: 193–200.

[12] Sahani D, Saini S, Pena C, et al. Using multidetector CT for preoperative vascular evaluation of liver neoplasms: technique and results. AJR Am J Roentgenol 2002;179:53–9.

[13] Kapoor V, Brancatelli G, Federle MP, et al. Multidetector CT arteriography with volumetric three-dimensional rendering to evaluate patients with metastatic colorectal disease for placement of a floxuridine infusion pump. AJR Am J Roentgenol 2003;181:455–63.

[14] Shanley CJ, Shah NL, Messina LM. Common splanchnic artery aneurysms: splenic, hepatic, and celiac. Ann Vasc Surg 1996;10:315–22.

[15] Katyal S, Oliver JH, Peterson MS, et al. Prognostic significance of arterial phase CT for prediction of response to transcatheter arterial chemoembolization in unresectable hepatocellular carcinoma: a retrospective analysis. AJR Am J Roentgenol 2000;175: 1665–72.

[16] Quiroga S, Sebastia C, Pallisa E, et al. Improved diagnosis of hepatic perfusion disorders: value of hepatic arterial phase imaging during helical CT. Radiographics 2001;21:65–81 [questionnaire 288–94].

[17] Gates J, Hartnell GG, Stuart KE, et al. Chemo-embolization of hepatic neoplasms: safety, complications, and when to worry. Radiographics 1999;19: 399–414.

[18] Sakamoto I, Aso N, Nagaoki K, et al. Complications associated with transcatheter arterial embolization for hepatic tumors. Radiographics 1998;18:605–19.

[19] Holbert BL, Baron RL, Dodd 3rd GD. Hepatic infarction caused by arterial insufficiency: spectrum and evolution of CT findings. AJR Am J Roentgenol 1996;166:815–20.

[20] Smith GS, Birnbaum BA, Jacobs JE. Hepatic infarction secondary to arterial insufficiency in native livers: CT findings in 10 patients. Radiology 1998; 208:223–9.

[21] Brancatelli G, Katyal S, Federle MP, et al. Three-dimensional multislice helical computed tomography with the volume rendering technique in the detection of vascular complications after liver transplantation. Transplantation 2002;73:237–42.

[22] Quiroga S, Sebastia MC, Margarit C, et al. Complications of orthotopic liver transplantation: spectrum of findings with helical CT. Radiographics 2001;21: 1085–102.

[23] Cheng YF, Huang TL, Lee TY, et al. Variation of the intrahepatic portal vein; angiographic demonstration and application in living-related hepatic transplantation. Transplant Proc 1996;28:1667–8.

[24] Pannu HK, Maley WR, Fishman EK. Liver transplantation: preoperative CT evaluation. Radiographics 2001;21 Spec no:S133–46.

[25] Kamel IR, Lawler LP, Fishman EK. Variations in anatomy of the middle hepatic vein and their impact on formal right hepatectomy. Abdom Imaging 2003; 28:668–74.

[26] Soyer P, Rabenandrasana A, Barge J, et al. MRI of Budd-Chiari syndrome. Abdom Imaging 1994;19: 325–9.

[27] Itai Y, Murata S, Kurosaki Y. Straight border sign of the liver: spectrum of CT appearances and causes. Radiographics 1995;15:1089–102.

[28] Chen WP, Chen JH, Hwang JI, et al. Spectrum of transient hepatic attenuation differences in biphasic helical CT. AJR Am J Roentgenol 1999;172:419–24.

[29] Gryspeerdt S, Van Hoe L, Marchal G, et al. Evaluation of hepatic perfusion disorders with double-phase spiral CT. Radiographics 1997;17:337–48.

[30] Danet IM, Semelka RC, Braga L, et al. Giant hemangioma of the liver: MR imaging characteristics in 24 patients. Magn Reson Imaging 2003;21:95–101.

[31] Hanafusa K, Ohashi I, Himeno Y, et al. Hepatic hemangioma: findings with two-phase CT. Radiology 1995;196:465–9.

[32] Yamashita Y, Ogata I, Urata J, et al. Cavernous hemangioma of the liver: pathologic correlation with dynamic CT findings. Radiology 1997;203:121–5.

[33] Kim S, Chung JJ, Kim MJ, et al. Atypical inside-out pattern of hepatic hemangiomas. AJR Am J Roentgenol 2000;174:1571–4.

[34] Jang HJ, Choi BI, Kim TK, et al. Atypical small hemangiomas of the liver: "bright dot" sign at two-phase spiral CT. Radiology 1998;208:543–8.

[35] Mitsudo K, Watanabe Y, Saga T, et al. Nonenhanced hepatic cavernous hemangioma with multiple calcifications: CT and pathologic correlation. Abdom Imaging 1995;20:459–61.

[36] Brancatelli G, Federle MP, Grazioli L, et al. Focal nodular hyperplasia: CT findings with emphasis on multiphasic helical CT in 78 patients. Radiology 2001; 219:61–8.

[37] Carlson SK, Johnson CD, Bender CE, et al. CT of focal nodular hyperplasia of the liver. AJR Am J Roentgenol 2000;174:705–12.

[38] Terayama N, Matsui O, Ueda K, et al. Peritumoral rim enhancement of liver metastasis: hemodynamics observed on single-level dynamic CT during hepatic arteriography and histopathologic correlation. J Comput Assist Tomogr 2002;26:975–80.

[39] Yu JS, Kim KW, Park MS, et al. Transient peritumoral enhancement during dynamic MRI of the liver: cavernous hemangioma versus hepatocellular carcinoma. J Comput Assist Tomogr 2002;26:411–7.

[40] Kamel IR, Liapi E, Fishman EK. Focal nodular hyperplasia: lesion evaluation using 16 slice multidetector row CT and 3D CT angiography. AJR Am J Roentgenol, in press.

[41] Hussain SM, Terkivatan T, Zondervan PE, et al. Focal nodular hyperplasia: findings at state-of-the-art MR imaging, US, CT, and pathologic analysis. Radiographics 2004;24:3–17 [discussion 18–9].

[42] Miyayama S, Matsui O, Ueda K, et al. Hemodynamics of small hepatic focal nodular hyperplasia: evaluation with single-level dynamic CT during hepatic arteriography. AJR Am J Roentgenol 2000;174: 1567–9.

[43] Ackerman NB, Lien WM, Kondi ES, et al. The blood supply of experimental liver metastases. I. The distribution of hepatic artery and portal vein blood to "small" and "large" tumors. Surgery 1969;66: 1067–72.

[44] Kemmerer SR, Mortele KJ, Ros PR. CT scan of the liver. Radiol Clin North Am 1998;36:247–61.

[45] Bonaldi VM, Bret PM, Reinhold C, et al. Helical CT of the liver: value of an early hepatic arterial phase. Radiology 1995;197:357–63.

[46] Hollett MD, Jeffrey Jr RB, Nino-Murcia M, et al. Dual-phase helical CT of the liver: value of arterial phase scans in the detection of small (< or =1.5 cm) malignant hepatic neoplasms. AJR Am J Roentgenol 1995;164:879–84.

[47] Lawler LP, Fishman EK. Multi-detector row CT of thoracic disease with emphasis on 3D volume rendering and CT angiography. Radiographics 2001;21: 1257–73.

[48] Dromain C, de Baere T, Elias D, et al. Hepatic tumors treated with percutaneous radio-frequency ablation: CT and MR imaging follow-up. Radiology 2002;223: 255–62.

[49] Lencioni R, Cioni D, Bartolozzi C. Percutaneous radiofrequency thermal ablation of liver malignancies: techniques, indications, imaging findings, and clinical results. Abdom Imaging 2001;26:345–60.

[50] Itai Y, Moss AA, Goldberg HI. Transient hepatic attenuation difference of lobar or segmental distribution detected by dynamic computed tomography. Radiology 1982;144:835–9.

[51] Colagrande S, Centi N, La Villa G, et al. Transient hepatic attenuation differences. AJR Am J Roentgenol 2004;183:459–64.

[52] Lee SJ, Lim JH, Lee WJ, et al. Transient subsegmental hepatic parenchymal enhancement on dynamic CT: a sign of postbiopsy arterioportal shunt. J Comput Assist Tomogr 1997;21:355–60.

[53] Lane MJ, Jeffrey Jr RB, Katz DS. Spontaneous intrahepatic vascular shunts. AJR Am J Roentgenol 2000;174:125–31.

[54] Genesca J, Esteban JI, Alter HJ. Blood-borne non-A, non-B hepatitis: hepatitis C. Semin Liver Dis 1991; 11:147–64.

[55] Dodd 3rd GD, Baron RL, Oliver 3rd JH, et al. Spectrum of imaging findings of the liver in end-stage cirrhosis: Part II, focal abnormalities. AJR Am J Roentgenol 1999;173:1185–92.

[56] Dodd 3rd GD, Baron RL, Oliver 3rd JH, et al. Spectrum of imaging findings of the liver in end-stage cirrhosis: part I, gross morphology and diffuse abnormalities. AJR Am J Roentgenol 1999;173:1031–6.

[57] Lim JH, Choi D, Cho SK, et al. Conspicuity of hepatocellular nodular lesions in cirrhotic livers at ferumoxides-enhanced MR imaging: importance of Kupffer cell number. Radiology 2001;220:669–76.

[58] Imai Y, Murakami T, Yoshida S, et al. Superparamagnetic iron oxide-enhanced magnetic resonance images of hepatocellular carcinoma: correlation with histological grading. Hepatology 2000;32:205–12.

[59] Kondo F, Ebara M, Sugiura N, et al. Histological features and clinical course of large regenerative nodules: evaluation of their precancerous potentiality. Hepatology 1990;12:592–8.

[60] Kim TK, Choi BI, Han JK, et al. Nontumorous arterioportal shunt mimicking hypervascular tumor in cirrhotic liver: two-phase spiral CT findings. Radiology 1998;208:597–603.

[61] Yu JS, Kim KW, Sung KB, et al. Small arterial-portal venous shunts: a cause of pseudolesions at hepatic imaging. Radiology 1997;203:737–42.

[62] Brancatelli G, Federle MP, Pealer K, et al. Portal venous thrombosis or sclerosis in liver transplantation candidates: preoperative CT findings and correlation with surgical procedure. Radiology 2001;220:321–8.

[63] Itai Y, Matsui O. Blood flow and liver imaging. Radiology 1997;202:306–14.

[64] Mulhern Jr CB, Arger PH, Coleman BG, et al. Nonuniform attenuation in computed tomography study of the cirrhotic liver. Radiology 1979;132: 399–402.

[65] Huet PM, Du Reau A, Marleau D. Arterial and portal blood supply in cirrhosis: a functional evaluation. Gut 1979;20:792–6.

[66] Popper H. Pathologic aspects of cirrhosis. A review. Am J Pathol 1977;87:228–64.

[67] Peterson MS, Baron RL, Marsh Jr JW, et al. Pretransplantation surveillance for possible hepatocellular carcinoma in patients with cirrhosis: epidemiology and CT-based tumor detection rate in 430 cases with surgical pathologic correlation. Radiology 2000;217:743–9.

[68] Kim T, Murakami T, Takahashi S, et al. Optimal phases of dynamic CT for detecting hepatocellular carcinoma: evaluation of unenhanced and triple-phase images. Abdom Imaging 1999;24:473–80.

[69] Baron RL, Oliver 3rd JH, Dodd 3rd GD, et al. Hepatocellular carcinoma: evaluation with biphasic, contrast-enhanced, helical CT. Radiology 1996;199: 505–11.

[70] Oliver 3rd JH, Baron RL. Helical biphasic contrast-enhanced CT of the liver: technique, indications, interpretation, and pitfalls. Radiology 1996;201:1–14.

[71] Murakami T, Kim T, Takamura M, et al. Hypervascular hepatocellular carcinoma: detection with double arterial phase multi-detector row helical CT. Radiology 2001;218:763–7.

[72] Tiribelli C, Melato M, Croce LS, et al. Prevalence of hepatocellular carcinoma and relation to cirrhosis: comparison of two different cities of the world— Trieste, Italy, and Chiba, Japan. Hepatology 1989;10: 998–1002.

[73] Nzeako UC, Goodman ZD, Ishak KG. Hepatocellular carcinoma in cirrhotic and noncirrhotic livers. A clinico-histopathologic study of 804 North American patients. Am J Clin Pathol 1996;105:65–75.

[74] Brancatelli G, Federle MP, Grazioli L, et al. Hepatocellular carcinoma in noncirrhotic liver: CT, clinical, and pathologic findings in 39 US residents. Radiology 2002;222:89–94.

[75] Smalley SR, Moertel CG, Hilton JF, et al. Hepatoma in the noncirrhotic liver. Cancer 1988;62:1414–24.

[76] Shimada M, Rikimaru T, Sugimachi K, et al. The importance of hepatic resection for hepatocellular carcinoma originating from nonfibrotic liver. J Am Coll Surg 2000;191:531–7.

[77] Ahmetoglu A, Kosucu P, Kul S, et al. MDCT cholangiography with volume rendering for the assessment of patients with biliary obstruction. AJR Am J Roentgenol 2004;183:1327–32.

[78] Breen DJ, Nicholson AA. The clinical utility of spiral CT cholangiography: pictorial review. Clin Radiol 2000;55:733–9.

[79] Izuishi K, Toyama Y, Nakano S, et al. Preoperative assessment of the aberrant bile duct using multislice computed tomography cholangiography. Am J Surg 2005;189:53–5.

[80] Baron RL, Tublin ME, Peterson MS. Imaging the spectrum of biliary tract disease. Radiol Clin North Am 2002;40:1325–54.

[81] Loperfido S, Angelini G, Benedetti G, et al. Major

early complications from diagnostic and therapeutic ERCP: a prospective multicenter study. Gastrointest Endosc 1998;48:1–10.

[82] Masci E, Toti G, Mariani A, et al. Complications of diagnostic and therapeutic ERCP: a prospective multicenter study. Am J Gastroenterol 2001;96: 417–23.

[83] Winick AB, Waybill PN, Venbrux AC. Complications of percutaneous transhepatic biliary interventions. Tech Vasc Interv Radiol 2001;4:200–6.

[84] Adamek HE, Albert J, Weitz M, et al. A prospective evaluation of magnetic resonance cholangiopancreatography in patients with suspected bile duct obstruction. Gut 1998;43:680–3.

[85] Greenberg M, Greenberg BM, Rubin JM, et al. Computed-tomographic cholangiography: a new technique for evaluating the head of the pancreas and distal biliary tree. Radiology 1982;144:363–8.

[86] Caoili EM, Paulson EK, Heyneman LE, et al. Helical CT cholangiography with three-dimensional volume rendering using an oral biliary contrast agent: feasibility of a novel technique. AJR Am J Roentgenol 2000;174:487–92.

[87] Sajjad Z, Oxtoby J, West D, et al. Biliary imaging by spiral CT cholangiography—a retrospective analysis. Br J Radiol 1999;72:149–52.

[88] Fleischmann D, Ringl H, Schofl R, et al. Three-dimensional spiral CT cholangiography in patients with suspected obstructive biliary disease: comparison with endoscopic retrograde cholangiography. Radiology 1996;198:861–8.

[89] Zeman RK, Berman PM, Silverman PM, et al. Biliary tract: three-dimensional helical CT without cholangiographic contrast material. Radiology 1995;196: 865–7.

[90] Kinami S, Yao T, Kurachi M, et al. Clinical evaluation of 3D-CT cholangiography for preoperative examination in laparoscopic cholecystectomy. J Gastroenterol 1999;34:111–8.

[91] Miller GA, Yeh BM, Breiman RS, et al. Use of CT cholangiography to evaluate the biliary tract after liver transplantation: initial experience. Liver Transpl 2004;10:1065–70.

[92] Yeh BM, Breiman RS, Taouli B, et al. Biliary Tract depiction in living potential liver donors: comparison of conventional MR, mangafodipir trisodium-enhanced excretory MR, and multi-detector row CT cholangiography—initial experience. Radiology 2004;230:645–51.

[93] Park SJ, Han JK, Kim TK, et al. Three-dimensional spiral CT cholangiography with minimum intensity projection in patients with suspected obstructive biliary disease: comparison with percutaneous transhepatic cholangiography. Abdom Imaging 2001; 26:281–6.

[94] Kim HC, Park SH, Park SI, et al. Three-dimensional reconstructed images using multidetector computed tomography in evaluation of the biliary tract. Abdom Imaging 2004;29:472–8.

[95] Johnson PT, Heath DG, Hofmann LV, et al. Multi-detector-row computed tomography with three-dimensional volume rendering of pancreatic cancer: a complete preoperative staging tool using computed tomography angiography and volume-rendered cholangiopancreatography. J Comput Assist Tomogr 2003;27:347–53.

[96] Zandrino F, Benzi L, Ferretti ML, et al. Multislice CT cholangiography without biliary contrast agent: technique and initial clinical results in the assessment of patients with biliary obstruction. Eur Radiol 2002;12: 1155–61.

[97] Zandrino F, Curone P, Benzi L, et al. MR versus multislice CT cholangiography in evaluating patients with obstruction of the biliary tract. Abdom Imaging 2004;30:77–85.

[98] Wang ZJ, Yeh BM, Roberts JP, et al. Living donor candidates for right hepatic lobe transplantation: evaluation at CT Cholangiography—initial experience. Radiology 2005;235:899–904.

[99] Chen JS, Yeh BM, Wang ZJ, et al. Concordance of second-order portal venous and biliary tract anatomies on MDCT angiography and MDCT cholangiography. AJR Am J Roentgenol 2005;184:70–4.

[100] Uchida M, Ishibashi M, Tomita N, et al. Hilar and suprapancreatic cholangiocarcinoma: value of 3D angiography and multiphase fusion images using MDCT. AJR Am J Roentgenol 2005;184:1572–7.

ELSEVIER
SAUNDERS

Radiol Clin N Am 43 (2005) 999 – 1020

RADIOLOGIC
CLINICS
of North America

Multidetector CT of the Pancreas

Raj Mohan Paspulati, MD*

Department of Radiology, University Hospitals of Cleveland, Case Western Reserve University, Cleveland, OH, USA

Imaging of the pancreas is challenging because of its anatomic location in the retroperitoneum and its intricate relationship with major blood vessels and bowel. CT has been the initial imaging modality of choice for evaluation of pancreatic pathology. Improvements in CT technology during the past decade, with fast image acquisition and improved spatial resolution, have increased the accuracy of CT for lesion detection and characterization. Axial CT images are not sufficient to demonstrate the complex anatomy of the pancreas and have made it mandatory to have multiphasic and multiplanar imaging of the pancreas. MRI had an advantage over single-detector CT in imaging the pancreas, because of its multiplanar capability and rapid serial dynamic image acquisition after administration of intravenous (IV) gadolinium. The introduction of multidetector CT (MDCT) in late 1990 has decreased these advantages of MRI over CT. The main advantages of MDCT are the enhanced speed of scan acquisition and the high spatial resolution because of the thin collimation (Box 1). This facilitates precise timing of multiphasic imaging and multiplanar reformations (MPR) using several reformation techniques, such as maximum intensity projections (MIP), volume rendering, and curved planar reconstructions (CPR). MDCT with various postprocessing techniques have contributed significantly to the diagnosis and staging of pancreatic carcinoma. This article reviews the technique, appli-

cations, and advantages of MDCT in the imaging of pancreatic diseases.

Technique

Careful attention to the CT technique is vital for accurate imaging of the pancreas. Patients drink approximately 500 to 1000 mL of water 1 hour before a scan. Another 300 to 500 mL of water is administered orally immediately before the scan. Water taken orally instead of radio-opaque contrast agents is used for better detection of common bile duct calculi in acute pancreatitis and for better delineation of the periampullary anatomy. Water also facilitates multiplanar imaging of the peripancreatic vessels. A right lateral decubitus position assumed before the scan improves duodenal distension and provides better evaluation of the periampullary anatomy. An initial unenhanced scan is performed from the level of the diaphragm to the iliac crest using a 5-mm slice thickness at 5-mm increments. An unenhanced scan demonstrates common bile duct calculi, pancreatic calcifications, and hemorrhage. It also demonstrates the craniocaudal extent of the pancreas to plan contrast-enhanced scans.

One hundred to 150 mL of nonionic IV contrast medium (300 mg of iodine/mL) is injected at the rate of 4 mL per second using a power injector. The contrast-enhanced scans are obtained in the pancreatic and portal venous phases as the pancreatic parenchyma, peripancreatic vessels, and liver are evaluated completely in these two phases [1]. An arterial phase is necessary only when CT angiography is required. In the pancreatic phase, the pancreas is imaged from the level of the celiac axis to the third

* Department of Radiology, University Hospitals of Cleveland, Case Western Reserve University, 11100 Euclid Avenue, Cleveland, OH 44106-5056.
   E-mail address: paspulati@uhrad.com

Box 1. Advantages of multidetector CT

Shorter scan duration
   Reduced motion artifacts
   Useful in acutely ill and in trauma
      patients
   Reduced dose of IV contrast medium
   Feasibility of multiphase contrast
      enhancement
Longer scan range
Thin collimation
   Increased spatial resolution
   MPR
   3-D volume rendering
*Ability to reconstruct images of a wide
   range of slice thickness from the same
   raw data*

---

stage of the duodenum in 35- to 40-second intervals after the initiation of IV contrast using a small field of view (20–25 cm), 1.25-mm collimation, and a pitch of 1.5. The portal venous phase begins 60 to 70 seconds after the IV contrast injection, and the scan range extends from the domes of the diaphragm to the iliac crests. Images are acquired using a large field of view, 2.5-mm collimation, and a pitch of 1.5 [2]. The pancreatic phase images are reconstructed at 0.5-mm intervals. The scanning technique may vary with the number of detectors and detector configuration. In the pancreatic phase, there is maximal enhancement not only of the pancreatic parenchyma but also of the peripancreatic arteries. In the portal venous phase, there is optimal enhancement of the hepatic parenchyma and superior mesenteric and portal veins. In the evaluation of acute pancreatitis, an unenhanced and post-IV contrast scan in the portal venous phase is sufficient for diagnosis of acute pancreatitis and associated complications.

Postprocessing imaging techniques

The large volume of data acquired as thin axial source images is transferred to a workstation for MPR. The common postprocessing techniques are coronal oblique reformations, MIP, minimum intensity projections, CPR, and volume rendering. These postprocessing techniques are useful especially in pancreatic carcinoma staging. The MIP and 3-D volume displays the peripancreatic vessels and their relationship to a pancreatic tumor. The CPR demonstrate the entire pancreatic duct or a particular pancreatic vessel in a single plane.

Normal anatomy

Pancreas

The pancreas is located in the anterior pararenal space of the retroperitoneum with an oblique orientation to the horizontal plane of approximately 20°. The shape, position, and orientation of the pancreas are variable depending on age, body habitus, and position of the spleen and left kidney. In patients who have abundant retroperitoneal fat, the peripancreatic planes are well delineated on CT scan. The pancreatic head bears a constant relationship with the second stage of the duodenum and the uncinate process with the third stage of the duodenum. The neck and body of the pancreas are related anteriorly to the stomach, from which they are separated by the potential space of the lesser sac. Adequate distension of the stomach and duodenum with water is necessary to display this intricate relationship of the pancreas to bowel in the staging of malignancy. The tail of the pancreas is intraperitoneal and is situated within the splenorenal ligament. It is variable in position depending on the location of the spleen and left kidney. The transverse mesocolon is attached to the anterior surface of the pancreas, and the root of small bowel mesentery is inferior to the body of the pancreas. MDCT with MPR can demonstrate the spread of inflammatory and neoplastic processes of the pancreas to the transverse mesocolon and small bowel mesentery.

Peripancreatic vessels

The arterial blood supply to the pancreas is derived from the branches of the celiac trunk and the superior mesenteric artery (SMA). The celiac trunk is located superior to the body of the pancreas, and the splenic artery courses along the superior margin of the pancreas. The SMA arises from the aorta posterior to the neck of pancreas at its origin and runs inferiorly, anterior to the uncinate process along with the superior mesenteric vein (SMV). This important relationship of the superior mesenteric vessels with the pancreas is displayed in sagittal MPR. The anterior and posterior superior pancreaticoduodenal branches of the gastroduodenal artery anastamose with the corresponding inferior pancreaticoduodenal branches of the SMA to form an arterial arcade around the head of the pancreas. The splenic vein runs along the posterior and superior aspects of the pancreas along with the splenic artery and forms an important landmark for the posterior surface of the pancreas. The splenic vein joins the SMV behind the neck of the pancreas to form the portal vein. Coronal oblique

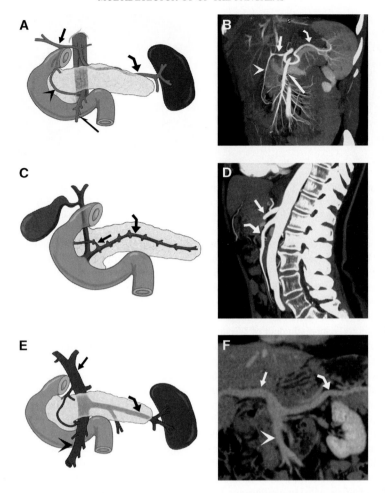

Fig. 1. Normal anatomy. (*A*) Line diagram of the peripancreatic arteries shows the hepatic artery (*straight arrow*), splenic artery (*curved arrow*), SMA (*half arrow*), and gastroduodenal artery (*arrowhead*). (*B*) Corresponding coronal MIP CT image of the peripancreatic arteries. (*C*) Line diagram demonstrates the distal common bile duct, main pancreatic duct (*curved arrow*), and accessory pancreatic duct (*straight arrow*). (*D*) Sagittal MIP CT image shows the celiac axis (*straight arrow*) and SMA (*curved arrow*). (*E*) Line diagram shows the main portal vein (*straight arrow*), splenic vein (*curved arrow*), and SMV (*arrowhead*). (*F*) Corresponding coronal oblique MIP of the peripancreatic veins.

MIP and CPR demonstrate the peripancreatic vessels in the staging of pancreatic carcinoma (Fig. 1).

Pancreatic and extrahepatic bile duct

The distal common bile duct courses inferiorly through the dorsal aspect of the head of the pancreas to meet the main pancreatic duct at the ampulla of Vater. The main pancreatic duct courses along the long axis of the pancreas and joins the distal common bile duct to form the ampulla of Vater, which opens into the second stage of the duodenum at the major papilla. The accessory pancreatic duct of Santorini opens into the duodenum at the minor papilla, which

is situated proximal to the major papilla (see Fig. 1C). The normal pancreatic duct measures 2 to 3 mm in diameter and may become wider in elderly individuals. CPR display the entire course of the pancreatic duct in a single image [3].

Clinical applications

Congenital anomalies of the pancreas

Pancreas divisum

Pancreas divisum is the most common developmental anomaly of the pancreas and is reported in

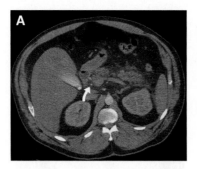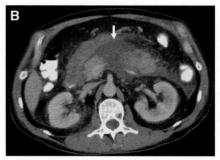

Fig. 2. Acute pancreatitis. (*A*) Axial CT image demonstrates the distal common bile duct calculus (*arrow*) and peripancreatic inflammation in a patient who had gallstone-induced acute pancreatitis. (*B*) Axial CT image in a patient who had acute necrotizing pancreatitis shows nonenhancing pancreatic parenchyma (*arrow*) representing pancreatic necrosis.

approximately 4% to 10% of the general population [4,5]. It is caused by the failure of the ventral and dorsal anlagen of the pancreas to fuse, thereby resulting in two separate pancreatic ductal systems draining the pancreas. The dorsal pancreatic duct of Santorini drains most of the pancreas through the minor papilla. The ventral pancreatic duct of Wirsung drains a portion of the head of the pancreas and uncinate process through the major papilla. Although controversial, pancreas divisum is associated with recurrent abdominal pain and pancreatitis [5]. In their series of 94 patients who had pancreas divisum, Morgan and colleagues report acute pancreatitis in 57% of their study population [6]. Endoscopic retrograde cholangiopancreatography (ERCP) and magnetic resonance cholangiopancreatography (MRCP) are proven imaging modalities for the diagnosis of pancreas divisum. Imaging with single-detector CT has low sensitivity for the detection of pancreas divisum [7]. MDCT with 1-mm collimation and CPR has a sensitivity of 90% and specificity of 98% in the detection of pancreas divisum [8].

Acute pancreatitis

Single-detector CT is an excellent imaging modality for detecting the severity of pancreatitis and its complications. Acute pancreatitis is classified as mild edematous or interstitial pancreatitis and severe, necrotizing pancreatitis. The role of imaging is not to diagnose acute pancreatitis but to demonstrate the presence and extent of pancreatic necrosis and the complications of acute pancreatitis. The presence and extent of pancreatic necrosis has excellent correlation with its morbidity and mortality rates. The extent of pancreatic necrosis cannot be judged by clinical and laboratory evaluation. Single-detector CT and MDCT are equally sensitive in demonstrating changes in acute pancreatitis and pancreatic necrosis. The CT

imaging features of acute pancreatitis include focal or diffuse enlargement of the pancreas, peripancreatic fat stranding, peripancreatic fascial thickening, and fluid collections (Fig. 2A). Pancreatic necrosis is defined as focal or diffuse areas of nonenhancing pancreatic parenchyma (see Fig. 2B). CT has an overall accuracy of 87% and sensitivity and specificity of 100% in the detection of pancreatic necrosis [9,10]. Pancreatic necrosis is defined better on CT 2 to 3 days after the onset of pancreatitis. As focal areas of interstitial edema and intrapancreatic fluid collections can be mistaken for pancreatic necrosis, follow-up CT is used for differentiation. Balthazar and colleagues [10] correlate the extent of pancreatic necrosis detected on CT with morbidity and mortality of acute pancreatitis. In their study, pancreatic necrosis of 50% or more is associated with 75% to 100% morbidity and 11% to 25% mortality. Central areas of parenchymal necrosis are more likely to disrupt the main pancreatic duct with a higher incidence of complications than the peripheral areas of necrosis [10].

Complications of acute pancreatitis

Pseudocysts

Pseudocysts are well-encapsulated fluid collections that develop approximately 4 to 6 weeks after an episode of acute pancreatitis. Pseudocysts result from the failure of resorption of peripancreatic fluid collections and disruption of the pancreatic duct caused by pancreatic parenchymal necrosis. Pseudocysts commonly are located in and around the pancreas but can occur any where in the abdomen and pelvis. Pseudocysts are of variable size and have a nonepithelialized wall derived from chronic inflammatory and fibrotic tissue. Contrast-enhanced CT demonstrates a well-defined cystic fluid collection with a uniformly thin, enhancing wall (Fig. 3A). A cystic pancreatic neoplasm must be considered when

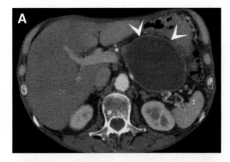

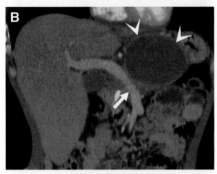

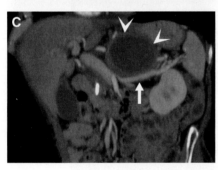

Fig. 3. Pseudocyst. (*A*) Axial CT image shows a pseudocyst (*arrowheads*) with a uniformly thin, enhancing wall, posterior to the stomach. (*B* and *C*) Coronal MPR CT images demonstrate the relationship of the pseudocyst with the superior mesenteric and splenic veins (*arrows*).

the cyst wall is thick and irregular and has mural nodules [11]. MDCT with MPR demonstrates the relationship of the pseudocyst with the pancreatic duct, peripancreatic vessels, and surrounding viscera (see Fig. 3B and C). Pseudocysts can resolve spontaneously by drainage into the pancreatic duct, rupture into the peritoneal cavity, or drainage into adjacent hollow viscera, such as the stomach and colon [12]. Complications of pseudocyst include hemorrhage; infection; rupture; and compression of bowel, extrahepatic bile duct, and peripancreatic vessels. Asymptomatic pseudocysts and pseudocysts less than 5 cm in diameter are managed conserva-

tively and are followed with CT. Symptomatic pseudocysts and those greater than 6 cm are managed either by CT-guided or surgical drainage procedures [9,13,14].

Pancreatic abscess

Pancreatic abscess develops in approximately 3% of patients who have acute pancreatitis [15]. Pancreatic abscess must be excluded in all patients who have acute pancreatitis presenting with sepsis. The risk of developing an abscess is reported to increase with the severity of pancreatitis [16], which manifests as ill-defined peripancreatic fluid collections The presence of gas bubbles in peripancreatic fluid collections is diagnostic of an abscess (Fig. 4). In the absence of gas bubbles, the diagnosis must be established by CT-guided aspiration after excluding other possible causes of sepsis. Pancreatic abscess is treated by either percutaneous drainage or surgical debridement [17].

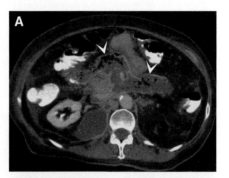

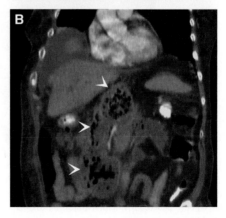

Fig. 4. Pancreatic abscess. (*A*) Axial CT image in a patient who had necrotizing pancreatitis shows a large abscess with mixed fluid and gas (*arrowheads*). (*B*) Coronal MPR CT image demonstrates the craniocaudal extent of the abscess (*arrowheads*).

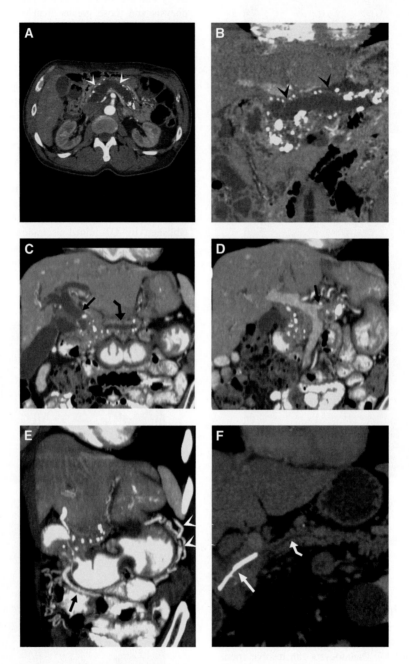

Fig. 5. Chronic pancreatitis. (*A*) Axial and (*B*) CPR CT images demonstrate the dilated pancreatic duct (*arrowheads*) with intraductal and parenchymal calcifications in atrophic pancreas. (*C*) Coronal oblique MPR CT image in a patient who had chronic calcific pancreatitis demonstrates the dilated CBD (*straight arrow*) and pancreatic duct (*curved arrow*). (*D*) Coronal oblique MPR CT image shows chronic splenic vein thrombosis (*arrow*). (*E*) Coronal MIP CT image of the same patient demonstrates dilated short gastric (*arrowheads*) and gastroepiploic collateral veins. (*F*) CPR in a patient who had chronic pancreatitis demonstrates a distal pancreatic duct stent (*arrow*) and upstream pancreatic duct (*curved arrow*).

Vascular complications

Extravasation of pancreatic enzymes and peripancreatic inflammation in acute pancreatitis causes vascular and hemorrhagic complications. Peripancreatic arteries and veins are affected. Venous thrombosis is the most common vascular complication affecting splenic, portal, and SMVs [18]. The splenic vein is thrombosed more commonly because of its close proximity to the pancreas. Mortele and coworkers report a 19% incidence of splenic vein thrombosis [19]. Splenic vein thrombosis is associated with dilated short gastric and gastroepiploic collateral veins (Fig. 5E) [20]. MDCT with MPR demonstrates the extent of splenic vein thrombosis and the presence of collateral veins. Gastric variceal bleeding occurs in 4% to 6% of patients who have pancreatitis-induced splenic vein thrombosis [21].

Pseudoaneurysm formation is a rare but important vascular complication of acute pancreatitis. It results from autodigestion of the arterial wall by extravasated pancreatic enzymes. The splenic, gastroduodenal, and pancreaticoduodenal arteries are affected more commonly. The left gastric, middle colic, hepatic arteries and small peripancreatic branches are affected less commonly. Hemorrhage from rupture of a pseudoaneurysm is the most dreaded complication and has a reported incidence of approximately 10% [22]. The most common presentation is rupture of a pseudoaneurysm into a pseudocyst [23]. Affected patients may present with upper gastrointestinal (GI) bleeding resulting from communication of the pseudocyst with the pancreatic duct; this is called hemosuccus pancreaticus [24]. Other less common sites of pseudoaneurysm rupture include the peritoneal cavity, retroperitoneum, duodenum, common bile duct, and colon. Contrast-enhanced CT has a sensitivity of 80% to 100% in detecting pseudoaneurysms [25]. They appear as well-defined, densely enhancing lesions in relation to a peripancreatic artery and either are isolated or in association with a pseudocyst. Three-dimensional volume-rendered images and MIP aid in demonstrating the contiguity of a pseudoaneurysm with peripancreatic arteries. Angiography is indicated for demonstration of small pseudoaneurysms and for treatment of pseudoaneurysms with embolization, which has a success rate of 75% to 100% [26,27]. Surgery is indicated in unstable patients and when initial treatment with embolization fails.

Chronic pancreatitis

Chronic panceatitis is a chronic inflammatory process with loss of normal functioning parenchyma and replacement with fibrosis. Alcohol intake is the leading cause of chronic pancreatitis and is responsible for nearly 70% of the cases of chronic pancreatitis in the United States. As the clinical diagnosis of chronic pancreatitis is difficult because of its nonspecific presentation, the diagnosis is established by imaging. For decades, CT has been the initial imaging modality for diagnosis of chronic pancreatitis. The diagnosis is based on morphologic changes of the pancreatic parenchyma and pancreatic duct. As early as 1979, Ferrucci and colleagues described pancreatic parenchymal atrophy, calcifications, and pancreatic ductal dilatation as hallmarks of chronic pancreatitis [28]. In 1989, Luetmer and coworkers reiterated the CT criteria of chronic pancreatitis [29]. In their study of 56 patients who had proven chronic pancreatitis, main pancreatic duct dilatation, parenchymal atrophy, and pancreatic calcification were the major CT findings. Other less common features of chronic pancreatitis are pseudocyst formation and alterations of the peripancreatic fascia and fat.

Advances in CT technology, including the current availability of MDCT, have not altered these CT features of chronic pancreatitis. Thin collimation and CPR with MDCT delineate the pancreatic duct morphology better (see Fig. 5A and B). Intraductal calcification, resulting from the accumulation of calcium carbonate within the proteinaceous plug, is a characteristic CT feature of chronic pancreatitis [30]. Pancreatic ductal dilatation, strictures, and intraductal calcifications are well displayed in CPR. Although parenchymal atrophy is characteristic of chronic pancreatitis, it may manifest occasionally with focal or diffuse pancreatic enlargement. This focal enlargement is indistinguishable from pancreatic carcinoma on CT or MRI [31]. Pancreatic atrophy and

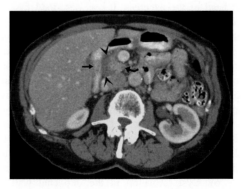

Fig. 6. Groove pancreatitis. Axial CT image in a patient who had biopsy-proven groove pancreatitis demonstrates a hypodense sheet-like mass (*arrowheads*) between the duodenum (*straight arrow*) and the normally enhancing pancreatic head (*curved arrow*).

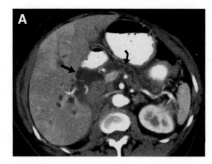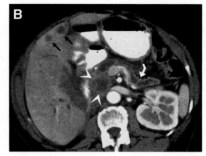

Fig. 7. Double-duct sign of pancreatic head carcinoma. (*A, B*) Contrast-enhanced axial CT images demonstrate a hypodense mass (*arrowheads*) in the head of pancreas, with dilated CBD (*straight arrow*) and pancreatic duct (*curved arrow*). Multiple hypodense lesions in the liver (*small straight arrows*) represent metastases.

ductal dilatation also are seen proximal to a pancreatic carcinoma obstructing the pancreatic duct. As chronic pancreatitis is associated with the increased risk of pancreatic cancer, diagnosis in these atypical cases must be established by imaging-guided biopsy. The dilated pancreatic duct in pancreatic carcinoma has a smooth contour compared with its irregular contour in chronic pancreatitis [32]. This holds true only when carcinoma is not associated with chronic pancreatitis.

Contrast-enhanced CT also detects complications of chronic pancreatitis, including pseudocysts, distal chronic bile duct (CBD) obstruction, pseudoaneurysms, and venous thrombosis (see Fig. 5C, D, E, and F). Chronic pancreatitis is the most common cause of splenic vein thrombosis, which is reported to occur in 45% of all cases of chronic pancreatitis [21,33].

Groove pancreatitis

This is a segmental form of chronic pancreatitis and is localized in the groove between the duodenum and head of the pancreas. It was described first by Becker in 1973, and its exact etiopathogenesis is unknown [34]. The pancreatic parenchyma and pancreatic duct do not show changes of chronic pancreatitis. Chronic inflammation and fibrosis may cause duodenal, common bile duct, and distal pancreatic duct stenosis [35]. The significance of groove pancreatitis is its clinical and imaging resemblance to periampullary or pancreatic carcinoma. Contrast-enhanced CT demonstrates a sheet-like mass with delayed enhancement effacing the pancreaticoduodenal groove, as is characteristic of fibrous tissue (Fig. 6). Cyst formation in the duodenal wall or pancreaticoduodenal groove also is described [36]. The key imaging feature of groove pancreatitis is demonstration of the normal enhancing pancreas and ductal morphology [37]. Tissue diagnosis is necessary when differentiation of groove pancreatitis from

periampullary or pancreatic carcinoma cannot be made by imaging [38].

Pancreatic carcinoma

Ductal adenocarcinoma is the most common neoplasm of the pancreas and the second most common malignancy of the digestive system after colorectal malignancy. Approximately 32,800 new cases of pancreatic carcinoma are estimated to be diagnosed in 2005 in the United States [39]. The 5-year survival rate of pancreatic carcinoma is 15% when it is confined to the pancreas and falls to 6.8% with peripancreatic invasion and 1.8% with distant metastases [40].

Surgical resection remains the only potentially curative therapy for carcinoma of the pancreas. With surgical resection, a 5-year survival rate of 20% is possible only when the tumor is small (<2 cm) and without peripancreatic invasion [41]. Unfortunately, only 10% to 15% of pancreatic carcinomas fall into this category, resulting in an overall poor survival rate [42]. Pancreatic surgery is associated with significant

---

Box 2. CT criteria for unresectability of pancreatic carcinoma

Peripancreatic vascular invasion
- Vascular occlusion
- Complete vascular encasement
- Contiguity of tumor with > 50% of the vascular circumference

Lymph nodal metastases beyond the regional peripancreatic chain

Hepatic metastases

Peritoneal implants and malignant ascitis

mortality and morbidity. Moreover, recurrence after surgical resection frequently is the result of residual tumor left behind [42]. This emphasizes the role of imaging in early detection and accurate staging of pancreatic carcinoma for select patients who benefit from surgery and to avoid unnecessary surgery in nonresectable tumors. Contrast-enhanced CT is the primary imaging modality for the diagnosis and staging of pancreatic carcinoma. Helical CT has a sensitivity of 89% to 97% for tumor detection and a positive predictive value of 89% to 100% for de-termining tumor unresectability. The accuracy of CT for detecting resectable tumors is low, with a negative predictive value (NPV) of 45% to 79% [43,44]. Increased spatial resolution and optimal pancreatic parenchymal and peripancreatic vascular enhancement with MDCT have a significant impact on accurate staging of pancreatic carcinoma and have improved detection of resectable tumors. Using the MDCT technique and CPR, Vargas and colleagues describe a NPV of 87% for resectabilty and a NPV of 100% for vascular invasion [45].

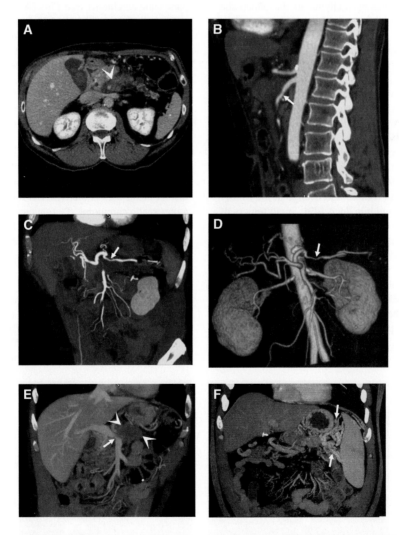

Fig. 8. Invasive pancreatic adenocarcinoma. (*A*) Axial contrast-enhanced CT image demonstrates a mass in the uncinate process (*arrowhead*) encasing the SMA. (*B*) Sagittal MIP image demonstrates focal narrowing of the SMA (*straight arrow*). (*C*) Coronal oblique MIP and (*D*) 3-D volume-rendered coronal image demonstrate focal narrowing (*straight arrow*) of the splenic artery resulting from tumor invasion. (*E*) Coronal MPR CT image demonstrates an invasive pancreatic body carcinoma (*arrowheads*) with splenic vein invasion (*straight arrow*) at the confluence of the portal and splenic veins. (*F*) Coronal MIP CT image shows dilated perigastric collateral veins (*straight arrows*).

The role of CT is to ensure tumor detection and accurate staging and to provide a vascular road map for the surgeon.

Tumor detection

Approximately 90% of pancreatic carcinomas present as a focal mass and the remaining 5% as a diffuse involvement of the gland. Approximately 60% to 65% of these focal carcinomas arise in the head, 20% in the body, and 5% in the tail [46]. The most frequent appearance of pancreatic carcinoma is a hypoattenuating mass relative to the normally enhancing pancreatic parenchyma in the pancreatic and portal venous phases of enhancement (Fig. 7B). The mean tumor to parenchymal attenuation difference is highest in the pancreatic phase but is adequate for tumor detection in the pancreatic and portal venous phases [1,47]. This decreased tumor attenuation is caused by fibroblastic proliferation and decreased vascularity. Bluemke and colleagues describe neointimal proliferation of the arterioles as a cause of decreased tumor vascularity [48]. A small percentage of pancreatic carcinomas is isoattenuating with pancreatic parenchyma, and diagnosis of these tumors is based on secondary signs, such as loss of normal lobular texture and contour and change in the caliber of the pancreatic and bile ducts [49]. Small tumors of the uncinate process are inconspicuous on CT and loss of contour may be the only abnormality. Tumors of the uncinate process have poor prognosis, because of their delayed clinical presentation, and early vascular involvement, because of their proximity to the superior mesenteric vessels [42].

Tumors in the head and body of the pancreas frequently cause pancreatic duct obstruction with upstream ductal dilatation and parenchymal atrophy (see Fig. 7B). Focal chronic pancreatitis can present as a mass with enhancing characteristics indistinguishable from those of a pancreatic carcinoma [31]. The nature of obstruction and degree of pancreatic ductal dilatation are the criteria to differentiate malignant obstruction from chronic pancreatitis. Abrupt amputation of the pancreatic duct associated with a focal mass favors pancreatic carcinoma [50]. Smooth dilatation of the pancreatic duct most often is a feature of malignant obstruction [32]. Pancreatic head tumors also cause bile duct obstruction. Combined bile duct and pancreatic duct obstruction represents the double duct sign, which is highly suggestive of but not diagnostic of pancreatic carcinoma (see Fig. 7A and B). Other less common causes of the double duct sign are cholangiocarcinoma, periampullary carcinoma, and chronic pancreatitis [50]. In pancreatic head carcinoma, combined bile duct and pancreatic duct dilatation is seen in 77%, isolated bile duct dilatation in 9%, and isolated pancreatic duct dilatation in 12% [51]. CPR through the extrahepatic bile duct and pancreatic duct demonstrate the entire course of the ducts and aid in the diagnosis of ductal obstruction [3].

Criteria for resectability

The absence of local peripancreatic extension and distant metastases is the criterion for respectability of a pancreatic carcinoma. Peirpancreatic vascular invasion, lymph node metastases, and hepatic and peritoneal metastases are the most common causes of tumor unresectability (Box 2) [48,52].

Vascular encasement

In the absence of distant metastases, vascular invasion is the most common cause of unresectability in pancreatic carcinoma. Lack of a distinct pancreatic capsule facilitates peripancreatic invasion. The accuracy of single-detector helical CT for the detection of

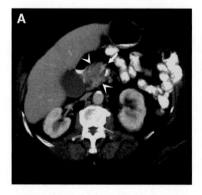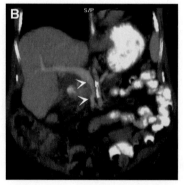

Fig. 9. Invasive pancreatic head carcinoma. (*A*) Axial contrast-enhanced CT image shows invasion of the SMV (*arrow*) by pancreatic head carcinoma (*arrowheads*). (*B*) Coronal oblique MPR CT image demonstrates the extent of SMV invasion (*arrowheads*).

vascular invasion is between 70% and 95% [43,44, 52,53]. Using MDCT and CPR, Vargas and colleagues report an accuracy of 99% and NPV of 100% in the detection of vascular invasion [45]. The major peripancreatic vessels commonly involved in pancreatic carcinoma are the celiac axis, SMA, portal vein, SMV, and splenic vein (Figs. 8–10). Lu and coworkers describe a grading system for peripancreatic vascular invasion based on the circumferential contiguity of the tumor to the vessel. They conclude that a tumor-to-vessel contact of more than 50% of the circumference is a highly specific sign of unresectability [43]. The SMV normally is in contact with the pancreas along its anterior and lateral margins. This results in an increased false positive rate of vascular invasion [45]. The teardrop appearance of the SMV described by Hough and colleagues is the result of tumor infiltration or peritumoral fibrosis and is a reliable sign of vascular invasion with a sensitivity of 91%, accuracy of 95%, and specificity of 98% (see Fig. 9A) [54]. There are reports of vascular invasion detection using MPR. Diehl and coworkers report a higher accuracy of 94% for venous invasion with MPR [52]. A higher accuracy rate of 92% to 96% for detecting vascular invasion can be obtained when axial images are interpreted along with MPR, compared with an accuracy of 70% when axial images are interpreted alone [53,55]. Dilatation of the small peripancreatic veins is an indirect sign of peripancreatic invasion and unresectability [56,57].

Lymph node metastases

CT is inaccurate for the detection of regional lymph node metastases [48,52,58]. The CT criteria of nodal involvement, based on size, are less reliable as large lymph nodes may be hyperplastic and normal-sized lymph nodes may have metastases. Using a short-axis diameter of more than 10 mm as the criterion for nodal involvement, Roche and colleagues attained a sensitivity of 14%, specificity of 85% and overall accuracy of 73% [59]. Valls and coworkers used 1.5 cm as the criterion and were able to identify lymph nodal involvement in only 16.7% of the patients. This low detection rate of lymph node involvement is of limited significance as peripancreatic lymph nodes are resected routinely at surgery. Regional lymph nodal metastasis is not a contraindication for surgical resection if there is no evidence of vascular invasion or distant metastases [58,59].

Metastases

Liver is a common site of metastases and an important cause of unresectability of pancreatic carcinoma [46,48,52,60,61]. The inability to identify small

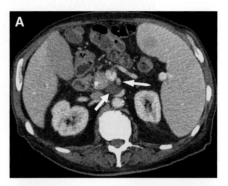
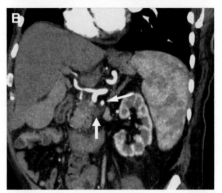
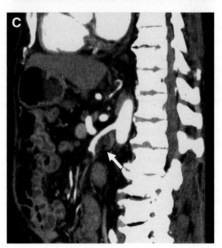

Fig. 10. Carcinoma of the uncinate process. (*A*) Axial contrast-enhanced CT image demonstrates a hypodense mass (*straight thick arrow*) of the uncinate process posterior to the SMA (*straight thin arrow*). (*B*) Coronal average intensity reformation clearly demonstrates the encasement of the SMA (*straight thin arrow*) by the uncinate process carcinoma (*straight thick arrow*). (*C*) Sagittal average intensity reformation demonstrates the extent of SMA invasion by the tumor (*straight arrow*).

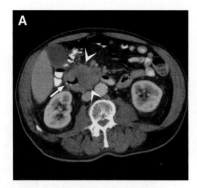 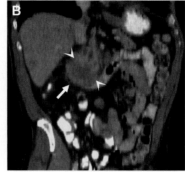

Fig. 11. Invasive pancreatic head carcinoma. (*A*) Axial and (*B*) coronal reformation contrast-enhanced CT images demonstrate pancreatic head carcinoma (*arrowheads*) invading the second stage of the duodenum (*straight arrow*).

hepatic metastases is the most common cause of understaging of pancreatic carcinoma. The hepatic metastases are hypovascular and are displayed best in the portal venous phase as hypodense lesions (see Fig. 7B). A 42% to 80% false negative staging of resectability because of undetected hepatic metastases is reported using single-detector CT [48,52]. The high spatial resolution of MDCT has improved the detection rate of small hepatic metastases. Catalano and colleagues, in their study of 46 patients who had pancreatic cancer, detected 83 of a total of 91 hepatic metastases using 1-mm thin-slice collimation compared with detection of 76 of hepatic metastases using 5-mm collimation [62]. Schima and coworkers correlated CT and MRI in the staging of pancreatic cancer and reported improved sensitivity of mangafodipir-trisodium–enhanced MR in the detection of small hepatic metastases [63].

Metastatic peritoneal implants are another important cause of unresectabilty. MDCT with thin-slice collimation has the ability to detect small implants. MPR confirms the presence of metastatic implants on liver, bowel, paracolic gutter, and cul-de-sac [64].

The stomach, duodenum, and transverse colon are the segments of the GI tract involved in pancreatic carcinoma (Fig. 11). The use of oral water as a contrast agent demonstrates the enhancing bowel wall better than radioopaque contrast agents; it also is used in 3-D imaging [65].

Neuroendocrine tumors

Neuroendocrine tumors (NET) are rare pancreatic neoplasms that arise from cells of the islets of Langerhans. Their overall incidence is 1 to 1.5 per 100,000 in the general population [66]. Although most islet cell tumors (ICT) occur sporadically, there is increased prevalence in patients who have von Hippel-Lindau syndrome and those affected with multiple endocrine neoplasia (MEN) type I. Half of NET are functioning with typical clinical presentation because of excess hormone secretion. The other half are nonfunctioning with delayed presentation because of mass effect and metastases. There are five types of functioning ICT: insulinomas, gastrinomas, glucagonomas, vasoactive-peptide secreting tumors (vipoma), and somatostatinomas. The types of NET and their clinical features are displayed in Table 1. Insulinoma is the most common functioning ICT of the pancreas. Insulinomas usually are solitary and small (<2 cm) and 90% of them are benign. Gas-

Table 1
Classification of neuroendocrine tumors of the pancreas: 50% functioning tumors

Type	Clinical features	Malignancy	Associated syndrome
Insulinoma	Hypoglycemic attacks	10%	—
Gastrinoma	Peptic ulcer, diarrhea, malabsorption	60%–85%	Zollinger-Ellison
Glucagonoma	4D syndrome[a]	—	—
Vipoma	Watery diarrhea, hypokalemia, and achlorydria (WDHA)	50%	WDHA or Verner-Morrison
Somatostatinoma	Abdominal pain, weight loss, diarrhea, and diabetes	—	Neurofibromatosis

[a] Diabetes, dermatitis (necrolytic migratory erythema), deep vein thrombosis, and depression.

trinomas are the second most common functional ICT and approximately 60% of them are malignant. They may be associated with Zollinger-Ellison syndrome, which is characterized by intractable peptic ulcer disease, elevated serum gastrin, and gastric hypersecretions. Other functioning ICT of the pancreas are rare. Approximately one third of gastrinomas are associated with MEN type 1. Gastrinomas associated with MEN type 1 are multifocal and approximately 50% of them are malignant. The gastrinomas can be in either intra- or extrapancreatic locations. The duodenum, lymph nodes, jejunum, and stomach are extrapancreatic locations with the duodenum the most common extrapancreatic location. Functioning and nonfunctioning pancreatic NET are hypervascular because of their rich capillary network and are hyperattenuating in the arterial and venous phase on contrast-enhanced CT (Fig. 12). The small size of the functioning tumors and their hypervascularity indicate the importance of thin-slice collimation and imaging early after the administration of contrast medium; this can be achieved with MDCT. Van Hoe and colleagues report an increased rate of detection of

these tumors in the arterial phase [67]. Fidler and colleagues report 63% sensitivity of multiphase CT for the detection of insulinomas; the pancreatic phase is more useful than the arterial phase for tumor detection [68]. The overall sensitivity of CT for the detection of functioning ICT varies from 71% to 82%. Imaging in the portal venous phase is essential, as some of these tumors show delayed enhancement in the venous phase [69]. CT and MRI have similar sensitivity in the localization of ICT. MPR differentiate hyperattenuating ICT from enhancing peripancreatic vasculature [70]. The nonfunctional tumors are large with heterogeneous enhancement and are associated with cystic degeneration and calcification [71]. Liver and lymph nodes are the common sites of metastases from malignant ICT and, like the primary tumor, are hypervascular. The metastases also are detected better in the arterial phase [72]. Endoscopic ultrasonography has higher sensitivity than CT for the detection of small functioning ICT. Anderson and coworkers report a sensitivity and accuracy of 93% and a specificity of 95% for the detection of NET of the pancreas by endoscopic ultrasonography [73].

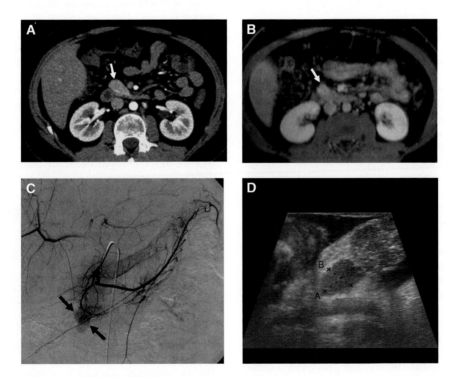

Fig. 12. Insulinoma in a 20-year-old man presenting with recurrent hypoglycemic attacks. (*A*) Contrast-enhanced axial CT and (*B*) contrast-enhanced axial MRI of the pancreatic head in the arterial phase demonstrate an enhancing lesion (*arrow*) in the head of the pancreas. (*C*) Selective celiac artery angiogram demonstrates a well-defined, focal, arterial blush (*arrows*), which corresponds to the enhancing lesion in the head of the pancreas. (*D*) Intraoperative ultrasonography demonstrates a well-defined hypoechoic mass (*cursors*) in the head of pancreas.

Table 2
Classification of cystic pancreatic tumors: nonfunctioning tumors

Type	Common location	Malignancy
Serious cyadenoma	Head and uncinate process	Benign
Mucinous cystadenoma	Body and tail	Potentially malignant
IMPT		
Branch duct type	Common in uncinate process and head of pancreas	Low-grade
Main duct type	—	Potentially malignant
Diffuse		
Segmental		
Combined	—	—
Solid and papillary epithelial neoplasm	Tail of pancreas	Low-grade
Miscellaneous	—	—
Lymphangioma		
Hemangioma		
Cystic neuro-endocrine tumors		
Cystic metastases		

Cystic pancreatic tumors

Approximately 10% of cystic pancreatic lesions are cystic tumors. One percent of these cystic pancreatic tumors are malignant [74]. Although inflammatory pseudocyst is the most common cystic lesion of the pancreas, a cystic pancreatic tumor must be excluded in all cystic pancreatic lesions. Most cystic pancreatic tumors are discovered incidentally as a result of the increased use of cross-sectional imaging. Serous cystadenomas, mucinous cystadenomas and carcinomas, and intraductal papillary mucinous tumors (IPMT) are the major cystic tumors of the pancreas (Table 2).

Serous cystadenomas (microcystic adenomas)

Serous cystadenoma is a benign neoplasm that constitutes approximately 1% to 2% of all pancreatic neoplasms. They occur commonly in women over 60 years of age with increased frequency in patients who have von Hippel-Lindau disease. They are more common in the head of the pancreas and vary in size from 2 to 25 cm [75]. They are characterized by multiple cysts measuring less than 2 cm within a dense fibrous stroma. The cysts are separated by fibrous septations, which radiate from the center of the mass. The fibrous bands form a central stellate scar, which may calcify. Their appearance on CT depends on the size of the cysts and the amount of the fibrous stroma

present in the tumor (Fig. 13). Tumors with predominantly fibrous stroma have a solid appearance.

Mucinous/macrocystic cystadenoma

Mucinous cystadenoma is a benign tumor with malignant potential and is the most common cystic neoplasm of the pancreas. There is increased prevalence in women between the fourth and sixth decades of age. These tumors commonly are located in the body and tail of the pancreas and generally are large at the time of diagnosis, with an average size of approximately 5 cm. They usually are multilocular with individual cystic spaces larger than 2 cm in diameter (Fig. 14A and B). Peripheral calcification of the cyst wall is reported in 10% to 25% of these tumors [76]. The presence of thick septations and mural nodules are indicators of a malignant neoplasm (see Fig. 14C).

Differentiation of serous and mucinous cystadenomas

The differentiation of serous from mucinous cystadenomas is important because of the malignant potential of mucinous tumors. As there are few reports regarding malignant serous cystadenocarcinoma, serous cystadenomas are managed expectantly with follow-up. There are reports of the sensitivity and accuracy of CT in differentiating serous from mucinous cystic tumors of the pancreas. Johnson and colleagues [77] report that serous tumors have more than six cysts, each cyst less than 2 cm in diameter, whereas mucinous tumors have fewer cysts greater than 2 cm in diameter. Curry and colleagues, however, report that CT cannot differentiate serous from mucinous tumors using the criteria of cyst number and size [76]. They conclude that the presence and location of tumor calcification are helpful in differ-

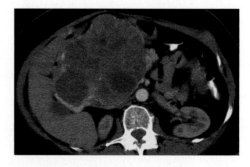

Fig. 13. Microcystic adenoma in a 60-year-old woman presenting with a palpable abdominal mass. Axial contrast-enhanced CT demonstrates a large, lobulated hypoattenuating mass arising from the head of the pancreas. The mass has a honeycomb appearance resulting from many small cysts within an enhancing stroma.

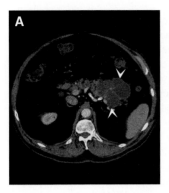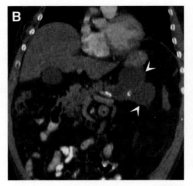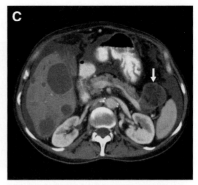

Fig. 14. Mucinous cyst neoplasms. (*A*) Axial and (*B*) coronal MPR, contrast-enhanced CT images in a patient who had proven mucinous cystadenoma demonstrate a multilocular cystic mass (*arrowheads*) in the tail of the pancreas with large loculations and no mural nodules. (*C*) Axial contrast-enhanced CT in a patient who had mucinous cystadenocarcinoma demonstrates a complex cystic mass (*arrow*) in the tail of the pancreas, with cystic hepatic metastases and ascitis.

entiating these tumors. Calcification in serous cystadenomas is central within the fibrous stroma and may have a sunburst appearance, whereas mucinous tumors have peripheral calcification [76]. A macrocystic variant of benign serous cystadenoma recently was described. It also is more common in the head of the pancreas and varies in size from 1.5 to 5.0 cm. It is a uni- or bilocular cyst with a thin (<2 mm) wall and lacks mural nodules or calcifications [11,78]. Its location in the head of the pancreas, lobulated contour, and lack of wall enhancement are the CT features of macrocystic serous cystadenoma and are helpful in distinguishing them from mucinous cystadenoma and pseudocyst [11].

When characterization of a pancreatic cyst is indeterminate with imaging, cyst fluid aspiration and analysis are useful. The fluid is analyzed for viscosity, mucin, and amylase and tumor markers CEA and CA 19.9 [79,80].

Intraductal papillary mucinous tumor

IPMT of the pancreas are rare and represent approximately 1% to 2% of the exocrine tumors of the pancreas. They arise from the epithelial lining of the pancreatic duct and typically produce a copious amount of mucin that may cause ductal dilatation and obstruction resulting from mucus plugs. Histologically, IPMT represent a spectrum ranging from hyperplasia to carcinoma, with approximately 40% to 80% malignant [81,82]. They have increased prevalence in men older than 60. Their clinical presentation is caused by pancreatic duct obstruction and mucin hypersecretion and mimics chronic pancreatitis. IPMT are classified according to the extent of pancreatic duct involvement into the main duct type, branch duct type, and combined type [82]. The branch duct type is

common in the uncinate process but may occur in the body and tail. The main duct type may be segmental or diffuse. The main duct type has a higher incidence of carcinoma and is treated with total pancreatectomy. MDCT in the pancreatic phase of enhancement with

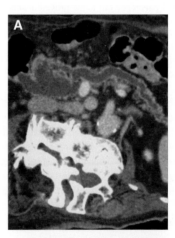

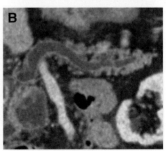

Fig. 15. (*A* and *B*) IPMT of the main duct type. CPR through the pancreatic duct demonstrate generalized dilatation of the main pancreatic duct and atrophic pancreas.

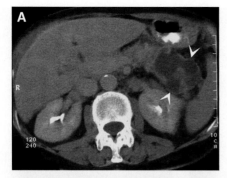

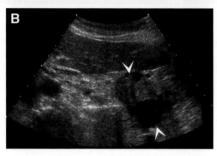

Fig. 16. A 45-year-old African American woman who had an incidental pancreatic tail mass, proved at surgery to be a solid and papillary epithelial neoplasm. (*A*) Axial contrast-enhanced CT shows a complex cystic mass (*arrowheads*) in the tail of the pancreas with mixed cystic and solid components. (*B*) Ultrasonography demonstrates the cystic and solid components of the mass (*arrowheads*).

thin collimation and CPR demonstrates the main pancreatic duct and the relationship of the cysts with the pancreatic duct [2,83]. The branch duct type appears as a cluster of cysts with a lobulated margin and thin septations. This closely resembles microcystic adenoma and is differentiated by demonstrating communication of the cysts with the pancreatic duct by ERCP. Fukukura and colleagues report a similar sensitivity of thin section helical CT and MRI in

demonstrating the communication between the cyst and the pancreatic duct [84]. The main pancreatic duct may be dilated in the branch duct type as a result of excess mucin production. The main duct type may have either diffuse or segmental dilatation of the pancreatic duct associated with parenchymal atrophy (Fig. 15). Intraductal papillary excrescences representing the papillary tumor and calcification of the impacted mucin may be seen. These imaging features of IPMT are difficult to differentiate from those of chronic pancreatitis. Demonstration of intraductal papillary nodules and a prominent duodenal papilla are helpful in differentiating IPMT from chronic pancreatitis. These are better demonstrated by ERCP, which is the imaging modality of choice for the diagnosis of IPMT. Fukukura and colleagues report an improved sensitivity of thin section helical CT in demonstrating the ductal communication of the cyst, intraductal mural nodules, and bulging duodenal papilla [85]. They were able to demonstrate ductal communication of the cyst in 76% of their patients and intraductal papillary tumors of 3 mm and larger. The differentiation of benign from malignant IPMT is important as the benign tumors are followed with imaging and malignant tumors are treated with pancreatectomy. The highly specific predictive signs of malignancy in IPMT include MPD dilatation greater than 10 mm, the presence of large mural nodules, diffuse or multifocal involvement, intraductal calcifications, and a bulging duodenal papilla [82,86,87]. Endoscopic ultrasonography and pancreatic juice analysis for atypical cells and CEA and CA19 tumor markers are helpful when the CT findings are indeterminate [88,89].

Solid papillary epithelial neoplasm

Solid and papillary epithelial neoplasms of the pancreas are uncommon pancreatic tumors with a low malignant potential. They are reported to be of higher incidence in young, African American, and Asian

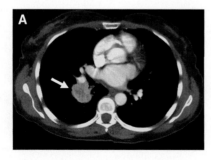

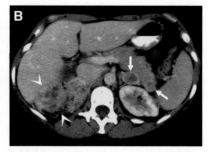

Fig. 17. A patient who had known bronchogenic carcinoma on follow-up CT. (*A*) Axial CT of the chest shows the primary lung carcinoma (*arrow*). (*B*) Contrast-enhanced axial CT of the abdomen demonstrates metastases in the right kidney (*arrowheads*), left adrenal gland, and pancreatic tail (*straight arrows*).

women. They are common in the tail of the pancreas with a mean size of 9 cm. They are well-encapsulated tumors with a variable internal architecture, depending on the degree of hemorrhage and cystic degeneration (Fig. 16) [90].

Pancreatic metastases

The common primary tumors that metastasize to the pancreas are from lung, breast, kidney, melanoma, colon, and ovary. Most of the affected patients have other evidence of metastatic disease (Fig. 17). The interval between diagnosis of the primary tumor and development of pancreatic metastases is variable. Pancreatic metastases from renal cell carcinoma frequently are detected several years after initial diagnosis [91]. Three distinct patterns of pancreatic metastases are de-scribed and include a solitary nodule, multiple nodules, and diffuse infiltration of the pancreas [92,93]. The enhancement characteristic of these nodules mimics that of the primary tumor. Most of the pancreatic metastases are hypodense relative to the pancreas. Hypervascular metastases from renal cell carcinoma and melanoma display enhancement [94].

Pancreas transplant

Improvements in the techniques of pancreas transplant surgery and immunosuppressive treatment have resulted in a 1-year patient survival rate greater than 95% and in a 1-year graft survival rate greater than 70% [95]. Nearly 90% of these transplants are performed as simultaneous pancreas-kidney transplantation from the same donor; the other less common

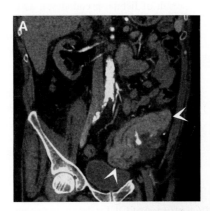
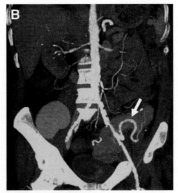
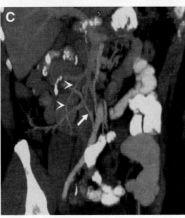

Fig. 18. Normal pancreas transplant. (*A*) Coronal oblique MPR demonstrates a normal pancreas transplant (*arrowheads*) in the left lower quadrant of the abdomen. (*B*) Coronal oblique MIP demonstrates the patent arterial supply (*arrow*) to the pancreas transplant from the left iliac artery. (*C*) Coronal oblique MIP in another patient who had a pancreas transplant in the midabdomen demonstrates a patent arterial supply (*straight arrow*) from the right common iliac artery and venous drainage (*arrowheads*) into the SMV.

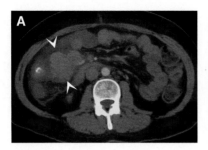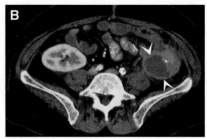

Fig. 19. (*A*) Acute pancreatitis of a pancreas transplant. Axial CT image of a patient who had pancreas transplant presenting with elevated serum amylase and lipase demonstrates an enlarged pancreas transplant (*arrowheads*) with peripancreatic inflammation. (*B*) Contrast-enhanced CT of the abdomen in another patient who had transplant pancreatitis demonstrates a pseudocyst (*arrowheads*).

techniques include pancreas after kidney transplantation and isolated pancreas transplantation. The more physiologic enteric drainage of exocrine secretions into the jejunum is replacing the older method of bladder drainage. The venous drainage is either into the systemic or more physiologic portal circulation. The systemic venous drainage involves anastamosis of the donor portal vein with the recipient iliac vein. The portal venous drainage is by anastamosis of the donor SMV with the recipient SMV or portal vein. The arterial reconstruction involves anastamoses of the donor splenic and SMAs with the recipient's common iliac or external iliac artery through an intervening donor Y-iliac artery extension graft. Knowledge of the surgical method and postoperative radiologic anatomy of a pancreas transplant is essential for follow-up of a transplant and diagnosis of complications (Fig. 18). Complications include vascular thrombosis, leakage of enteric anastamosis, hematoma, abscess, pancreatitis, pesudocyst formation, rejection and post-transplant lymphoproliferative disorder (Fig. 19). In contrast to hepatic and renal transplants, ultrasonography of the pancreas transplant is hampered by superimposed bowel gas [96]. Contrast-enhanced MDCT in the arterial and venous phases with 3-D reconstruction of the vascular anatomy is the preferred imaging technique [97]. MRI is indicated in patients who have impaired renal function [98]. CT also is used in the placement of percutaneous drainage catheters in peripancreatic fluid collections and in pancreatic graft biopsy.

Pancreas trauma

Pancreatic injury is uncommon and occurs in 2% of penetrating injuries and in 5% to 12% of blunt abdominal injuries [99,100]. Most of the deaths associated with pancreatic injuries occur within the first 48 hours after injury and are caused by hemorrhage from injury to the major peripancreatic vessels. The delayed mortality and morbidity are the result of fistula, pseudodcyst, and abscess formation from pancreatic duct disruption [101,102]. It is important to assess the integrity of the pancreatic duct in all cases of pancreatic injury, as pancreatic injuries with ductal disruption are treated surgically or by endoscopic stent placement, whereas injuries without ductal involvement are treated conservatively [103]. The primary signs of pancreatic parenchymal injury are contusion, laceration, and transaction. Peripancreatic fat stranding, hematoma, and fluid collections are important secondary signs. The sensitivity of single-detector CT is reported to be low for detecting pancreatic ductal disruption. MDCT with good spatial resolution and CPR is likely to improve the efficacy of CT for detecting pancreatic ductal injuries [104]. ERCP is the gold standard for the diagnosis of pancreatic ductal injury and is therapeutic in stenting the pancreatic duct. MRCP shows promising results for the detection and exclusion of pancreatic ductal injury [105,106].

Summary

The advantages of MDCT, which include high spatial resolution, rapid data acquisition and various postprocessing techniques, are suited perfectly for imaging of the pancreas and the complex peripancreatic anatomy. Excellent visualization of the pancreatic parenchyma in various phases of contrast enhancement facilitates early detection of small pancreatic lesions. Postprocessing techniques not only facilitate accurate staging of pancreatic cancer but also provide a vascular road map for the operating surgeon.

Acknowledgments

The author thanks Bonnie Hami, MA (Department of Radiology, University Hospitals of Cleveland), for her editorial assistance in preparing this article. The author also thanks Elena Dupont for the line diagrams and Joseph Molter for his assistance in preparing the images for this article.

References

[1] McNulty NJ, Francis IR, Platt JF, et al. Multi-detector row helical CT of the pancreas: effect of contrast-enhanced multiphasic imaging on enhancement of the pancreas, peripancreatic vasculature, and pancreatic adenocarcinoma. Radiology 2001;220:97–102.

[2] Nino-Murcia M, Tamm EP, Charnsangavej C, et al. Multidetector-row helical CT and advanced postprocessing techniques for the evaluation of pancreatic neoplasms. Abdom Imaging 2003;28:366–77.

[3] Nino-Murcia M, Jeffrey Jr RB, et al. Multidetector CT of the pancreas and bile duct system: value of curved planar reformations. AJR Am J Roentgenol 2001;176:689–93.

[4] Delhaye M, Engelholm L, Cremer M. Pancreas divisum: congenital anatomic variant or anomaly? Contribution of endoscopic retrograde pancreatography. Gastroenterology 1985;89:951–8.

[5] Agha FP, Williams KD. Pancreas divisum: incidence, detection, and clinical significance. Am J Gastroenterol 1987;82:315–20.

[6] Morgan DE, Logan K, Baron TH, et al. Pancreas divisum: implications for diagnostic and therapeutic pancreatography. AJR Am J Roentgenol 1999;173: 193–8.

[7] Zeman RK, McVay LV, Silverman PM, et al. Pancreas divisum: thin-section CT. Radiology 1988;169: 395–8.

[8] Soto JA, Lucey BC, Stuhlfaut JW. Pancreas divisum: depiction with multi-detector row CT. Radiology 2005;235:503–8.

[9] Yassa NA, Agostini JT, Ralls PW. Accuracy of CT in estimating extent of pancreatic necrosis. Clin Imaging 1997;21:407–10.

[10] Balthazar EJ. Acute pancreatitis: assessment of severity with clinical and CT evaluation. Radiology 2002;223:603–13.

[11] Cohen-Scali F, Vilgrain V, Brancatelli G, et al. Discrimination of unilocular macrocystic serous cystadenoma from pancreatic pseudocyst and mucinous cystadenoma with CT: initial observations. Radiology 2003;228:727–33.

[12] Gumaste VV, Pitchumoni CS. Pancreatic pseudocyst. Gastroenterologist 1996;4:33–43.

[13] Yeo CJ, Bastidas JA, Lynch-Nyhan A, et al. The natural history of pancreatic pseudocysts documented by computed tomography. Surg Gynecol Obstet 1990;170:411–7.

[14] Pitchumoni CS, Agarwal N. Pancreatic pseudocysts. When and how should drainage be performed? Gastroenterol Clin North Am 1999;28:615–39.

[15] Katsohis CD, Jardinoglou E, Basdanis G, et al. Pancreatic abscess following acute pancreatitis. Am Surg 1989;55:427–34.

[16] Ranson JH, Balthazar E, Caccavale R, et al. Computed tomography and the prediction of pancreatic abscess in acute pancreatitis. Ann Surg 1985;201: 656–65.

[17] vanSonnenberg E, Wittich GR, Chon KS, et al. Percutaneous radiologic drainage of pancreatic abscesses. AJR Am J Roentgenol 1997;168:979–84.

[18] Belli AM, Jennings CM, Nakielny RA. Splenic and portal venous thrombosis: a vascular complication of pancreatic disease demonstrated on computed tomography. Clin Radiol 1990;41:13–6.

[19] Mortele KJ, Mergo PJ, Taylor HM, et al. Peripancreatic vascular abnormalities complicating acute pancreatitis: contrast- enhanced helical CT findings. Eur J Radiol 2004;52:67–72.

[20] Moody AR, Poon PY. Gastroepiploic veins: CT appearance in pancreatic disease. AJR Am J Roentgenol 1992;158:779–83.

[21] Heider TR, Azeem S, Galanko JA, et al. The natural history of pancreatitis- induced splenic vein thrombosis. Ann Surg 2004;239:876–80.

[22] Balthazar EJ, Fisher LA. Hemorrhagic complications of pancreatitis: radiologic evaluation with emphasis on CT imaging. Pancreatology 2001;1:306–13.

[23] Carr JA, Cho JS, Shepard AD, et al. Visceral pseudoaneurysms due to pancreatic pseudocysts: rare but lethal complications of pancreatitis. J Vasc Surg 2000; 32:722–30.

[24] Dasgupta R, Davies NJ, Williamson RC, et al. Haemosuccus pancreaticus: treatment by arterial embolization. Clin Radiol 2002;57:1021–7.

[25] Pitkaranta P, Haapiainen R, Kivisaari L, et al. Diagnostic evaluation and aggressive surgical approach in bleeding pseudoaneurysms associated with pancreatic pseudocysts. Scand J Gastroenterol 1991;26: 58–64.

[26] Savastano S, Feltrin GP, Antonio T, et al. Arterial complications of pancreatitis: diagnostic and therapeutic role of radiology. Pancreas 1993;8:687–92.

[27] de Perrot M, Berney T, Buhler L, et al. Management of bleeding pseudoaneurysms in patients with pancreatitis. Br J Surg 1999;86:29–32.

[28] Ferrucci JT, Wittenberg J, Black EB, et al. Computed body tomography in chronic pancreatitis. Radiology 1979;130:175–82.

[29] Luetmer PH, Stephens DH, Ward EM. Chronic pancreatitis: reassessment with current CT. Radiology 1989;171:353–7.

[30] Remer EM, Baker ME. Imaging of chronic pancreatitis. Radiol Clin North Am 2002;40:1229–42.

[31] Kim T, Murakami T, Takamura M, et al. Pancreatic

mass due to chronic pancreatitis: correlation of CT
and MR imaging features with pathologic findings.
AJR Am J Roentgenol 2001;177:367–71.

[32] Karasawa E, Goldberg HI, Moss AA, et al. CT pan-
creatogram in carcinoma of the pancreas and chronic
pancreatitis. Radiology 1983;148:489–93.

[33] Weber SM, Rikkers LF. Splenic vein thrombosis and
gastrointestinal bleeding in chronic pancreatitis.
World J Surg 2003;27:1271–4.

[34] Rey P, Carrere C, Tissier S, et al. Groove pancreatitis.
Diagnostic impact of dynamic radiology. Presse Med
2003;32:1705–6.

[35] Becker V, Mischke U. Groove pancreatitis. Int J
Pancreatol 1991;10:173–82.

[36] Itoh S, Yamakawa K, Shimamoto K, et al. CT findings in groove pancreatitis: correlation with histo-
pathological findings. J Comput Assist Tomogr 1994;
18:911–5.

[37] Stolte M, Weiss W, Volkholz H, et al. A special form
of segmental pancreatitis: "groove pancreatitis."
Hepatogastroenterology 1982;29:198–208.

[38] Yamaguchi K, Tanaka M. Groove pancreatitis mas-
querading as pancreatic carcinoma. Am J Surg 1992;
163:312–6.

[39] Estimated new cancer cases and deaths by sex for
all sites, US, 2005. Cancer facts and figures 2005.
Atlanta (GA): American Cancer Society; 2005.

[40] Cooperman AM. Pancreatic cancer: the bigger
picture. Surg Clin North Am 2001;8:557–74.

[41] Tsiotos GG, Farnell MB, Sarr MG. Are the results
of pancreatectomy for pancreatic cancer improving?
World J Surg 1999;23:913–9.

[42] Beger HG, Rau B, Gansauge F, et al. Treatment
of pancreatic cancer: challenge of the facts. World J
Surg 2003;27:1075–84.

[43] Lu DS, Reber HA, Krasny RM, et al. Local staging
of pancreatic cancer: criteria for unresectability of
major vessels as revealed by pancreatic-phase, thin-
section helical CT. AJR Am J Roentgenol 1997;168:
1439–43.

[44] O'Malley ME, Boland GW, Wood BJ, et al. Adenocarcinoma of the head of the pancreas: determination of surgical unresectability with thin-section
pancreatic-phase helical CT. AJR Am J Roentgenol
1999;173:1513–8.

[45] Vargas R, Nino-Murcia M, Trueblood W, et al.
MDCT in pancreatic adenocarcinoma: prediction
of vascular invasion and resectability using a multiphasic technique with curved planar reformations.
AJR Am J Roentgenol 2004;182:419–25.

[46] Freeny PC, Traverso LW, Ryan JA. Diagnosis and
staging of pancreatic adenocarcinoma with dynamic
computed tomography. Am J Surg 1993;165:600–6.

[47] Fletcher JG, Wiersema MJ, Farrell MA, et al.
Pancreatic malignancy: value of arterial, pancreatic,
and hepatic phase imaging with multi-detector row
CT. Radiology 2003;229:81–90.

[48] Bluemke DA, Cameron JL, Hruban RH, et al. Potentially resectable pancreatic adenocarcinoma: spiral

CT assessment with surgical and pathologic correlation. Radiology 1995;197:381–5.

[49] Prokesch RW, Chow LC, Beaulieu CF, et al. Isoattenuating pancreatic adenocarcinoma at multidetector row CT: secondary signs. Radiology 2002;
224:764–8.

[50] Zeman RK, Silverman PM, Ascher SM, et al. Helical
(spiral) CT of the pancreas and biliary tract. Radiol
Clin North Am 1995;33:887–902.

[51] Freeny PC, Marks WM, Ryan JA, et al. Pancreatic
ductal adenocarcinoma: diagnosis and staging with
dynamic CT. Radiology 1988;166:125–33.

[52] Diehl SJ, Lehmann KJ, Sadick M, et al. Pancreatic
cancer: value of dual-phase helical CT in assessing
resectability. Radiology 1998;206:373–8.

[53] Lepanto L, Arzoumanian Y, Gianfelice D, et al. Helical CT with CT angiography in assessing periampullary neoplasms: identification of vascular invasion.
Radiology 2002;222:347–52.

[54] Hough TJ, Raptopoulos V, Siewert B, et al. Teardrop
superior mesenteric vein: CT sign for unresectable
carcinoma of the pancreas. AJR Am J Roentgenol
1999;173:1509–12.

[55] Raptopoulos V, Steer ML, Sheiman RG, et al. The use
of helical CT and CT angiography to predict vascular
involvement from pancreatic cancer: correlation with
findings at surgery. AJR Am J Roentgenol 1997;168:
971–7.

[56] Yamada Y, Mori H, Kiyosue H, et al. CT assessment of the inferior peripancreatic veins: clinical significance. AJR Am J Roentgenol 2000;174:
677–84.

[57] Hommeyer SC, Freeny PC, Crabo LG. Carcinoma of
the head of the pancreas: evaluation of the pancreaticoduodenal veins with dynamic CT—potential for
improved accuracy in staging. Radiology 1995;196:
233–8.

[58] Valls C, Andia E, Sanchez A, et al. Dual-phase helical
CT of pancreatic adenocarcinoma: assessment of
resectability before surgery. AJR Am J Roentgenol
2002;178:821–6.

[59] Roche CJ, Hughes ML, Garvey CJ, et al. CT and
pathologic assessment of prospective nodal staging
in patients with ductal adenocarcinoma of the head
of the pancreas. AJR Am J Roentgenol 2003;180:
475–80.

[60] Tabuchi T, Itoh K, Ohshio G, et al. Tumor staging
of pancreatic adenocarcinoma using early- and late-
phase helical CT. AJR Am J Roentgenol 1999;173:
375–80.

[61] Warshaw AL, Fernandez-del Castillo C. Pancreatic
carcinoma. N Engl J Med 1992;326:455–65.

[62] Catalano C, Laghi A, Fraioli F, et al. Pancreatic car-
cinoma: the role of high- resolution multislice spiral
CT in the diagnosis and assessment of resectability.
Eur Radiol 2003;13:149–56.

[63] Schima W, Fugger R, Schober E, et al. Diagnosis and
staging of pancreatic cancer: comparison of mangafodipir trisodium-enhanced MR imaging and contrast

enhanced helical hydro-CT. AJR Am J Roentgenol 2002;179:717–24.

[64] Pannu HK, Bristow RE, Montz FJ, et al. Multidetector CT of peritoneal carcinomatosis from ovarian cancer. Radiographics 2003;23:687–701.

[65] Horton KM, Eng J, Fishman EK. Normal enhancement of the small bowel: evaluation with spiral CT. J Comput Assist Tomogr 2000;24:67–71.

[66] Delcore R, Friesen SR. Gastrointestinal neuroendocrine tumors. J Am Coll Surg 1994;178:187–211.

[67] Van Hoe L, Gryspeerdt S, Marchal G, et al. Helical CT for the preoperative localization of islet cell tumors of the pancreas: value of arterial and parenchymal phase images. AJR Am J Roentgenol 1995; 165:1437–9.

[68] Fidler JL, Fletcher JG, Reading CG, et al. Preoperative detection of pancreatic insulinomas on multiphasic helical CT. AJR Am J Roentgenol 2003;18: 775–80.

[69] Ichwaka T, Peterson MS, Federle MP, et al. Islet cell tumor of the pancreas: biphasic CT versus MR imaging in tumor detection. Radiology 2000;216:163–71.

[70] Sheth S, Hruban RK, Fishman EK. Helical CT of islet cell tumors of the pancreas: typical and atypical manifestations. AJR Am J Roentgenol 2002;179: 725–30.

[71] Buetow PC, Parrino TV, Buck JL, et al. Islet cell tumors of the pancreas: pathologic-imaging correlation among size, necrosis and cysts, calcification, malignant behavior, and functional status. AJR Am J Roentgenol 1995;165:1175–9.

[72] Stafford-Johnson DB, Francis IR, Eckhauser FE, et al. Dual-phase helical CT of nonfunctioning islet cell tumors. J Comput Assist Tomogr 1998;22:335–9.

[73] Anderson MA, Carpenter S, Thompson NW, et al. Endoscopic ultrasound is highly accurate and directs management in patients with neuroendocrine tumors of the pancreas. Am J Gastroenterol 2000;95: 2271–7.

[74] Gasslander T, Arnelo U, Albiin N, et al. Cystic tumors of the pancreas. Dig Dis 2001;19:57–62.

[75] Buck JL, Hayes WS. From the Archives of the AFIP. Microcystic adenoma of the pancreas. Radiographics 1990;10:313–22.

[76] Curry CA, Eng J, Horton KM, et al. CT of primary cystic pancreatic neoplasms: can CT be used for patient triage and treatment? AJR Am J Roentgenol 2000;175:99–103.

[77] Johnson CD, Stephens DH, Charboneau JW, et al. Cystic pancreatic tumors: CT and sonographic assessment. AJR Am J Roentgenol 1988;151:1133–8.

[78] Khurana B, Mortele KJ, Glickman J, et al. Macrocystic serous adenoma of the pancreas: radiologic-pathologic correlation. AJR Am J Roentgenol 2003; 181:119–23.

[79] Hammel P, Levy P, Voitot H, et al. Preoperative cyst fluid analysis is useful for the differential diagnosis of cystic lesions of the pancreas. Gastroenterology 1995;108:1230–5.

[80] Lewandrowski KB, Warshaw AL, Compton CC, et al. Variability in cyst fluid carcinoembryonic antigen level, fluid viscosity, amylase content, and cytologic findings among multiple loculi of a pancreatic mucinous cystic neoplasm. Am J Clin Pathol 1993; 100:425–7.

[81] Farrell JJ, Brugge WR. Intraductal papillary mucinous tumor of the pancreas. Gastrointest Endosc 2002;55:701–14.

[82] Sugiyama M, Atomi Y. Intraductal papillary mucinous tumors of the pancreas: imaging studies and treatment strategies. Ann Surg 1998;228:685–91.

[83] Desser TS, Sommer FG, Jeffrey Jr RB. Value of curved planar reformations in MDCT of abdominal pathology. AJR Am J Roentgenol 2004;182:1477–84.

[84] Fukukura Y, Fujiyoshi F, Hamada H, et al. Intraductal papillary mucinous tumors of the pancreas. Comparison of helical CT and MR imaging. Acta Radiol 2003;44:464–71.

[85] Fukukura Y, Fujiyoshi F, Sasaki M, et al. Intraductal papillary mucinous tumors of the pancreas: thinsection helical CT findings. AJR Am J Roentgenol 2000;174:441–7.

[86] Taouli B, Vilgrain V, Vullierme MP, et al. Intraductal papillary mucinous tumors of the pancreas: helical CT with histopathologic correlation. Radiology 2000;217:757–64.

[87] Sugiyama M, Izumisato Y, Abe N, et al. Predictive factors for malignancy in intraductal papillary-mucinous tumours of the pancreas. Br J Surg 2003; 90:1244–9.

[88] Kubo H, Chijiiwa Y, Akahoshi K, et al. Intraductal papillary-mucinous tumors of the pancreas: differential diagnosis between benign and malignant tumors by endoscopic ultrasonography. Am J Gastroenterol 2001;96:1429–34.

[89] Kawai M, Uchiyama K, Tani M, et al. Clinicopathological features of malignant intraductal papillary mucinous tumors of the pancreas: the differential diagnosis from benign entities. Arch Surg 2004;139: 188–9.

[90] Buetow PC, Buck JL, Pantongrag-Brown L. Solid and papillary epithelial neoplasm of the pancreas: imaging-pathologic correlation on 56 cases. Radiology 1996;199:707–11.

[91] Ghavamian R, Klein KA, Stephens DH, et al. Renal cell carcinoma metastatic to the pancreas: clinical and radiological features. Mayo Clin Proc 2000;75: 581–5.

[92] Ferrozzi F, Bova D, Campodonico F, et al. Pancreatic metastases: CT assessment. Eur Radiol 1997;7: 241–5.

[93] Maeno T, Satoh H, Ishikawa H, et al. Patterns of pancreatic metastasis from lung cancer. Anticancer Res 1998;18:2881–4.

[94] Ng CS, Loyer EM, Iyer RB, et al. Metastases to the pancreas from renal cell carcinoma: findings on three-phase contrast-enhanced helical CT. AJR Am J Roentgenol 1999;172:1555–9.

[95] Gruessner AC, Sutherland DE. Pancreas transplant outcomes for United States (US) and non-US cases as reported to the United Network for Organ Sharing (UNOS) and the International Pancreas Transplant Registry (IPTR) as of May 2003. Clin Transpl 2003:21–51.

[96] Dachman AH, Newmark GM, Thistlethwaite Jr JR, et al. Imaging of pancreatic transplantation using portal venous and enteric exocrine drainage. AJR Am J Roentgenol 1998;171:157–63.

[97] Neri E, Cappelli C, Boggi U, et al. Multirow CT in the follow-up of pancreas transplantation. Transplant Proc 2004;36:597–600.

[98] Freund MC, Steurer W, Gassner EM, et al. Spectrum of imaging findings after pancreas transplantation with enteric exocrine drainage: part 2, posttransplantation complications. AJR Am J Roentgenol 2004; 182:919–25.

[99] Fischer JH, Carpenter KD, O'Keefe GE. CT diagnosis of an isolated blunt pancreatic injury. AJR Am J Roentgenol 1996;167:1152.

[100] Ilahi O, Bochicchio GV, Scalea TM. Efficacy of computed tomography in the diagnosis of pancreatic injury in adult blunt trauma patients: a single-institutional study. Am Surg 2002;68:704–7.

[101] Bradley 3rd EL, Young Jr PR, Chang MC, et al. Diagnosis and initial management of blunt pancreatic trauma: guidelines from a multiinstitutional review. Ann Surg 1998;227:861–9.

[102] Akhrass R, Yaffe MB, Brandt CP, et al. Pancreatic trauma: a ten-year multi- institutional experience. Am Surg 1997;63:598–604.

[103] Cirillo Jr RL, Koniaris LG. Detecting blunt pancreatic injuries. J Gastrointest Surg 2002;6:587–98.

[104] Shanmuganathan K. Multi-detector row CT imaging of blunt abdominal trauma. Semin Ultrasound CT MR 2004;25:180–204.

[105] Fulcher AS, Turner MA, Yelon JA, et al. Magnetic resonance cholangiopancreatography (MRCP) in the assessment of pancreatic duct trauma and its sequelae: preliminary findings. J Trauma 2000;48: 1001–7.

[106] Ragozzino A, Manfredi R, Scaglione M, et al. The use of MRCP in the detection of pancreatic injuries after blunt trauma. Emerg Radiol 2003;10:14–8.

RADIOLOGIC CLINICS
of North America

Radiol Clin N Am 43 (2005) 1021 – 1047

Renal Multidector Row CT

Ercan Kocakoc, MD[a], Shweta Bhatt, MD[b], Vikram S. Dogra, MD[b,*]

[a]*Department of Radiology, Faculty of Medicine, Firat University, Elazig, Turkey*
[b]*Department of Imaging Sciences, University of Rochester School of Medicine and Dentistry, Rochester, NY, USA*

Multidetector—(also known as multislice, multi-channel, or multisection)—CT (MDCT) is the most recent advance in CT technology. It uses a multiple-row detector array instead of the single-row detector array used in helical CT [1]. These new CT scanners, with reduced gantry rotation times (0.5 s or less for one 360° rotation), allow 2 to 25 times faster scan times than helical CT with the same or better image quality [2–4]. These faster scan times result in decreased breath-hold times with reduced motion artifact and more diagnostic images. Increased volume coverage is combined with thinner slice thickness to obtain better quality volume data sets for workstation analysis, either in 2-D axial, multiplanar reformation (MPR), or three-dimensional (3-D) imaging. Moreover, by using MDCT, different image thickness can be obtained from the same acquisition data set [3].

Helical noncontrast CT is used widely for evaluation of the kidneys and urinary collecting system, especially to detect urinary calculi. MDCT allows images to be obtained in multiple phases of renal parenchymal enhancement and excretion in the collecting system after administration of a single bolus of intravenous (IV) contrast material. Therefore, detection and characterization of small renal masses, display of the arterial and venous supply of the kidney similar to conventional angiography, and demonstration of the collecting system's abnormalities using different 3-D display techniques are possible with MDCT. This review discusses the advantages, techniques, and clinical value of MDCT in kidney imaging.

Advantages of multidetector row CT

The main advantages of MDCT are faster scanning time, increased volume coverage, and improved spatial and temporal resolution [5]. These advantages also result in an increased number of slices obtained within a certain amount of time, which depends on the number of rows or channels.

Increased number of slices

As MDCT uses multiple rows of detectors, it allows for registration of more than one channel per gantry rotation, whereas single-detector helical CT allows registration of only one channel of image information of the scanned body part per gantry rotation [6]. The number of slices obtained per unit time depends on the scanner's number of rows (or channels) and on the gantry rotation time. The number of slices obtained per second can be as many as 38 for a 16-slice CT with a 0.4-second rotation time [6].

Increased temporal resolution

Current MDCT scanners have a very fast gantry rotation time that is equal to or less than 0.4 seconds. This reduced examination time creates advantages, especially in examinations affected by voluntary or involuntary patient motion, such as pediatric, geriatric, trauma, and cardiac studies. Decreased gantry rotation time provides reduced scanning times and

* Corresponding author. Department of Imaging Sciences, University of Rochester Medical Center, 601 Elmwood Avenue, Box 648, Rochester, NY 14642.
E-mail address: vikram_dogra@urmc.rochester.edu (V.S. Dogra).

increased coverage along the z-axis [3,7]. Therefore, image acquisitions in multiple phases of renal parenchymal enhancement and contrast excretion in the collecting system after administration of a single bolus of IV contrast media are possible [8].

Isotropic data acquisition and increased spatial resolution

Isotropic data acquisition is defined as obtaining images with equal voxel size in three axes [7]. MDCT scanners permit acquisition of thin sections with isotropic voxel size [7,8]. Their effective section thickness is between 0.75 and 1.6 mm [5]. MDCT scanners permit reconstruction of images at various thicknesses different from that chosen before the scan [7,8]. Isotropic imaging minimizes the importance of patient positioning and obviates obtaining axial, coronal, and sagittal planes directly [6]. Increased temporal resolution and acquisition of thin slices with isotropic voxel allows excellent quality MPR images to be obtained and 3-D rendering of

virtually any plane [7,9]. Optimal imaging of the renal hilar anatomy requires small slice widths and isotropic or near-isotropic MDCT data sets [10,11].

Examination technique and imaging protocols of multidetector row CT of the kidney

Imaging protocols and parameters vary depending on the type of MDCT scanner (number of detectors and name of manufacturer). Every imaging department should optimize its imaging protocols and parameters. The CT examination phases of the kidney are precontrast (noncontrast), arterial, angionephrographic (corticomedullary or venous), nephrographic, and delayed (excretory or urographic) (Fig. 1) [8,12].

Noncontrast CT

Noncontrast scans are obtained to locate the kidneys, evaluate urolithiasis, detect acute hematoma,

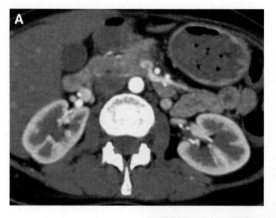
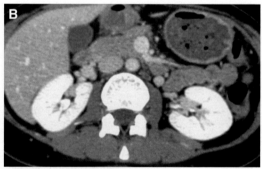
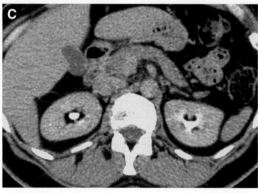

Fig. 1. Contrast-enhanced phases of the kidney on MDCT. (*A*) Arterial-phase image shows dense cortical enhancement. (*B*) Nephrographic-phase image shows homogeneous parenchymal enhancement. (*C*) Delayed-phase (10 minutes) axial CT demonstrates calyceal opacification.

and obtain baseline density measurements of renal masses [12,13]. Noncontrast CT is accepted as primary imaging to detect urinary calculi [14].

Contrast-enhanced CT

Oral contrast medium

In the evaluation of urolithiasis, dense oral contrast medium in the bowel can make detection of ureteral stones more difficult [15]. In addition, for 3-D CT angiography, positive oral contrast medium should not be given to improve postprocessing image quality and to avoid major overlay in postprocessed images [16]. Some investigators suggest drinking 500 to 750 mL of water over a 15- to 20-minute period before the start of a renal CT examination [17]. In CT angiography, the use of a saline chase bolus after contrast medium injection is essential to provide a compact contrast bolus and to push it toward the right atrium [18]. The authors do not use oral contrast medium for renal MDCT.

Administration of intravenous contrast medium

For the contrast-enhanced phases, the optimal timing depends on the volume of the contrast medium, the rate of its administration, and patients' cardiac output.

The difference between the start of contrast medium injection and the start of scanning is referred to as delay time. For specific vascular imaging studies, such as CT angiography, a fixed scanning delay is recommended, especially in patients who have cardiovascular disorders. If the delay is not chosen properly, the bolus may be missed completely with the short acquisition time. With MDCT, the delay time must be adjusted properly relative to patients' contrast transit time. This can be determined easily using a test bolus injection or automatic bolus triggering [5]. The test bolus technique requires the additional injection of a small amount of contrast medium (10–20 mL) before the acquisition of the CT angiography data, followed by the use of the same injection parameters (eg, flow rate) [16]. Using the bolus triggering (or bolus tracking) method, a region of interest is placed into the target vessel on an unenhanced image, and the attenuation level is monitored online within the region-of-interest during a single-level dynamic scan. Bolus tracking allows for the initial injection of the entire contrast medium volume, whereas the start of the data acquisition is triggered based on automated detection of the contrast bolus arrival using preassigned trigger thresholds (eg, 100–120 HU) [5,16].

The authors routinely use 100 to 120 mL of nonionic contrast at an infusion rate of 2 to 3 mL per second for routine renal imaging, 3 mL per second for CT urography, and 4 mL per second for CT angiography. Contrast is injected through an 18-gauge angiocatheter placed in the antecubital vein followed by 250 mL of saline infusion to provide better visualization of the collecting system.

Phases of renal enhancement

There are four phases of renal enhancement.

Arterial-phase imaging, performed to evaluate the arterial anatomy, is a short phase that occurs after a delay time of approximately 15 to 25 seconds [12,17]. In the late arterial phase, the renal veins usually also opacify [17]. The authors prefer a bolus-triggering method (aorta threshold value 120 HU) rather than a standard delay for arterial-phase imaging.

The angionephrographic (corticomedullary or venous) phase, performed to evaluate the venous anatomy, begins approximately 30 to 40 seconds after the start of contrast medium injection and continues for approximately 60 seconds [12,17,19]. In this phase, intense enhancement of the renal cortex can be observed while the medulla remains relatively less enhanced [17].

The nephrographic phase refers to the time during which the renal cortex and medulla are enhanced uniformly and contrast medium has not yet entered the renal collecting system. This phase begins 75 to 100 seconds after the start of contrast medium injection and is optimal for the detection of focal masses arising in the cortex or medulla and for evaluation of the renal parenchyma [12,17]. The authors use a standard 100-second delay to obtain nephrographic-phase images of the kidney.

The delayed phase (the excretory or urographic phase), used to evaluate renal collecting system and ureters, begins 3 minutes after the start of contrast medium injection. In this phase, while the intensity of the nephrogram declines, excretion of the contrast medium permits opacification of the calyces, renal pelvises, and ureters [17]. The authors obtain excretory-phase images at 10 minutes routinely.

Image processing and postprocessing techniques

Axial 3- to 5-mm, reconstructed slices are obtained to examine entire kidneys and the collecting system. The authors use a 3-mm slice thickness routinely for flank pain evaluation and a 5-mm slice thickness for nonspecific abdominal pain evaluation.

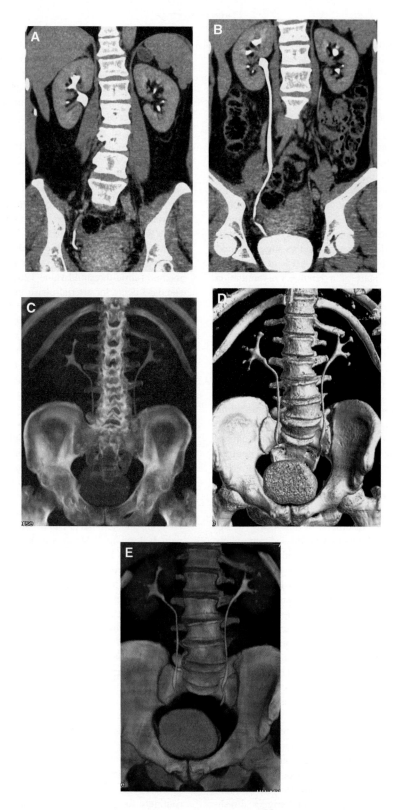

Fig. 2. Image post processing. The figures demonstrate the reconstructed images using the following techniques: (*A*) MPR; (*B*) CPR; note that the visualization of the ureter is facilitated; (*C*) MIP; (*D*) SSD; and (*E*) VRT.

The smaller collimation allows better quality MPR of the renal parenchyma and collecting system.

Four main 3-D visualization techniques currently are used on clinical 3-D workstations: MPR, maximum intensity projections (MIP), shaded surface displays (SSD), and a volume-rendering technique (VRT) [20].

Multiplanar reformation

MPR is the postprocessing technique used most commonly [21] and represents a simple reordering of the image voxels [10]. A known limitation of MPR is that visualized structures must be in a same plane. Because most structures of interest are not within a single plane, a MPR cannot be created that demonstrates an entire structure (Fig. 2A). As structures course in and out of the MPR, pseudostenoses are created. To solve this problem, curved planar reformations (CPR) are used. CPR have a single-voxel–thick tomogram, but it is capable of demonstrating an uninterrupted longitudinal cross-section as the display plane curves along the structure of interest (Fig. 2B) [20]. CPR images can be obtained manually by drawing a line over a structure of interest or it can be produced automatically or semiautomatically by dedicated software. CPR provide the most useful luminal assessment (such as of blood vessels, airways, and bowel) and are useful in improving the visualization of vessels of small diameter or tortuous anatomy [22]. CPR have an important limitation in that they are highly dependent on the accuracy of the curve [20].

Maximum intensity projection

MIP displays the maximum voxel intensity along a line of viewer projection in a given volume [17]. High-density structures, such as contrast-filled vessels and the collecting system, are demonstrated nicely in images, such as angiograms or urograms (Fig. 2C). The main disadvantage of MIP is that it obscures the area of interest by high-density material, such as bone, calcium, and oral contrast medium. With the MIP technique, a 3-D effect can be obtained with rotational viewing of multiple projections, but it lacks depth orientation [23].

Shaded surface displays

SSD enable accurate 3-D representations of anatomy, relying on the gray scale to encode surface reflections from an imaginary source of illumination (Fig. 2D) [24,25]. SSD images are limited by their dependence on user-selected threshold settings [13]. The 12-bit CT data is reduced to binary data, each pixel either within or outside of the threshold range [20]. Because of this, it can overestimate or underestimate stenosis.

Volume-rendered technique

With this technique, all attenuation values within a voxel are used to obtain the final image (that each voxel contributes brightness, color, and opacity to the final image) [23]. Anatomic structures with different levels of opacity (eg, renal parenchyma, renal veins and arteries, and the collecting system) can be demonstrated simultaneously [17]. VRT is an excellent 3-D technique for presentation that provides a roadmap for surgery and summary picture for the referring physician [22]. The most important limitation of VRT is its need for more powerful computers and costly workstations [17]. Using editing techniques, structures overlying the area of interest can be removed for better visualization and desired orientation (Fig. 2E) [20,23].

Normal CT anatomy

The kidneys are surrounded by perinephric fat and renal fascia. The anterior renal fascia (fascia of Gerota) covers the kidney anteriorly, whereas the posterior renal fascia (Zuckerkandl's fascia) covers the kidney posteriorly. These fascial layers divide the general retroperitoneal space into three compartments extending from the diaphragm to the pelvic brim (ie, the anterior pararenal space, the perinephric space, and the posterior pararenal space) [26]. MDCT is able to demonstrate the normal anatomy of the kidney (ie, the renal fascia and the major extraperitoneal compartments) not only in the axial plan but also in the sagittal and coronal planes, thereby making it possible to define the exact location and extension of lesions. The 3-D VR images nicely demonstrate the location of the kidney in relation to adjacent structures (Fig. 3A).

Renal arteries

The renal arteries usually arise from the aorta at the level of L2 below the origin of the superior mesenteric artery (Fig. 3B). The renal arteries enter

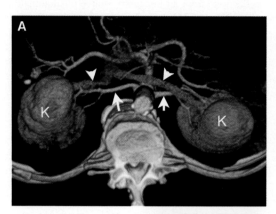
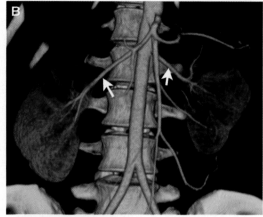
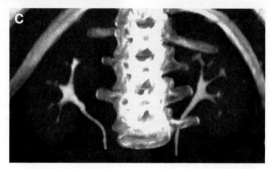

Fig. 3. Normal CT anatomy. (*A*) Axial view of the VRT demonstrates the renal arteries (*arrows*) and the renal veins (*arrowheads*). (*B*) Coronal CT angiogram in a renal donor demonstrates renal arterial anatomy; arrows point to renal arteries. (*C*) Contrast-enhanced CT with MIP reformation demonstrates normal kidneys and their calyceal systems. K, kidneys.

the renal hilus anterior to the renal pelvis. The main renal arteries divide into segmental arteries next to the renal hilum. The first branch usually is the posterior branch; following this branch, anterior segmental (ie, apical, upper, middle, and lower) arteries are visible. The segmental arteries divide into the lobar arteries. Further divisions are the interlobar, arcuate, and interlobular arteries. MDCT (16 slice) clearly demonstrates the interlobar artery level of the renal arterial anatomy.

Renal veins

The renal cortex drains into the arcuate and interlobar veins. The lobar veins join to form the main renal vein. The renal veins usually are anterior to the renal artery. The left renal vein is approximately 3 times longer than the right renal vein. Several branches drain into the left renal vein before joining the inferior vena cava (IVC). These branches are the left adrenal vein superiorly, the left gonadal vein inferiorly, and a lumbar vein posteriorly. MDCT enables visualization these veins [23].

Renal collecting system

The first radiologically visible structure and the distal part of the renal collecting system is the minor calyx. The minor calyces have a narrow neck, called the infundibulum, and at this point minor calyces join to form three major calyces, which form the renal pelvis at the renal hilus. The renal pelvis is continuous with the ureter. The excretory phase of MDCT can demonstrate the anatomy and pathology of these collecting systems (Fig. 3C).

CT urography

Until recently, intravenous urography (IVU) or excretory urography was used as the traditional imaging technique for the radiologic evaluation of the kidneys, pelvicaliceal systems, ureters, and bladder. IVU has lower sensitivity in detecting small renal masses and can detect only 21% of masses smaller than 2 cm, 52% of masses between 2 and 3 cm, and 82% of masses 3 cm or larger [27]. Noncontrast CT has 97% sensitivity and 96% specificity for the detection of renal calculi [14]. For detecting urinary calculi, the sensitivity and specificity of IVU are 52% and 59%, respectively [28].

One of the advantages of IVU over CT is its ability to detect intraluminal filling defects and mucosal abnormalities in the renal collecting systems and ureters [29]. Excretory-phase collecting system opacification obtained during CT urography was found by McNicholas and colleagues to be comparable to collecting system opacification obtained during IVU [30]. With advances in CT technology, the technique of CT urography is used to evaluate the entire urinary system [29,31].

MDCT enables faster data acquisition and higher resolution images than single-detector helical CT with very thin (approximatley 1-mm) slices The entire urinary system (ie, kidneys, ureters, and bladder) are visualized in one breath-hold on MDCT. Its initial thin data acquisition enables better quality reconstructed and reformatted coronal images similar to those of IVU [32]. CT urography can demonstrate not only urinary tract lumen but also the walls of the urinary tract and its surrounding structures.

CT urography techniques

The ideal technique for CT urography is unclear and evolving [29,31,33]; however, there are two major approaches for CT urography. One of them, a hybrid technique, combines the use of axial CT images with some projection radiographs (conventional film-screen abdominal radiographs, computed digital radiographs, or CT scanned projection radiographic [SPR] images) after IV contrast medium administration [33,34]. This method combines the strengths of CT and IVU into a single comprehensive examination [34]. The second approach is CT-only CT urography, which combines conventional axial CT with thin-section, excretory-phase, axial CT images and is reviewed as 2-D and 3-D reformatted images [29,31].

CT hybrid urography

This technique combines the advantages of CT in imaging the kidneys with those of contrast radiography in imaging the urinary collecting system; the advantage of this technique is that it does not need CT postprocessing procedures [35]. If CT topography is used, the image quality of a CT topogram to view the urothelium is questionable. If conventional radiography is obtained after the CT scan, patients must undergo imaging in two different locations.

Movement of patients between different procedure rooms requires additional time and resources, which can cause scheduling conflicts and may affect the level of pyelocalyceal distention at the time of the radiography adversely [34,35].

An alternative approach, developed at the Mayo Clinic, solves this problem. An MDCT scanner configured with a special tabletop apparatus is used to obtain CT and radiographic images without moving patients [36]. This tabletop is capable of receiving a combined slip-on grid and standard film cassette. This system requires the installation of a ceiling-mounted x-ray tube above the CT table and the attachment of an auxiliary CT tabletop with a hollow bay under the patient surface in which to place the radiographic cassette [34–36].

With this technique, an abdominal radiograph, an unenhanced renal CT, and a multiphasic, contrast-enhanced, renal CT scan followed by overhead excretory urographic and postvoid radiographs can be obtained [36]. This method permits high spatial resolution IVU film images to be obtained at various times before and after the CT acquisitions, and there is no need to transfer patients between radiography and CT suites [34]. An alternative method of obtaining projection images, without moving patients from the CT table, is the use of the CT SPR technique (scout view, topogram, or scanogram). The spatial resolution of CT SPR is inferior to that of conventional radiography, whereas the contrast resolution of opacified structures is similar to that of conventional radiography [37]. This CT urography approach, the combination of helical CT scans and enhanced CT SPR urographic images, is attractive because modification of the CT tabletop and installation of a ceiling-mounted x-ray tube are unnecessary; therefore, this technique can be performed with any MDCT equipment [34].

With this technique, some investigators recommend bowel preparation using a mild laxative to reduce gas and fecal material. To visualize the intrarenal collecting system and ureter better, IVU abdominal compression is applied after the IV contrast medium injection. It is important to use a low-osmolar, iodinated contrast medium [38]. The ureters generally are well visualized on 10-minute decompressed film images. Twenty-minute and postvoiding films are optional but may be useful for bladder evaluation [34].

CT-only CT urography

This approach is based on the acquisition of unenhanced and enhanced CT scans of the abdomen and pelvis, including the essential acquisition of thin-section helical CT scans of the urinary tract during the excretory phase of enhancement [34]. No bowel preparation is necessary for this type of CT urography. Multiplanar 2-D and 3-D reformation images can be generated on workstations from axial source images obtained during the excretory phase. Detection of urothelial abnormalities with excretory-phase CT requires visualization of the optimally distended and opacified collecting system. Some studies show that CT with abdominal compression improves opacification of the collecting system when compared with CT scans without compression [30,39]. Caoili and coworkers [29] describe four-phase MDCT urography performed using an unenhanced scan, a nephrographic-phase scan with abdominal compression, and two excretory-phase scans, one obtained 200 seconds after the injection of contrast material with compression and the other 300 seconds after release of compression. They easily identified all congenital anomalies on transverse and 3-D reformatted images. Renal, pelvic, ureteral, and bladder abnormalities are visualized better on compression-release excretory-phase images. Three-dimensional images are helpful particularly in the diagnosis of papillary abnormalities, such as renal tubular ectasia and papillary necrosis.

Alternative techniques can be used to achieve optimal visualization of the collecting systems, such as normal saline infusion and diuretic injection. CT urography with supplemental saline administration can improve opacification of the distal ureters significantly. Patient position (supine or prone) during CT examination does not affect ureteral visualization [31]. CT depicts the high attenuation produced by contrast material easily; dilution of the contrast material does not affect perceived opacification and may minimize potential beam-hardening artifacts associated with dense contrast material in the intrarenal collecting system [40]. The distal ureters are the most difficult segments to opacify; they opacify more reliably if a saline infusion technique is used (250 mL saline chase after the IV contrast administration). Using IV injection of low-dose diuretics (10 mg of furosemide) before IV contrast injection allows less dense, homogeneous opacification of the collecting system [40]. Some investigators use oral water (1000 mL within 15 to 20 minutes) before the examination, as this allows sufficient opacification of the calyces and ureters in most instances [17]. The authors do not use an oral bowel contrast agent or water routinely in CT urography protocols. Evaluation of axial CT images (source images) with a wide window setting is important for accurate diagnosis, and these images can be assessed at a workstation. Coronal or oblique MPR images help to define the location and extent of the lesions shown on axial images. MIP images resemble conventional IVU images (Fig. 4A). CPR allow a single image to outline the course of ureterectasis to the point where an obstructing process, such as a calculus or tumor, is present [41].

The authors' CT urography protocol

The standard CT urography protocol at the authors' institution is demonstrated in Table 1. The

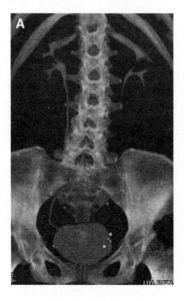 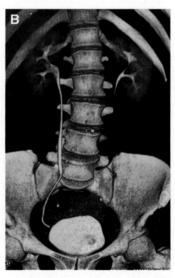

Fig. 4. CT urography: (*A*) coronal MIP image and the corresponding coronal VRT (*B*) demonstrating the CT urographic image.

Table 1
Protocol of CT urography

		Phase		
	Noncontrast	Nephrographic	Pyelographic	
	From diaphragm to			
Criteria	Symphysis pubis	Iliac crest	Symphysis pubis	Additional film
Slice collimation	16 × 1.5	16 × 1.5	16 × 1.5	—
Slice thickness (mm)	3	2	2	—
Increment (mm)	1	1	1	—
Pitch	0.75	0.5	0.5	—
Rotation time (s)	0.5	0.5	0.5	—
kVp	120	120	120	—
Mas	245	245	245	—
$CTDI_{vol}$ (mGy)	16.3 for 450 mm	~Noncontrast	16.7 for 450 mm	—
Oral contrast medium	None	None	None	—
IV saline infusion	None	250 mL	—	—
IV contrast medium (injection rate)	None	100–120 mL (3 mL/s)	—	—
Scan delay	None	100 s	10 min	
Additional image	None	None	None	CT scout view at 10 min
3-D technique	None	MPR, VRT, and MIP	MPR, VRT, and MIP	—

The 16-detector M × 8000 IDT (Philips Medical Systems, Cleveland, Ohio) was used.
Abbreviation: $CTDI_{vol}$, CT dose index of scanned volume.

first phase is precontrast imaging of the abdomen from the dome of the liver to the pubic symphysis using a 3-mm section thickness. The second phase is the nephogram phase that includes imaging from the diaphragm to the iliac crest area with a 2-mm section thickness 100 seconds after starting IV contrast medium followed by 250-mL saline administration. The third phase is the delayed or excretory phase obtained 10 minutes after contrast media administration. After this phase, a scout abdominal CT view

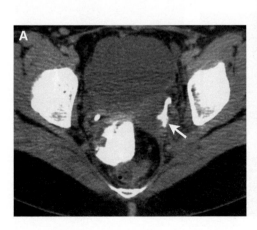
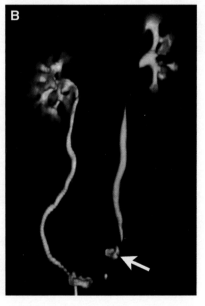

Fig. 5. Iatrogenic ureteral trauma. (*A*) Excretory-phase axial CT image of the pelvis shows contrast medium extravasations in the left distal ureter (*arrow*). Corresponding coronal VRT (*B*) CT urogram demonstrates contrast leak (*arrow*) in the left distal ureteral segment.

similar to IVU also is obtained. The authors routinely use MPR, MIP, and 3-D VRT postprocessing techniques to assess the acquired axial data. MIP and 3-D VRT images resemble IVU and are preferred by referring physicians (Fig. 4B). Oblique MIP and VRT images are useful for demonstrating distal or tortuous ureteral segments and the ureterovesical junction.

Using oblique MIP imaging, phleboliths are easily distinguished from ureteral calculi.

Evaluation of urinary trauma with multidector CT urography

Delayed images may be useful for trauma patients if there is renal laceration or perinephric fluid suggesting hematoma or urinoma. The delayed scan usually is performed approximately 10 minutes after

contrast injection. Delayed or excretory images may detect renal hemorrhage or urinoma that is not visible on routine images [15,42]. Traumatic or iatrogenic ureteral injuries also are demonstrated clearly on delayed-phase images (Fig. 5).

Evaluation of ureteropelvic junction obstruction with CT urography

Ureteropelvic junction obstruction (UPJO) is defined as functional or anatomic obstruction of urine flow from the renal pelvis into the ureter at their anatomic junction [10,43]. Large parapelvic cysts located closely to the ureter can mimic UPJO on early-phase contrast-enhanced imaging [10], but UPJO opacifies on late-phase CT urography (Fig. 6). With a very large extrarenal pelvis, the collecting

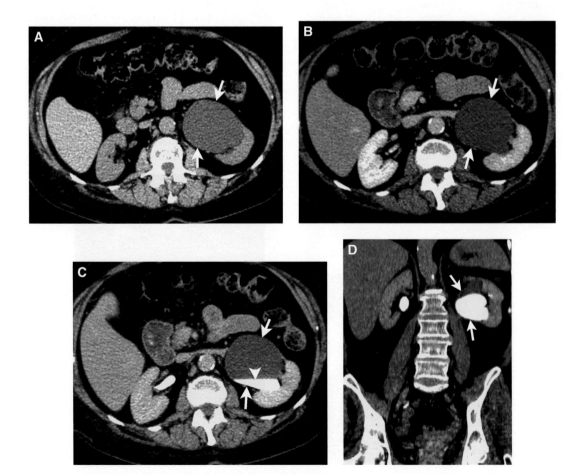

Fig. 6. UPJO: nonenhanced CT (*A*) and corresponding nephrographic phase (*B*), excretory phase (*C*), and coronal MPR excretory phase (*D*) demonstrate the dilated left renal pelvis (*arrows*) secondary to uretero pelvic junction obstruction; arrowhead in the excretory-phase image points to the contrast layering in the dilated pelvis.

system and ureter may not be fully opacified in some cases. Vessels crossing the ureter or renal pelvis can be demonstrated easily by MDCT angiography. MDCT with 3-D reconstruction shows the classic inverted teardrop shape of the hydronephrosis in patients who have UPJO [10].

Vascular pathologies and renal donor evaluation (CT angiography)

The main indications for renal artery imaging include the evaluation of patients who have suspected renal hypertension to exclude hemodynamically significant renal artery stenosis (RAS) and a complete preoperative assessment for renal transplant candidates [44].

MDCT angiography of the renal arteries is obtained using a high-resolution protocol (thickness of 1–1.25 mm or less). Contrast medium injection timing is important for obtaining high-quality CT angiograms. With four channel scanners, the injection duration usually is equal to the acquisition time, whereas with faster scanners, the injection duration may be somewhat longer. The injection duration should match the acquisition time. Faster acquisitions require less total contrast medium volume [5]. Using

a large-bore IV line, 120 to 150 mL of contrast medium should be given at a rate of at least 3 mL per second (preferably 4 mL/s or more) [23]. The images are obtained during the arterial plateau of contrast enhancement.

Renal donor evaluation

To evaluate potential renal donors, the scan area begins above the origin of the superior mesenteric artery and extends to the bifurcation of the common iliac arteries to include potential accessory renal arteries. Images are obtained in the arterial and venous phases of enhancement to demonstrate the arterial and venous anatomy. The authors do not obtain dedicated renal venous phase routinely because the renal veins usually can be seen on arterial phase. The gonadal and lumbar veins enhance more slowly and are visualized well on nephrographic phase. Therefore, the authors prefer the nephrographic phase instead of a dedicated venous phase. This is followed by a scout urogram obtained at 4 to 5 minutes [17]. Thin collimation with 4-mm × 1-mm detectors, 1.25-mm section collimation, and an overlapping reconstruction interval of 1 mm creates high-quality 3-D images [17]. A section width of 1 mm should be used for the arterial- and nephrographic-phase examinations,

Table 2
Protocol of CT angiography for renal donor evaluation

Criteria	Phase		Noncontrast[a]
	Arterial	Nephrographic	
	Top of the kidney to		
	Iliac crest		Symphisis pubis
Slice collimation	16 × 1.5	16 × 1.5	16 × 1.5
Slice thickness (mm)	2	2	3
Increment (mm)	1	1	1
Pitch	0.5	0.5	0.75
Rotation time (s)	0.5	0.5	0.5
kVp	120	120	120
Mas	250	250	250
$CTDI_{vol}$ (mGy)	16.7	16.7	16.3
Oral contrast medium	None	None	None
IV saline infusion	None	None	None
IV contrast medium (injection rate)	120–320 mL (4 mL/s)		None
Scan delay	Bolus tracking after aorta level 120 HU reached	75 s	None
Additional image	None	None	None
3-D technique	VRT and MIP	VRT, MPR, and MIP	None

The 16-detector M × 8000 IDT (Philips Medical Systems, Cleveland, Ohio) was used.
Abbreviation: $CTDI_{vol}$, CT dose index of scanned volume.
[a] Unless specifically ordered, noncontrast study of the kidney for CT angiography should not be obtained.

because accessory renal arteries and lumbar veins can be small and missed easily when thicker sections are used [12].

With a 16-detector scanner, higher quality reconstructions can be obtained. For postprocessing, MIP and VRT often are used. Table 2 demonstrates the authors' MDCT protocol for renal donor evaluation. Although a five-phase CT examination may be possible with an MDCT scanner, the authors use two- or three-phase CT examinations routinely in an attempt to reduce the radiation dose to the patients who generally are young, healthy adults.

MDCT of the kidney allows delineation of the size, number, and course of the renal arteries and veins, evaluation of the renal parenchyma and collecting system, and diagnosis of unsuspected conditions that preclude organ donation [17]. CT angiography can depict 100% of the main renal arteries and veins [45]. For surgical planning, it is important to identify occult lesions and anatomic anomalies, such as accessory renal arteries (Fig. 7A and B), prehilar renal

arterial branching (Fig. 7C), multiple renal veins, renal artery aneurysms or occlusive disease, and duplicated renal collecting systems. Because of the small diameter of the vessels of interest and their parallel or near parallel course to the imaging plane, thin nominal section thickness of 1 to 1.25 mm and overlapping reconstruction are necessary [46]. It is important that all vessels arising from the kidney be traced to their origin and, similarly, all vessels arising from the abdominal aorta between the SMA and the common iliac bifurcation should be followed to their terminus. This evaluation process ideally is performed at a workstation with the capability of scrolling through images in a cine display mode [46].

Multiple renal arteries are present in approximately one third of all examined kidneys. Accessory renal arteries can arise from the aorta or the iliac arteries [17]. Compared with surgical findings, the accuracy of MDCT angiography for detecting the number of renal arteries is as high as 93% [11]. In a recent study, Kawamoto and colleagues found super-

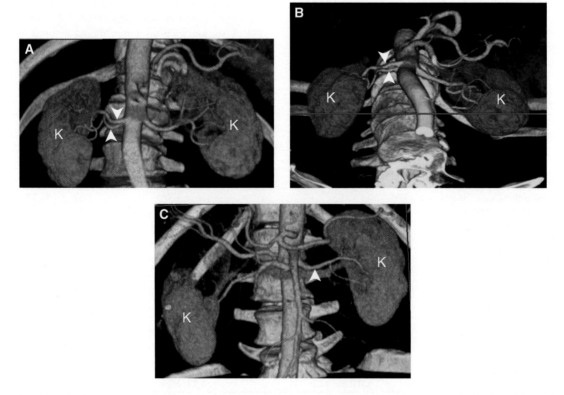

Fig. 7. Renal CT angiography. Coronal (*A*) and the corresponding oblique (*B*) VRT demonstrates right-sided, double renal artery (*arrowheads*). (*C*) Coronal VRT of CT angiography in another patient shows an early branching left renal artery (*arrowhead*). K, kidneys.

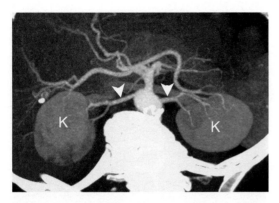

Fig. 8. Axial MIP image of a CT angiography demonstrates the origin of the renal arteries (*arrowheads*). K, kidneys.

numerary renal arteries in 24% of the donor kidneys, early branching of the renal artery in 19%, and left renal vein anomalies in 11% [11].

Surgeons need complete details of the venous anatomy, because venous bleeding potentially is a serious complication of laparoscopic surgery and sometimes requires the conversion of a laparoscopic procedure to an open one [12]. Approximately 15% of healthy subjects have more than one renal vein [12,17]. MDCT can demonstrate venous variants easily, including multiple veins, right-sided gonadal and adrenal veins draining into the renal vein, and left retroaortic, circumaortic, and partially duplicated veins [12]. The location and number of gonadal, adrenal, and lumbar veins should be defined. The left renal anatomy is critical particularly because it is the

preferred side for resecting the kidney. The most common anomaly of the left renal venous system is the circumaortic renal vein, seen in as many as 17% of all patients [11,23]. A less common venous anomaly is the completely retroaortic renal vein, seen in 2% to 3% of patients [23,47].

The MIP technique is preferred for well-defined structures, such as arteries (Fig. 8), whereas MPR is the preferred technique for analysis of small, less well opacified veins [12]. More accurate measurement of these vascular structures can be obtained on CPR images.

Assessment of the collecting system also is important in detecting unexpected anatomic variants or urolithiasis, and precontrast study combined with late-phase scout view provides sufficient information regarding the collecting system. MDCT can be used to display the transplant kidney anatomy and transplant-related complications (Fig. 9). MDCT angiography also can be used to confirm or rule out artery stenosis after kidney transplantation [16].

Evaluation of renal hypertension

RAS is responsible for approximately 5% of all cases of hypertension. Atherosclerotic disease is the most common cause (approximately 90%) of RAS. Fibromuscular dysplasia (FMD) is the second most common cause (approximately 10%) of RAS. Atherosclerotic disease generally involves the ostium and the proximal third of the main renal arteries, whereas FMD usually affects the distal two thirds of the main

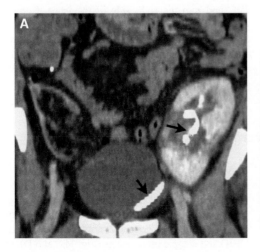

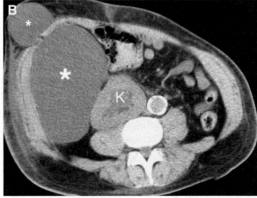

Fig. 9. Transplant kidney. (*A*) Coronal MPR demonstrates the left transplant kidney with a ureteric stent (*arrows*) in situ. (*B*) Axial nonenhanced CT image in a different patient demonstrates a right transplant kidney (K), with a large peritransplant loculated fluid collection (*) extending into the abdominal wall.

renal or renal artery branches [48]. Neurofibromato-
sis, Takayasu's arteritis, and radiation are rare causes
of renal hypertension [17].

The sensitivity and specificity of CT angiography
for the detection of hemodynamically significant
RAS are as high as 90% and 97%, respectively [49].
Willmann and colleagues report [50] 92% and 99%
sensitivity and specificity, respectively, for the detection of hemodynamically significant arterial stenosis of the aortoiliac and renal arteries by using MDCT
scanner and a 1-mm nominal section thickness.

MIP and VRT have similar sensitivities for demonstrating significant stenosis, but the VRT can display calcified atherosclerotic plaques and the lumen
simultaneously [17]. If patients have extensive calcification, stenosis can be obscured by the MIP techniques, and attentive assessment with VR images
then is needed [24].

Indirect signs of RAS are poststenotic dilatation
and have an 85% predictive value of significant
stenosis [24] Other indirect signs of RAS are a small
kidney with a smooth contour, thinning of the renal
cortex, and the presence of a delayed and prolonged
nephrogram [51]. Volume-rendered MDCT angiography enables high-quality 3-D evaluation of the patency of implanted renal artery stents.

Renal artery aneurysms

The most common cause of renal artery aneurysm
is atherosclerosis. Pregnancy, FMD, and neurofibro-
matosis are other causes of renal artery aneurysms.
Pseudoaneurysm and arteriovenous fistulas usually
are posttraumatic, iatrogenic, or inflammatory [52].

Diagnosis of crossing vessels in ureteropelvic junction obstruction

Vessels crossing a UPJ contribute to the degree of
hydronephrosis in up to 46% of patients presenting
with UPJ obstruction [17]. Demonstration of these
vessels and their localization anterior or posterior to
the obstruction facilitates surgical planning and limits
potentially serious complications [17].

Renal vein thrombosis

The renal vein with thrombosis is distended and
filled with thrombus that appears hypodense. Delayed
images may be helpful to confirm the presence of

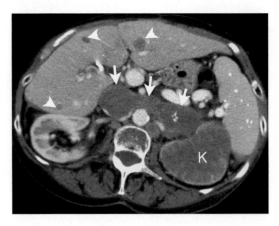

Fig. 10. Contrast-enhanced CT image demonstrates a left
adrenal tumor invading the left kidney (K), extending into
the left renal vein, and IVC (*arrows*). Incidentally, three
metastatic foci (*arrowheads*) are seen in the liver.

thrombus and to exclude a false-positive finding
caused by mixing of poorly opacified blood from the
lower extremities [52]. The most important cause of
renal vein thrombosis is tumor thrombus from renal
cell carcinoma (RCC) or, in rare cases, from adrenal
carcinoma (Fig. 10). Demonstrating the extent and
location of renal vein involvement by tumor is crucial
in planning the surgical approach for removing the
renal tumor [23]. Over time, the thrombus may con-
tract and extensive collateral vessels may develop.
CT angiography also can demonstrate secondary
signs of renal vein thrombosis, including delay in
the renal cortical nephrogram and global renal enlargement. Tumoral thrombus can extend into the
IVC and into the right side of the heart. Complete
opacification of the IVC usually requires a second
helical acquisition performed 90 to 120 seconds after
injection of contrast material; this additional scanning is recommended in patients who have known
tumors [23].

Congenital abnormalities and normal variants

Various types of vascular, parenchymal, and urinary tract anomalies, including accessory renal arteries, aberrant renal artery origins, anomalous renal
veins, ptotic malrotated and horseshoe kidney
(Fig. 11A and B), urinary tract duplication, and
UPJO and ectopic ureteroceles (Fig. 11C and D), may
be detected incidentally during MDCT studies.

CT angiography for vascular abnormalities or CT
urography for ureteral and collecting system abnor-

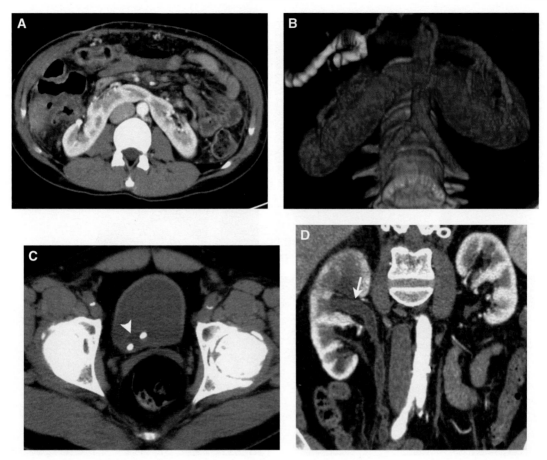

Fig. 11. Contrast-enhanced CT axial (*A*) image and corresponding oblique VRT (*B*) demonstrate a horseshoe kidney. (*C*) Axial CT image of the bladder demonstrates a right-sided ureterocele (*arrowhead*) in the bladder containing two stones. (*D*) Coronal CPR image in another patient demonstrates a right-sided duplicated collecting system with a dilated upper pole moiety (*arrow*).

malities, with 3-D VRT or MIP reconstruction, can demonstrate these abnormalities nicely.

Evaluation of flank pain and urinary calculi

After the first report by Smith and colleagues [14] of the use of unenhanced CT for detection of urinary tract calculi, helical noncontrast CT became the standard method of evaluating flank pain and suspected urinary lithiasis [53]. Its reported sensitivity and specificity are as high as 97% and 96%, respectively [14].

Using MDCT, thin-collimation (3- to 5-mm), noncontrast scans are obtained through the abdomen from the superior aspect of the kidneys (or from the dome of the liver) through the inferior aspect of the

bladder base or pubic symphysis. This technique is simple and does not require any patient preparation or administration of oral or IV contrast.

If CT does not display evidence of stones, subsequent imaging with IV contrast is needed. Regardless of their calcium content, almost all urinary tract calculi are radio-opaque on noncontrast CT. The stones that form in 4% of patients who have HIV and who are treated with indinavir therapy may not be radio-opaque [54].

Reconstructed images, such as MPR or CPR, are useful in demonstrating the exact location of stones and their relationship to the ureter (Fig. 12A and B). Noncontrast CT also is helpful in detecting nonobstructing calculi in patients who have hematuria. Stone size is the single most reliable indicator of stone passage and can be measured accurately on CT [55].

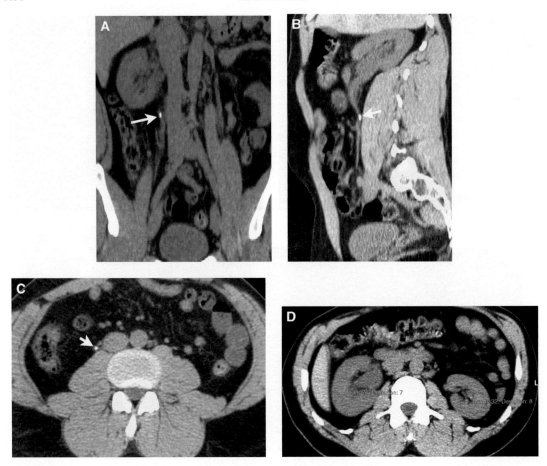

Fig. 12. Urolithiasis. (A) Coronal MPR and their corresponding sagittal CPR image (B) and a nonenhanced axial CT image (C) demonstrate a right ureteral stone (arrow) with minimal dilation of the collecting system as seen in (A) and (B). (D) Density measurement in the kidneys demonstrates mild right renal edema secondary to obstruction.

The most specific diagnostic finding of urolithiasis is the identification of a stone within the ureter (Fig. 12C). The second important finding is the "rim sign," seen as 1 to 2 mm of soft tissue thickening around the stone secondary to ureteral wall edema at the site of stone impaction. The specificity of this sign is reported as 92% [56]. Other secondary CT findings of urolithiasis are dilatation of the ureter or collecting system, asymmetric enlargement or decreased density of the kidney, and perinephric stranding. Perinephric stranding can be seen in nonobstructed kidneys for various reasons; if it is not asymmetric and ipsilateral to patients' symptoms, it may not be significant [53]. It is a common finding, particularly in older patients. Renal edema from obstruction results in loss of the hyperdense pyramid (white pyramid sign) and the attenuation of the parenchyma on the obstructed side is 5 to 14 HU less than on the normal side, an objective finding of obstruction (Fig. 12D) [57].

Some degree of ureteral edema and thickening can be seen if a stone already has passed into the bladder. To decide whether or not a distal ureteral stone is in the ureterovesical junction or in the bladder, prone position imaging can be useful [53].

Pelvic phleboliths, arterial vascular calcification, calcified vas deferens, and a calcified appendicolith can be considered a differential diagnosis of ureteric calculi [19]. Phleboliths often show a central lucency, whereas true calculi are as dense or more dense at the center than at the periphery [58]. Another useful sign for diagnosing phlebolith is the comet-tail sign, which is a linear or curvilinear soft tissue structure represented by the noncalcified vessel, extending from an abdominal or pelvic calcification; its positive predictive value for phlebolith is 100% [59].

Comparison with prior CT scans can be useful because phleboliths remain stable in position, whereas calculi tend to move [53].

Sometimes CT may permit alternative diagnoses, such as appendicitis, diverticulitis, hemorrhagic ovarian cyst, ruptured abdominal aortic aneurysm, and biliary colic [19].

Inflammatory lesions of the kidney

The majority of patients who have urinary tract infection require no imaging studies. In patients who have acute infection unresponsive to antibiotic therapy, CT scanning may be used to detect intrarenal or perirenal abscess, particularly in patients who have diabetes or those who have known xanthogranulomatous disease [19].

The main purpose of renal imaging is to obtain information regarding the nature and extent of the disease process and to identify any significant complications, such as gas-forming infection, abscess, and urinary obstruction [60]. Gas, calculi, parenchymal calcifications, and hemorrhage are demonstrated well with noncontrast CT.

Imaging features of inflammatory disease of the kidney seen on MDCT are similar to those on single-detector CT [8]. MDCT is more useful than IVU or ultrasonography for the assessment of renal infection [35].

Acute pyelonephritis and abscess

The diagnosis of acute pyelonephritis is based on clinical and laboratory findings in most cases, and routine imaging, therefore, is unnecessary. When a definite diagnosis of acute renal infection is not established or patients present with recurrent episodes of infection, renal imaging is indicated because of an increased possibility of stones, obstruction, abscess, or a congenital anomaly [61]. After noncontrast CT, a contrast-enhanced study is essential, including angionephrographic or corticomedullary and nephrographic phases, for a complete evaluation of patients who have renal inflammatory disease to demonstrate alterations in the renal parenchymal perfusion and excretion of contrast material that may occur as a result of the inflammatory process [61].

The most common CT finding of acute pyelonephritis is ill defined, wedge-shaped lesions of decreased attenuation radiating from the papilla to the cortical surface, with or without swelling (Fig. 13A) [61]. This finding may be subtle in the cortico-medullary phase. This perfusion abnormality is detected best in the nephrographic phase (Fig. 13B) [17]. Another characteristic finding of acute pyelonephritis is a striated nephrogram on contrast-enhanced CT, consisting of linear bands of alternating hypoattenuation and hyperattenuation oriented parallel to the axes of the tubules and collecting ducts (Fig. 13C) [35,61]. Diminished concentration of contrast material in the tubules, caused by tubular obstruction by inflammatory cells and debris, ischemia, and interstitial edema, results in this characteristic CT finding [17,61].

Other useful secondary CT findings of acute pyelonephritis are global or focal enlargement of the kidney, thickening of the pelvicalyceal wall, obliteration of the renal sinus and perinephric fat planes, focal calyceal obliteration, and thickening of the fascia of Gerota [17,61].

Scarring resulting from pyelonephritis may be demonstrated by MDCT as focal thinning of the cortex or extensive contour abnormalities (Fig. 13D). VRT images may be useful for demonstrating focal defects resulting from abscess foci related to pyelonephritis.

Severe renal inflammation sometimes causes multiple small suppurative foci that ultimately may coalesce into a larger focal collection of pus or an acute renal abscess [61]. Perinephric abscess may result from rupture of a renal abscess into the perirenal space or develop directly from acute pyelonephritis. Perinephric abscess can extend through the fascia of Gerota to the pararenal space. Abscesses also may involve the psoas muscle and extend into the pelvis and groin [61]. MDCT may demonstrate the origin and extent of these pathologies (Fig. 13E).

Xanthogranulomatous pyelonephritis

Xanthogranulomatous pyelonephritis is a rare chronic infection caused by long-standing urinary tract obstruction by a urinary stone. *Eschericia coli* and *Proteus mirabilis* are the most common agents [62]. This infection is most common in middle-aged women and the usual clinical presentations are flank pain, fever, and a history of recurrent low-grade urinary tract infection [17]. MDCT usually demonstrates an enlarged nonfunctioning kidney, staghorn calculus, and multiple, round, hypodense masses resulting from a markedly hydronephrotic collecting system (Fig. 14) [17,61]. Extension of the inflammatory process to the perirenal and pararenal spaces and adjacent organs, such as the pancreas and spleen, is common [17,61]. Cutaneous and renocolic fistulas also may be present [61].

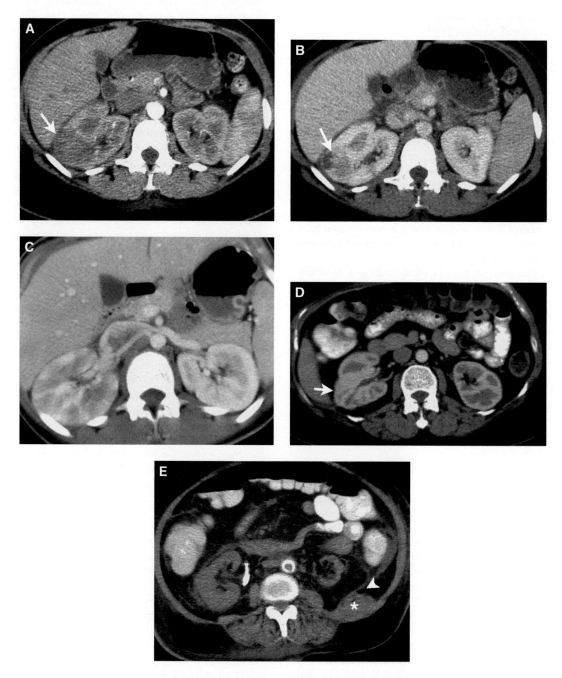

Fig. 13. Acute pyelonephritis and abscess. (*A*) Arterial-phase axial image shows subtle hypodensity (*arrow*) in the posterior region of the right kidney. Corresponding nephrographic-phase (*B*) image confirms the peripheral hypodensity to be related to acute pyelonephritis. (*C*) Contrast-enhanced CT axial image demonstrates a striated nephrogram in the right kidney resulting from early acute pyelonephritis. Culture confirmed pyelonephritis caused by *Escherichia coli*. (*D*) Contrast-enhanced CT image of the kidneys shows right renal contour abnormalities (*arrow*). (*E*) Nonenhanced axial CT image in another patient demonstrates left renal atrophy and an ipsilateral posterior pararenal abscess (*) with a focus of air (*arrowhead*).

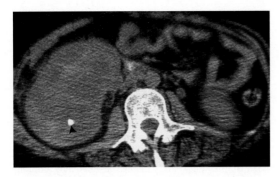

Fig. 14. Xanthogranulomatous pyelonephritis: nonenhanced CT image of the kidneys demonstrates an enlarged right kidney with multiple hypodense areas and a stone (*arrowhead*).

Hydatid cysts

Renal involvement is rare in patients who have hydatid disease and represents only 2% to 3% of all patients who have hydatid cysts [63]. Clinical presentation usually is nonspecific and includes a flank mass, renal colic, persistent fever, hematuria, dysuria, pyuria, renal stones, or hypertension [64]. Renal involvement usually is single and located in the cortex. The CT findings usually are of unilocular or multilocular cysts. Accompanying mural calcification and the presence of daughter cysts help differentiate unilocular cysts from simple renal cysts [63,64]. A multiseptated cystic appearance is more typical of hydatid cyst, especially in endemic areas (Fig. 15).

Other inflammatory lesions

Emphysematous pyelonephritis is a fulminant gas-forming infection of the kidney parenchyma and usually occurs in patients who have uncontrolled diabetes or severe immunosuppression [17,61]. Classic emphysematous pyelonephritis (type I) is characterized by parenchymal destruction with mottled or streaky region of gas within the parenchyma and with little or no fluid. The second form (type II) is characterized by large renal or perirenal fluid collections with associated bubbly or loculated gas. Patients who have the type II pattern of imaging have a better prognosis than those who have type I [65].

In renal tuberculosis, the genitourinary system is the second most common site of tuberculous infection. CT findings depend on the stage of infection. Infundibular strictures cause proximal calyceal dilatation. Hydronephrosis may be caused by ureteral strictures [61]. In the late phase of disease, cavities that communicate with the collecting system, large caseating granulomas, focal or diffuse cortical scarring, and dystrophic amorphous calcifications, are present.

In end-stage disease, a small, calcified nonfunctioning renal remnant representing autonephrectomy may be seen. MDCT also may be helpful in the evaluation of other chronic inflammatory processes, such as chronic pyelonephritis and fungal infections.

Benign renal tumors and cysts

Renal cyst

Benign renal cysts are a common incidental finding and may be seen on CT in up to 27% of patients more than 50 years of age [66]. The CT criteria for the diagnosis of simple cysts are well

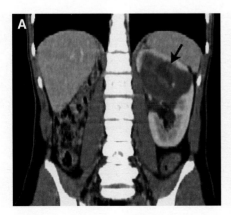
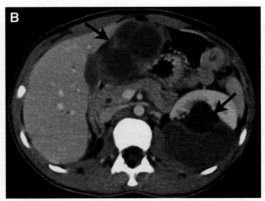

Fig. 15. (*A*) Contrast-enhanced coronal CT demonstrates a well-defined, multilocular hypodense cystic mass (*arrow*) consistent with hydatid cyst in the left kidney. (*B*) Axial contrast-enhanced CT image in another patient demonstrates septated cysts (*arrows*) in liver and left kidney. (Courtesy of M. Emin Sakarya, MD, and Omer Etlik, MD, Firat University, Elazig, Turkey.)

established and include an imperceptible wall, absence of internal septations, unenhanced attenuation of less than 20 HU, and no enhancement or enhancement of less than 10 HU after administration of IV contrast medium [66,67]. A phenomenon described as pseudoenhancement, however, is observed in intrarenal cysts of less than 2 cm examined during the nephrographic phase of enhancement. This phenomenon is believed secondary to beam-hardening artifact [19,65]. Although HU elevation may reach up to 15 HU in older CT scanners, when using newer scanners this value is limited to 10 HU [65]. Therefore, a renal cystic lesion that measures in the range of 0 to 20 HU on a precontrast study may have HU values up to 35 HU if the lesion is intrarenal and is examined during the nephrographic phase [8].

Cystic renal masses usually are characterized according to the Bosniak classification system (Fig. 16) [67]. Category I lesions are simple benign cysts with thin walls; they do not contain septa or calcification.

Category II lesions are slightly more complicated and may contain a few thin septa, thin calcifications, or high-attenuation fluid. Category III lesions are indeterminate masses that may contain foci of wall calcifications or septal thickening. Enhancement of the wall or septa can be appreciated clearly. Category IV lesions are malignant cystic masses that have solid enhancing areas or thick, irregular enhancing walls or septa [67,68]. Category IIF lesions cannot be differentiated as category II or category III lesions and need a follow-up study. These lesions may contain an increased amount of calcification that may be thicker and nodular [68]. The size criteria demarcating category IIF from category II cysts is 3 cm.

A cystic renal mass with one or two septations thinner than 3 mm with thin peripheral or septal calcifications, a nonenhancing hyperdense cyst, and an obviously infected renal cyst or abscess all are considered benign; therefore, no further imaging or follow-up is recommended [67,69]. If a cystic renal

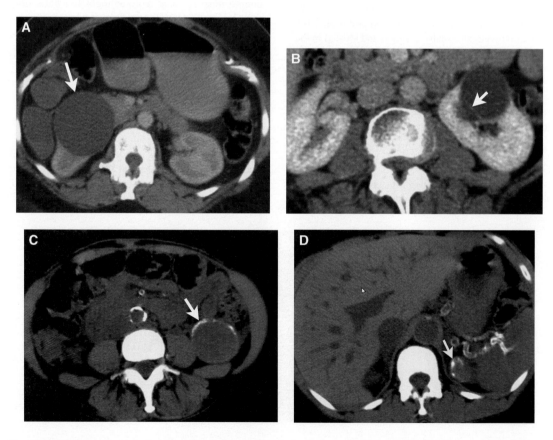

Fig. 16. Bosniak classification of renal cysts. (*A*) Category I, simple renal cyst (*arrow*). (*B*) Category II, cyst with a thin septa (*arrow*). (*C*) Category IIF, cyst greater than 3 cm with peripheral calcification (*arrow*). (*D*) Category III, cyst with chunky calcification (*arrow*). (Category IV cyst is demonstrated in Fig. 17B.)

mass contains milk of calcium, it also is accepted as benign. Follow-up renal CT is recommended in 3 to 6 months if the findings are suspicious or equivocal [69].

Angiomyolipoma

Angiomyolipoma (AML) is a benign hamartoma composed of blood vessels, smooth muscle, and fatty tissue. AML is seen either sporadically or associated with tuberous sclerosis. AMLs usually are seen on CT as in well-defined renal masses. The presence of intratumoral fat is diagnostic of AMLs (Fig. 17A). As AML is a benign mass with a low risk of hemorrhage when it is smaller than 4 cm, it usually is not removed surgically [69]. Three contiguous measurements of fat density less than −20 HU are diagnostic of fat and AMLs [70].

Oncocytoma

Oncocytomas are benign epithelial tumors with a generally benign course. They are usually single,

well-defined, uniformally expansile masses. These tumors are hypervascular and in 80% of cases show a spoke-and-wheel pattern of enhancement with a central stellate scar of low-CT attenuation [13].

Renal cystic disease associated with renal tumors (hereditary syndromes)

Renal cystic diseases associated with renal tumors include acquired cystic kidney disease, von Hippel-Lindau disease, and tuberous sclerosis.

In acquired cystic kidney disease, RCC occurs at a three- to sixfold increased incidence, may be multiple and bilateral, and often arise from the cyst wall but also can occur in areas not involved by cysts [71]. MDCT improves the characterization of hyperdense cysts and the detection of small RCCs in areas not involved by the cysts.

Patients who have von Hippel-Lindau disease are at the highest risk for developing of multicentric, intracystic RCCs, which occur in 40% of these patients [69]. If these patients have even very small renal cysts without malignant features, they should

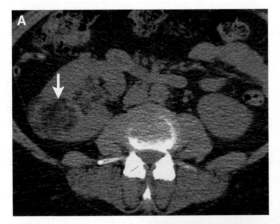
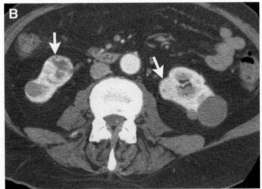
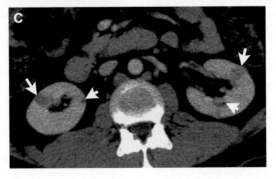

Fig. 17. (A) Right renal AML (arrow). (B) Contrast-enhanced CT axial image demonstrates bilateral RCC (arrows) in a known case of von Hippel-Lindau disease. (C) Axial contrast-enhanced CT image in a patient who had tuberous sclerosis demonstrates bilateral renal AML (arrows).

be followed with CT because the cysts may contain malignant foci [69,71]. Multiple bilateral renal cysts and cystic and solid neoplasms are the most common renal manifestation of von Hippel-Lindau disease (see Fig. 17B).

Renal manifestations of tuberous sclerosis include multiple cysts, AMLs, and RCCs. The AMLs usually are small (less than 1 cm), multiple, and bilateral (Fig. 17C). The combination of renal cysts and AMLs is strongly suggestive of tuberous sclerosis. Patients who have tuberous sclerosis have an increased risk of bilateral RCCs [71]. MDCT is useful in demonstrating perinephric extension and hemorrhage.

Malignant tumors of the kidney

RCC is the most common primary tumor of the kidney. With the widespread use of cross-sectional imaging, many tumors are discovered incidentally and most of them are small, early-stage lesions [72].

For optimal evaluation of a renal mass with MDCT, multiphase imaging is necessary [72]. For all renal imaging, the use of thin (5 mm or less) collimation is essential [69]. When a renal mass is suspected, CT without contrast should be obtained to serve as the baseline for measurements of enhancement on images obtained after contrast material administration.

The most common appearance of an RCC is a solid noncalcified lesion with an attenuation value of 20 HU or greater on unenhanced CT [73]. Although larger lesions tend to be more heterogeneous because of hemorrhage or necrosis, small (3 cm or less) tumors usually have a homogeneous appearance [72].

The first phase of contrast enhancement is the corticomedullary phase that is essential for accurate staging of RCC. Maximal opacification of the renal arteries and veins allows confident diagnosis of venous extension of tumoral tissue. Accurate demonstration of the arterial anatomy is useful in selected cases to plan nephron-sparing surgery [72].

The nephographic phase is the most useful for detecting renal masses and for characterizing indeterminate lesions [17,72]. In this phase, the renal mass enhances relatively less than the normal renal parenchyma [42].

As most RCCs have a rich vascular supply, they enhance significantly after contrast administration on the nephrographic phase (Fig. 18). Enhancement values of more than 20 HU are considered suspicious for malignancy [73]. Some less vascular RCC masses enhance 10 to 20 HU, and this level of enhancement is seen more frequently with cystic RCC. Sometimes this level of enhancement can be

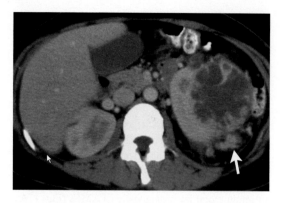

Fig. 18. RCC; nephrographic-phase image shows a large necrotic tumor in the left kidney with perinephric infiltration (*arrow*).

seen in some benign lesions, such as complicated cysts [73]. All renal masses enhance less than the surrounding renal parenchyma.

The excretory phase is useful to delineate the relationship of a centrally located mass with the collecting system better and to define potential involvement of the calyces and the renal pelvis [72]. This phase also is useful for detecting transitional cell carcinoma. Measurement of washout of contrast material from a lesion at 15 minutes may allow differentiation between hyperdense cysts and renal neoplasms [74].

Location of the tumors may be helpful in the diagnosis of solid renal masses. RCC originates in the renal cortex and, therefore, frequently is located at the periphery or near the corticomedullary junction of the kidney. Transitional cell carcinoma and other tumors arise from the urothelium, and spread into the kidney from the renal pelvicaliceal system. These occur more centrally in the kidney and usually displace surrounding renal sinus fat [69].

Three-dimensional CT combined with CT angiography has the potential to provide all the critical information needed to plan the required surgical procedure. These images can be viewed in multiple planes and orientations to define the tumor and its relationship to the renal surface, the collecting system, and adjacent organs [72]. A 3-D CT angiogram can display the renal arterial and venous anatomy.

Perinephric spread of tumor and local extension

Spread of tumoral tissue within the perinephric fat cannot always be diagnosed reliably, and differentiation between stage T2 and T3a tumors is problematic. Perinephric stranding may be caused by edema, vascular engorgement, or previous inflammation, and perinephric stranding does not indicate tumoral spread reliably and is found in approximately half the patients who have localized T1 and T2 tumors [72].

The use of a high-resolution protocol during the vascular phase allows better detection of small enhancing nodules as typical features of perinephric involvement and assessment of edema and venous engorgement as benign causes of perirenal stranding [75].

Venous spread of tumors

The evaluation of renal vein and IVC thrombosis is crucial for treatment planning. Venous extension optimally is shown during the corticomedullary phase. The most specific sign of venous extension is the presence of a hypodense filling defect within the vein. A sudden change in the caliber of the renal vein and the presence of a clot within collateral veins are useful ancillary signs [72]. Direct continuity of the thrombus with the primary tumor and heterogeneous enhancement of the thrombus with contrast medium indicate tumoral thrombus [72].

Miscellaneous conditions

Reflux of contrast medium from the left renal vein into the left ovarian vein often is seen during the corticomedullary phase and is a common finding in asymptomatic women. In a recent study, reflux into the left ovarian vein was found in 44% of parous women (most of them multiparous) and in 5% of

nulliparous women [76]. Reflux into the left ovarian vein and the associated parauterine varices often are seen in asymptomatic multiparous women [76].

Ovarian reflux also can be a sign of disease (eg, pelvic congestion syndrome) and can be associated with chronic pelvic pain. Pelvic congestion syndrome is characterized by chronic pelvic pain of at least 6 months' duration without any identifiable organic cause [77]. Most patients who have pelvic congestion syndrome are multiparous women. Ovarian venous dilatation sometimes occurs as a result of tumoral compression, such as RCC. MDCT can demonstrate these abnormalities accurately (Fig. 19).

Enlarged left gonadal veins that empty into the inferior left renal vein have been observed and are associated with varicoceles in men [23]. The relationship between the retroaortic left renal vein and associated varicoceles in men also are demonstrated in a recent study [47].

Rarely, abnormal diaphragm attachment may mimic renal tumor because of its nodular appearance. Viewing subsequent images is useful to differentiate these pseudomasses from real ones.

Radiation dose of multidector row CT

CT is a significant source of radiation to the population and is responsible for more than 40% of all medical sources of radiation [78].

Most CT urography protocols use at least two CT scans resulting in significantly higher radiation dose to patients than does IVU [35]. In a recent study, McTavish and colleagues find that skin doses of three-scan MDCT urography protocol are similar to

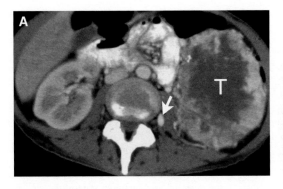
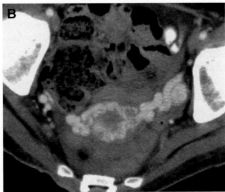

Fig. 19. (*A*) Contrast-enhanced CT axial image of the kidneys shows a large, left renal tumor (T) and a dilated left lumbar vein (*arrow*) (*B*) with extensive left gonadal vein dilatation secondary to a large left RCC extending in left renal vein (not shown).

IVU, but the effective dose of MDCT urography is approximately 1.5 times higher than that of IVU [31].

There are new CT scanner software programs that permit CT doses to be reduced by lowering the tube current based on body width and tissue absorption [35,79].

The effective dose of radiation is directly proportional to the tube current (eg, milliampere) and, thus, increases linearly with tube current. The relationship between the effective dose and the tube potential (eg, peak kilovoltage) is nonlinear and more complex because at higher peak kilovoltage values, more x-rays pass through the body and cause less absorption [80]. The relationship between pitch and radiation dose is different in single-slice CT and in MDCT. For the MDCT system, the measured radiation doses for all slice combinations essentially are the same regardless of the pitch [81]. Keeping the noise level constant, the tube current must be increased to compensate for the higher pitch. The effective dose is independent of pitch at constant noise levels [80]. Alternatively, for the single-slice helical CT system, as pitch increases, the measured radiation dose decreases proportionately [81].

There are two alternative ways to reduce patient doses; in one of these, the user selects the appropriate protocol and scanning parameters for all CT examinations. For example, reduced miliampere seconds allows detection of most stones with less radiation [82], but performing multiple series with thinner collimation significantly increases the dose. As patients who have urolithiasis usually are relatively young and suffer from nonmalignant disease, every attempt should be made to limit the radiation dose and perform CT only when indicated [53]. Another option for reducing patient radiation dose is to develop dose efficiency systems by the manufacturer. For this purpose, automatic tube current modulation systems are used. This system allows automatic adjustment of the tube current in the x-y plane (angular modulation) or along the z-axis (z-axis modulation) according to the size and attenuation characteristics of the body part being scanned, thereby achieving constant CT image quality with lower radiation exposure [79]. Using this method, initial results show a 20% to 60% dose reduction depending on the anatomic region scanned and patient habitus with improved image quality [79,83].

It is important to evaluate the benefits versus the risks to patients of any imaging study or CT-guided procedure to avoid unnecessary exposure to radiation [84].

Initial studies show that MDCT results in higher radiation dosages if techniques similar to those of single-detector helical CT are used. Similar quality images with similar dosimetry, however, can be obtained using lower milliampere and kilovolt (peak) settings [15]. Proper adjustment of the imaging parameters and using automatic tube current techniques can reduce patients' radiation dose.

Summary

MDCT is the most recent advance in CT technology. An increased number of detector rows and more powerful x-ray tubes result in faster scanning time, increased volume coverage, and improved spatial and temporal resolution. MDCT technology allows superior image quality, decreased examination time, and the ability to perform complex multiphase vascular and 3-D examinations.

Using MDCT, complete evaluation of the kidney and urinary system can be performed. Examinations should be tailored to answer specific clinical questions to reduce patient radiation dose. Multiphase contrast-enhanced studies are possible within seconds on MDCT. In the near future, CT urography rather than IVU will be used to evaluate patients who have hematuria. Proper use of the scanning technique and scan parameters is critical for high-quality images.

Acknowledgments

The authors would like to thank Bonnie Hami, MA, University Hospitals Cleveland, for her editorial assistance in the preparation of this manuscript.

References

[1] McCollough CH, Zink FE. Performance evaluation of a multi-slice CT system. Med Phys 1999;26:2223–30.

[2] Rydberg J, Buckwalter KA, Caldemeyer KS, et al. Multisection CT: scanning techniques and clinical applications. Radiographics 2000;20:1787–806.

[3] Hu H, He HD, Foley WD, et al. Four multidetector row helical CT: image quality and volume coverage speed. Radiology 2000;215:55–62.

[4] Prokop M. General principles of MDCT. Eur J Radiol 2003;45(Suppl 1):S4–10.

[5] Napoli A, Fleischmann D, Chan FP, et al. Computed tomography angiography: state-of-the-art imaging using multidetector-row technology. J Comput Assist Tomogr 2004;28:S32–45.

[6] Rydberg J, Liang Y, Teague SD. Fundamentals of

multichannel CT. Radiol Clin North Am 2003;41: 465–74.

[7] Kalra MK, Maher MM, D'Souza R, et al. Multidetector computed tomography technology: current status and emerging developments. J Comput Assist Tomogr 2004;28(Suppl 1):S2–6.

[8] Foley WD. Special focus session: multidetector CT: abdominal visceral imaging. Radiographics 2002;22: 701–19.

[9] Jakobs TF, Becker CR, Wintersperger BJ, et al. CT angiography of the coronary arteries with a 16-row spiral tomograph. Effect of spatial resolution on image quality. Radiologe 2002;42:733–8.

[10] Lawler LP, Jarret TW, Corl FM, et al. Adult ureteropelvic junction obstruction: insights with three-dimensional multi-detector row CT. Radiographics 2005;25:121–34.

[11] Kawamoto S, Montgomery RA, Lawler LP, et al. Multidetector CT angiography for preoperative evaluation of living laparoscopic kidney donors. AJR Am J Roentgenol 2003;180:1633–8.

[12] Rydberg J, Kopecky KK, Tann M, et al. Evaluation of prospective living renal donors for laparoscopic nephrectomy with multisection CT: the marriage of minimally invasive imaging with minimally invasive surgery. Radiographics 2001;21 Spec no:S223–36.

[13] Tunaci A, Yekeler E. Multidetector row CT of the kidneys. Eur J Radiol 2004;52:56–66.

[14] Smith RC, Rosenfield AT, Choe KA, et al. Acute flank pain: comparison of non-contrast-enhanced CT and intravenous urography. Radiology 1995;194:789–94.

[15] Lockhart ME, Smith JK. Technical considerations in renal CT. Radiol Clin North Am 2003;41:863–75.

[16] Wintersperger BJ, Nikolaou K, Becker CR. Multidetector-row CT angiography of the aorta and visceral arteries. Semin Ultrasound CT MR 2004;25:25–40.

[17] Sheth S, Fishman EK. Multi-detector row CT of the kidneys and urinary tract: techniques and applications in the diagnosis of benign diseases. Radiographics 2004;24(2):e20.

[18] Haage P, Schmitz-Rode T, Hubner D, et al. Reduction of contrast material dose and artifacts by a saline flush using a double power injector in helical CT of the thorax. AJR Am J Roentgenol 2000;174: 1049–53.

[19] Foley WD. Renal MDCT. Eur J Radiol 2003; 45(Suppl 1):S73–8.

[20] Rubin GD. 3-D imaging with MDCT. Eur J Radiol 2003;45(Suppl 1):S37–41.

[21] Mortele KJ, McTavish J, Ros PR. Current techniques of computed tomography. Helical CT, multidetector CT, and 3D reconstruction. Clin Liver Dis 2002;6: 29–52.

[22] Cademartiri F, Luccichenti G, van Der Lugt A, et al. Sixteen-row multislice computed tomography: basic concepts, protocols, and enhanced clinical applications. Semin Ultrasound CT MR 2004;25:2–16.

[23] Urban BA, Ratner LE, Fishman EK. Three-dimensional volume-rendered CT angiography of the renal arteries

and veins: normal anatomy, variants, and clinical applications. Radiographics 2001;21:373–86.

[24] Rubin GD, Dake MD, Napel S, et al. Spiral CT of renal artery stenosis: comparison of three-dimensional rendering techniques. Radiology 1994;190:181–9.

[25] Magnusson M, Lenz R, Danielsson PE. Evaluation of methods for shaded surface display of CT volumes. Comput Med Imaging Graph 1991;15:247–56.

[26] Meyers MA. Dynamic radiology of the retroperitoneum. Normal and pathologic anatomy. Acta Gastroenterol Belg 1983;46:273–88.

[27] Warshauer DM, McCarthy SM, Street L, et al. Detection of renal masses: sensitivities and specificities of excretory urography/linear tomography, US, and CT. Radiology 1988;169:363–5.

[28] Grossfeld GD, Litwin MS, Wolf Jr JS, et al. Evaluation of asymptomatic microscopic hematuria in adults: the American Urological Association best practice policy—part II: patient evaluation, cytology, voided markers, imaging, cystoscopy, nephrology evaluation, and follow-up. Urology 2001;57:604–10.

[29] Caoili EM, Cohan RH, Korobkin M, et al. Urinary tract abnormalities: initial experience with multidetector row CT urography. Radiology 2002;222: 353–60.

[30] McNicholas MM, Raptopoulos VD, Schwartz RK, et al. Excretory phase CT urography for opacification of the urinary collecting system. AJR Am J Roentgenol 1998;170:1261–7.

[31] McTavish JD, Jinzaki M, Zou KH, et al. Multi-detector row CT urography: comparison of strategies for depicting the normal urinary collecting system. Radiology 2002;225:783–90.

[32] Kundra V, Silverman PM. Impact of multislice CT on imaging of acute abdominal disease. Radiol Clin North Am 2003;41:1083–93.

[33] Kawashima A, Glockner JF, King Jr BF. CT urography and MR urography. Radiol Clin North Am 2003;41: 945–61.

[34] Kawashima A, Vrtiska TJ, LeRoy AJ, et al. CT urography. Radiographics 2004;24(Suppl 1):S35–54.

[35] Akbar SA, Mortele KJ, Baeyens K, et al. Multidetector CT urography: techniques, clinical applications, and pitfalls. Semin Ultrasound CT MR 2004;25:41–54.

[36] Vrtiska TJ, King BF, LeRoy AJ, et al. CT urography: description of a novel technique using a modified multi-detector-row CT scanner [abstract]. Radiology 2000;217(P):225.

[37] McCollough CH, Bruesewitz MR, Vrtiska TJ, et al. Image quality and dose comparison among screen-film, computed, and CT scanned projection radiography: applications to CT urography. Radiology 2001; 221:395–403.

[38] Dyer RB, Chen MY, Zagoria RJ. Intravenous urography: technique and interpretation. Radiographics 2001;21:799–821.

[39] Caoili EM, Cohan RH, Korobkin M, et al. Effectiveness of abdominal compression during helical renal CT. Acad Radiol 2001;8:1100–6.

[40] Nolte-Ernsting CC, Wildberger JE, Borchers H, et al. Multi-slice CT urography after diuretic injection: initial results. Rofo 2001;173:176–80.

[41] Chow LC, Sommer FG. Multidetector CT urography with abdominal compression and three-dimensional reconstruction. AJR Am J Roentgenol 2001;177: 849–55.

[42] Yuh BI, Cohan RH. Different phases of renal enhancement: role in detecting and characterizing renal masses during helical CT. AJR Am J Roentgenol 1999; 173:747–55.

[43] Park JM, Bloom DA. The pathophysiology of UPJ obstruction. Current concepts. Urol Clin North Am 1998;25:161–9.

[44] Kim JK, Park SY, Kim HJ, et al. Living donor kidneys: usefulness of multi-detector row CT for comprehensive evaluation. Radiology 2003;229:869–76.

[45] Rankin SC, Jan W, Koffman CG. Noninvasive imaging of living related kidney donors: evaluation with CT angiography and gadolinium-enhanced MR angiography. AJR Am J Roentgenol 2001;177:349–55.

[46] Chow LC, Rubin GD. CT angiography of the arterial system. Radiol Clin North Am 2002;40:729–49.

[47] Arslan H, Etlik O, Ceylan K, et al. Incidence of retroaortic left renal vein and its relationship with varicocele. Eur Radiol 2005;15(8):1717–20.

[48] Safian RD, Textor SC. Renal-artery stenosis. N Engl J Med 2001;344:431–42.

[49] Kim TS, Chung JW, Park JH, et al. Renal artery evaluation: comparison of spiral CT angiography to intra-arterial DSA. J Vasc Interv Radiol 1998;9:553–9.

[50] Willmann JK, Wildermuth S, Pfammatter T, et al. Aortoiliac and renal arteries: prospective intraindividual comparison of contrast-enhanced three-dimensional MR angiography and multi-detector row CT angiography. Radiology 2003;226:798–811.

[51] Prokop M. Protocols and future directions in imaging of renal artery stenosis: CT angiography. J Comput Assist Tomogr 1999;23(Suppl 1):S101–10.

[52] Kawashima A, Sandler CM, Ernst RD, et al. CT evaluation of renovascular disease. Radiographics 2000;20:1321–40.

[53] Kenney PJ. CT evaluation of urinary lithiasis. Radiol Clin North Am 2003;41:979–99.

[54] Blake SP, McNicholas MM, Raptopoulos V. Nonopaque crystal deposition causing ureteric obstruction in patients with HIV undergoing indinavir therapy. AJR Am J Roentgenol 1998;171:717–20.

[55] Olcott EW, Sommer FG, Napel S. Accuracy of detection and measurement of renal calculi: in vitro comparison of three-dimensional spira CT, radiography, and nephrotomography. Radiology 1997;204: 19–25.

[56] Heneghan JP, Dalrymple NC, Verga M, et al. Soft-tissue "rim" sign in the diagnosis of ureteral calculi with use of unenhanced helical CT. Radiology 1997; 202:709–11.

[57] Georgiades CS, Moore CJ, Smith DP. Differences of renal parenchymal attenuation for acutely obstructed and unobstructed kidneys on unenhanced helical CT: a useful secondary sign? AJR Am J Roentgenol 2001; 176:965–8.

[58] Traubici J, Neitlich JD, Smith RC. Distinguishing pelvic phleboliths from distal ureteral stones on routine unenhanced helical CT: is there a radiolucent center? AJR Am J Roentgenol 1999;172:13–7.

[59] Guest AR, Cohan RH, Korobkin M, et al. Assessment of the clinical utility of the rim and comet-tail signs in differentiating ureteral stones from phleboliths. AJR Am J Roentgenol 2001;177:1285–91.

[60] Kawashima A, Sandler CM, Goldman SM, et al. CT of renal inflammatory disease. Radiographics 1997;17: 851–66.

[61] Kawashima A, LeRoy AJ. Radiologic evaluation of patients with renal infections. Infect Dis Clin North Am 2003;17:433–56.

[62] Chuang CK, Lai MK, Chang PL, et al. Xanthogranulomatous pyelonephritis: experience in 36 cases. J Urol 1992;147:333–6.

[63] Kiresi DA, Karabacakoglu A, Odev K, et al. Uncommon locations of hydatid cysts. Acta Radiol 2003;44: 622–36.

[64] Odev K, Kilinc M, Arslan A, et al. Renal hydatid cysts and the evaluation of their radiologic images. Eur Urol 1996;30:40–9.

[65] Wan YL, Lee TY, Bullard MJ, et al. Acute gasproducing bacterial renal infection: correlation between imaging findings and clinical outcome. Radiology 1996;198:433–8.

[66] Coulam CH, Sheafor DH, Leder RA, et al. Evaluation of pseudoenhancement of renal cysts during contrast-enhanced CT. AJR Am J Roentgenol 2000; 174:493–8.

[67] Bosniak MA. The current radiological approach to renal cysts. Radiology 1986;158:1–10.

[68] Israel GM, Bosniak MA. Calcification in cystic renal masses: is it important in diagnosis? Radiology 2003; 226:47–52.

[69] Zagoria RJ. Imaging of small renal masses: a medical success story. AJR Am J Roentgenol 2000;175: 945–55.

[70] Takahashi K, Honda M, Okubo RS, et al. CT pixel mapping in the diagnosis of small angiomyolipomas of the kidneys. J Comput Assist Tomogr 1993;17: 98–101.

[71] Schreyer HH, Uggowitzer MM, Ruppert-Kohlmayr A. Helical CT of the urinary organs. Eur Radiol 2002; 12:575–91.

[72] Sheth S, Scatarige JC, Horton KM, et al. Current concepts in the diagnosis and management of renal cell carcinoma: role of multidetector CT and three-dimensional CT. Radiographics 2001;21 Spec no: S237–54.

[73] Silverman SG, Lee BY, Seltzer SE, et al. Small (< or =3 cm) renal masses: correlation of spiral CT features and pathologic findings. AJR Am J Roentgenol 1994;163:597–605.

[74] Macari M, Bosniak MA. Delayed CT to evaluate renal

masses incidentally discovered at contrast-enhanced CT: demonstration of vascularity with deenhancement. Radiology 1999;213:674–80.

[75] Catalano C, Fraioli F, Laghi A, et al. High-resolution multidetector CT in the preoperative evaluation of patients with renal cell carcinoma. AJR Am J Roentgenol 2003;180:1271–7.

[76] Hiromura T, Nishioka T, Nishioka S, et al. Reflux in the left ovarian vein: analysis of MDCT findings in asymptomatic women. AJR Am J Roentgenol 2004; 183:1411–5.

[77] Beard RW, Reginald PW, Wadsworth J. Clinical features of women with chronic lower abdominal pain and pelvic congestion. Br J Obstet Gynaecol 1988;95: 153–61.

[78] Charles M. UNSCEAR report 2000: sources and effects of ionizing radiation. United Nations Scientific Comittee on the Effects of Atomic Radiation. J Radiol Prot 2001;21:83–6.

[79] Kalra MK, Maher MM, Toth TL, et al. Techniques and applications of automatic tube current modulation for CT. Radiology 2004;233:649–57.

[80] Saini S. Multi-detector row CT: principles and practice for abdominal applications. Radiology 2004;233: 323–7.

[81] Mahesh M, Scatarige JC, Cooper J, et al. Dose and pitch relationship for a particular multislice CT scanner. AJR Am J Roentgenol 2001;177:1273–5.

[82] Spielmann AL, Heneghan JP, Lee LJ, et al. Decreasing the radiation dose for renal stone CT: a feasibility study of single- and multidetector CT. AJR Am J Roentgenol 2002;178:1058–62.

[83] Suess C, Chen X. Dose optimization in pediatric CT: current technology and future innovations. Pediatr Radiol 2002;32:729–34.

[84] Haaga JR. Radiation dose management: weighing risk versus benefit. AJR Am J Roentgenol 2001;177: 289–91.

RADIOLOGIC
CLINICS
of North America

Radiol Clin N Am 43 (2005) 1049–1062

Multislice CT Colonography: Current Status and Limitations

Matthew A. Barish, MD*, Tatiana C. Rocha, MD

Department of Radiology, 3D & Image Processing Center, Brigham and Women's Hospital, Harvard Medical School, Boston, MA, USA

Colorectal cancer is the third most fatal cancer in men and women and is the second most common cause of cancer death among men aged 40 to 79 years [1]. Most colorectal cancers are believed to arise within benign adenomatous polyps that develop slowly over the course of many years [2,3]. Screening has been shown to save lives by detection and removal of premalignant polyps and early stage cancer [4,5]. Nevertheless, despite this evidence and screening guidelines [6–9], about one half of the average-risk population of the United States eligible for colorectal cancer screening does not pursue this test [10,11]. Many individuals avoid screening because current tests are invasive, expensive, or embarrassing.

Since the introduction of CT colonography (CTC) or virtual colonoscopy in 1994, significant progress has occurred in the development and clinical implementation of this new technique. Currently, CTC is performed on an elective basis at countless institutions around the world. A recent advance in CTC is the application of multislice CT (MSCT) technology. By combining the multi-row detector with increased gantry rotation speed, MSCT can acquire 64 slices per second, and this number is expected to increase in the future. MSCT makes high spatial resolution feasible at shorter acquisition times, increasing the sensitivity of the scan to smaller lesions. In addition, recent advances in the software used for interpretation have made time-efficient interpretation

possible using combined two-dimensional (2-D), three-dimensional (3-D), and endoluminal "fly-through." This article summarizes the technique, ongoing research, limitations, and other issues in the use of MSCT colonography.

Technique

Numerous scanning techniques have been described for CTC [12,13], all of which apply the same basic principles of patient preparation and imaging. Patient preparation consists of cleansing the patient's colon with a laxative bowel preparation and insufflating the colon with room air or carbon dioxide. Thin section helical CT of the abdomen and pelvis in the prone and supine position is then performed. Interpretation is facilitated by image processing of the CT data set using specialized computer software to improve inspection of the colonic wall. The use of stool-tagging agents, electronic cleansing, intravenous contrast, spasmolytics, low-dose MSCT, translucency rendering 3-D and other advanced 3-D image processing techniques has been considered in attempts to improve the accuracy of CTC.

Bowel preparation

The accuracy of CTC is directly related to the adequacy of colon cleansing. Residual stool (Figs. 1–3) and fluid interfere with image interpretation and are a significant cause of false-positive and false-negative interpretations. Retained stool can simulate polyps, decreasing specificity, whereas retained fluid can obscure polyps, resulting in decreased sensitivity. Full

---
* Corresponding author. Department of Radiology, 3D & Image Processing Center, Brigham and Women's Hospital, Harvard Medical School, 75 Francis Street, Boston, MA 02115.

E-mail address: mabarish@partners.org (M.A. Barish).

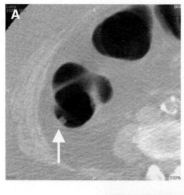
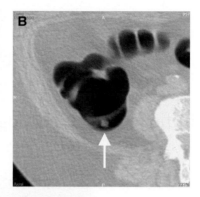

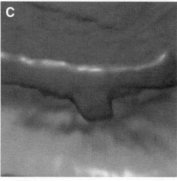

Fig. 1. Fecal material is identified based on morphology (cubic shape). Axial CTC images in the supine position (*A*) and prone position (*B*) show a geometric cube of soft-tissue density (*arrows*). A polyp would not be expected to demonstrate such a shape. (*C*) The corresponding 3-D endoluminal image is shown.

colonic cleansing with cathartics is required to achieve acceptable results.

Multiple laxative regimens have been used for CTC, including polyethylene glycol (GoLYTELY), magnesium citrate (LOSOL), and sodium phosphate laxative solution (Fleet Prep No. 1) [14]. The standard optical colonoscopy preparation (polyethylene glycol electrolyte solution) tends to result in more retained fluid; therefore, most investigators prefer magnesium citrate or sodium phosphate, which results in less retained fluid [15,16]. Macari and coworkers [16] compared the polyethylene solution with the sodium phosphate laxative solution and concluded that, on average, sodium phosphate laxative solution provided significantly less residual fluid. In a study by Barish and coworkers [14], 66% of CTC experts preferred sodium phosphate solution (single or double dose) to polyethylene glycol.

Even following a full-dose bowel cleansing regiment, residual stool can cause problems for interpretation. Methods to label or "tag" residual stool to improve CTC accuracy have been investigated (Fig. 3). Stool-tagging agents composed of iodine or barium are administered orally with meals during the 1 or 2 days before the CTC examination. These agents are designed to mix with enteric contents, altering the attenuation of stool so it can be distinguished from polyps or cancer. The soft-tissue attenuation of the polyp can be differentiated from the high attenuation of the labeled stool [17]. The tagging material can mark solid and fluid fecal contents, enabling solid fecal material to be differentiated from polyps and cancers and helping to detect polyps submerged in opacified fluid. In one study, Fletcher and coworkers [18] found no benefit in using orally administered iodinated contrast as a stool-tagging agent before scanning. Lefere and coworkers [19] adopted a combined regimen of oral contrast, a low-residue diet, and mild bowel cleansing in the day preceding CT examination and achieved a sensitivity of 85% in a feasibility study of 50 patients. In addition, some experts [20,21] have attributed the excellent results achieved by Pickhardt and coworkers [22] to the use of fluid and fecal tagging with excellent laxative cleansing. The same group performed a similar study [20] adding electronic cleansing of the luminal fluid to the stool tagging and reported good results when used together with colon purgation.

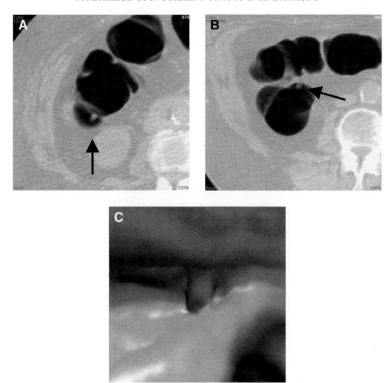

Fig. 2. Fecal material showing mobility. Fecal material changes position when supine axial CTC images (*A*) are compared with prone (*B*) images (*arrows*). (*C*) The corresponding 3-D endoluminal image is shown.

The requirement of a laxative for bowel cleansing in CTC is one of the major barriers for patient compliance with screening [23]. Edwards and coworkers [24] showed that the bowel preparation and the associated diet were the major reasons why patients had a negative experience with CTC. Efforts to eliminate or minimize the need for a rigorous bowel cleansing are under investigation. Approaches to reducing the burden of bowel cleansing include allowing the patient to consume a structured low-fiber diet instead of clear liquids, reducing the laxative dose by adding fecal/fluid tagging [25], or eliminating completely the laxative by using fecal/fluid tagging combined with electronic stool subtraction [26–30].

Many investigators have attempted to eliminate the need for laxative cathartic preparation completely with the use of fecal tagging. Lefere and coworkers [30] used a combination of a dedicated low-residue diet, hydration control, and barium as the sole tagging agent with no cathartic bowel cleansing and achieved an almost completely dry colon with efficient tagging of fecal residue. Callstrom and coworkers [28] using multiple doses of diluted barium sulfate and a 48-hour lead time showed that the

sensitivity for polyp detection in patients with adequate stool labeling approached the sensitivity for polyp detection in colons prepared with cathartics. Bielen and coworkers [31] evaluated the feasibility of a dry bowel preparation without a laxative and with stool tagging and reported a good fecal tagging with a good patient acceptance. Iannaccone and coworkers [29] obtained a sensitivity of 95.5% for polyps 8 mm or larger using iodinated contrast without cathartic bowel preparation when comparing CTC and optical colonoscopy for the detection of colorectal polyps.

Once the stool has been labeled adequately, interpretation can be improved by electronically removing the tagged fecal material before inspection by a radiologist [20,26,27]. This technique has been termed *electronic cleansing* or *digital stool subtraction*. This automated technique has been shown to be useful when fecal tagging is used in addition to cathartic bowel cleansing [20], and also when tagging is used as a complete replacement for cathartic cleansing [26,27]. Clearly, methods that would reduce discomfort and inconvenience, or methods that would eliminate the need for preparation, would address an

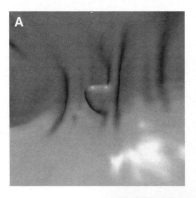
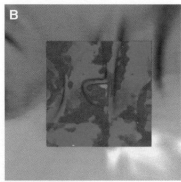
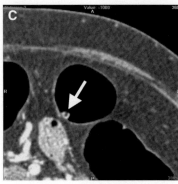

Fig. 3. Fecal material: use of density and fecal tagging. The 3-D endoluminal image (*A*) shows a polypoid lesion. (*B*) Translucency rendering is applied to the 3-D image, showing a green center (air) with a white tip (barium) representing tagged stool. The axial CTC image (*C*) demonstrates the high density of the fecal material with central lucency (*arrow*).

important obstacle for widespread colorectal cancer screening [23,24].

Colonic insufflation

A well-distended colon is mandatory for proper evaluation by CTC. Determination of adequate insufflation can be assessed by volume, pressure, or the patient's tolerance. Use of the volume-limited method suggests that the patient should receive approximately 2 L of room air or CO_2. This limit can be accomplished by counting the number of insufflator bulb compressions (when room air is used) or by volume gauge measurement (when CO_2 is used). The pressure method is usually used in conjunction with CO_2, and the pressure is typically set to 25 mm Hg.

No consensus is apparent regarding the use of CO_2 versus room air [14]. The main benefit of CO_2 is based on the absorption of the gas through the colonic wall, which is believed to improve the patient's comfort after the procedure. The benefits of room air are that it is readily available at no cost and requires no special equipment to deliver [14]. A CT scout image

is routinely checked for the adequacy of distension before the actual CTC scan is performed. If the distention is not adequate, more gas can be insufflated to the patient's tolerance.

Some investigators have recommended the routine use of spasmolytics to prevent unwanted colonic collapse and spasm, a problem encountered most commonly in the sigmoid colon. Glucagon (1 mg before colon insufflation) or an anticholinergic agent (hyoscine N-butylbromide, 20 mg) is typically used; however, the benefit of spasmolytic agents is controversial [14,32–35]. Yee and coworkers [32] compared colonic distension in 60 patients who were scanned in the supine and prone positions and reported no beneficial effect from routine glucagon administration. Furthermore, owing to its effect on the ileocecal valve, glucagon can cause unwanted reflux of air into the small bowel and can secondarily reduce colonic distention. Morrin and coworkers [33] found no benefits of using intravenous glucagon, whereas Taylor and coworkers [34] found that hyoscine N-butylbromide improved colonic distention during CTC and recommended that it should be administered routinely where available. Currently, most experts believe that spasmolytics are not routinely necessary [14].

CT scan acquisition

MSCT offers several advantages over single slice CT and has improved the diagnostic performance of CTC [36–38]. Large body areas can be scanned with high spatial resolution in short periods, increasing the sensitivity for polyp detection and helping to prevent motion artifacts owing to voluntary and involuntary movements. Thin slices using MSCT produce high-quality 3-D images that may aid interpretation and increase reader confidence, even if a high positive predictive value for small lesions is not possible because of retained stool or other factors [39].

Typical MSCT imaging parameters include a collimation of 3 mm or less, a table speed of 20 to 25 mm/s, 80 mAs, 120 kVp, and a 512×512 matrix. An acquisition of the abdomen and pelvis is obtained within a single breath hold in the supine position and is repeated with the patient in the prone position. The use of supine and prone helical CT data sets is a consensus among experienced CTC radiologists, and most agree with the use of a minimum of 3-mm collimation [14]. The use of both positions helps differentiate mobile stool from fixed pathology such as cancers and polyps, allows redistribution of the air with better assessment of poorly distended segments, and improves visualization of segments of the colon obscured by intraluminal fluid [18,33,40–42]. Fletcher and coworkers [18] found that the prone scan permitted better distension of the sigmoid colon in a significant number of cases, and Morrin and coworkers [33] demonstrated that turning the patient from supine to prone positioning improved colonic distention, particularly in the rectum and left colon, where two thirds of colorectal cancers occur. The use of an additional prone scan seems to improve accuracy; studies using supine and prone views tend to produce greater accuracy in polyp detection than do studies using only the supine view [13,33,41,42].

The total time required for the CT acquisition is typically less than 10 minutes. Unlike in optical colonoscopy, sedation is not required, and patients are immediately discharged from the CT suite without the need for extended observation or recovery time. The patient's ability to return immediately to activities of daily living is an important societal advantage of CTC over conventional colonoscopy.

The use of intravenously administered contrast material with CTC may improve reader confidence in the assessment of bowel wall and the ability of CTC to depict medium-sized polyps in suboptimally prepared colons [43] (Fig. 4). Nevertheless, the risks of intravenous contrast administration may warrant restricting its use to discretionary cases, such as patients undergoing diagnostic CTC (ie, patients with symptoms of colorectal disease or with known colorectal cancers). Contrast-enhanced CTC is also useful for other applications of CTC, such as detecting local tumor recurrence, metachronous disease, and distant metastases in patients with prior invasive colorectal carcinoma [44], but it cannot predict the malignant differentiation of colorectal neoplasms based on the enhancement values [45].

Radiation dose

The patient's exposure to radiation during CTC is a major concern and disadvantage when this method is proposed as a potential screening tool in the prevention of colorectal cancer [46]. In most cases, CTC can be performed at a reduced radiation dose when compared with conventional CT. For colorectal screening, the dose may be 40% to 50% of the typical dose for CT of the abdomen and pelvis.

Hara and coworkers [47] compared a low-dose setting of 70 mA (5 mm collimation, 3 mm interval, 1.3 pitch) with a standard body setting of 140 mA and found no difference in diagnostic efficacy. The effective dose equivalent for a supine acquisition in Hara's study was 1.87 mGy for men and 2.85 mGy for women, which doubles with the use of an additional prone scan. Nevertheless, the dose for both scans is still 20% lower than the typical dose for a double-contrast barium enema (4.53 mGy for men and 7.45 mGy for women). Some studies have found a similar comparison in dose between CTC and double-contrast barium enema [48], and others have concluded that low-dose multislice CTC performs as well as standard dose multislice CTC in diagnosing polyps measuring 5 mm or more [49] and 6 mm or more [46,50]. MSCT increases the dose efficiency of the x-ray beam, resulting in an even smaller radiation dose to the patient. At a dose of 30 mAs (3.6 mSv), polyp detection remains unimpaired, although image quality decreases significantly [51,52]. A narrow detector collimation with thin section imaging (4 × 1.0 mm detector collimation, 1.25 mm section thickness) is a prerequisite for low-dose (10 mAs) multislice CTC [53]. A full-dose, contrast-enhanced CT is often used for patients who present with symptoms. The full dose is desirable to combine polyp detection with a full review of the organs contained within the abdomen and pelvis.

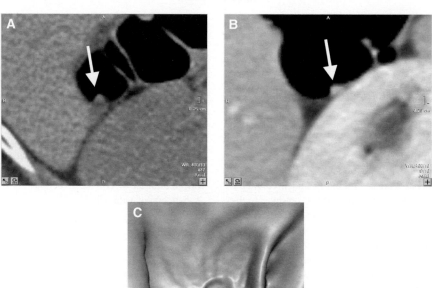

Fig. 4. Enhancing adenoma. Axial CTC images (*A*) before and (*B*) after intravenous contrast. (*A*) A 5-mm adenomatous polyp is seen in the ascending colon (*arrow*). (*B*) After contrast, the lesion enhances intensely (*arrow*). (*C*) 3-D endoluminal image of the same lesion.

Image display

Following image acquisition, the CT data are sent to an off-line workstation and can be viewed using a variety of techniques [54–61]. The goal of computer workstations and display techniques in CTC is to reduce perceptive errors by demonstrating data in a fashion that facilitates interpretation for the observer and reduces interpretation time [17]. Some studies suggest the advantage of supplementing axial views with post-processed reformats and 3-D views. Dachman and coworkers [62] of the University of Chicago using axial 2-D CT images with limited 3-D endoluminal reconstructions for problem solving in 44 patients with 22 proven polyps reported a sensitivity of 83% and a specificity of 100% for polyps 8 mm or larger. Although most experts in CTC (as of 2004) interpret virtual colonoscopy studies using a primary 2-D approach at the lung window setting, with the 3-D approach reserved for problem solving, a growing minority prefer a primary 3-D approach [14]. Most studies to date have used the primary 2-D interpretation method [18,19,28,29,46,49,50,62–68]; however, some recent studies have achieved excellent

results with a primary 3-D approach [22,68]. The main role of post-processed 3-D views is to help differentiate polyps from complex colonic folds, which may have a similar profile on an axial view [69,70]. Alternatively, 3-D views can be used as a primary review method, with 2-D views reserved for differentiating stool or lipomas from polyps (Fig. 5).

Few studies have directly compared primary 2-D methods against primary 3-D methods. Dachman and coworkers [62] concluded that endoluminal views should be used only when necessary to help distinguish normal folds from fixed lesions. Macari and coworkers [63] reported that results with combined axial and 3-D orthogonal views were no better than with axial views alone. Although the test performance of 3-D CTC is likely to improve as a result of thinner slabs, shorter acquisition time, fewer image artifacts, and superior z-axis resolution, many investigators agree that review of 2-D images at lung windows settings is sufficient for detection of abnormalities. Nevertheless, Pickhardt and coworkers [22] showed that CTC using the 3-D approach was an effective and accurate method for detecting relevant lesions in asymptomatic patients.

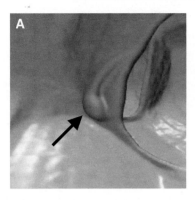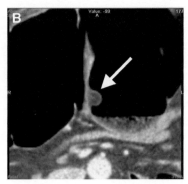

Fig. 5. Use of 2-D problem solving to image lipoma. (*A*) The 3-D endoluminal image shows a polyp on the ileocecal valve (*arrow*). (*B*) The 2-D axial image shows the fatty content of the lesion (*arrow*).

New software algorithms have been developed to supplement or replace traditional 2-D and endoluminal 3-D views. The virtual gross pathology provides mathematically straightened or "unraveled" views of the colon. The colon-straightening method opens the colon along its longitudinal axis, allowing inspection of gross pathology in a flat rather than tubular form [60,61] (Fig. 6). Another display method is the unfolded cube. This projectional format displays the endoluminal view of the colon as if it were flattened onto a six-sided cube, providing a full 360-degree view (including a rear projection). The unfolded cube display has been found to be a time efficient and highly accurate method, improving the 3-D display for CTC [69].

Other viewing techniques focus on methods to provide additional information to differentiate polyps from stool. Translucency rendering adds information below the colonic surface to describe the density of the lesion. Translucency rendering 3-D images have the ability to differentiate benign lesions, improving polyp specificity and increasing overall diag-

nostic confidence, especially when stool tagging is used (Fig. 3) [71].

Computer-aided detection (CAD) automatically detects polyps and masses on CT images of the colon and provides a marker of the location of the suspicious lesions to radiologists [72]. All CAD schemes rely on three main steps: (1) extraction of the colonic wall, (2) identification of potential polyp candidates, and (3) elimination of false-positive findings as far as possible [73]. CAD can act as a second reader, increasing the radiologist's diagnostic performance and decreasing variability among readers [72]. It has been proposed as a means of improving the consistency of CTC interpretations and increasing sensitivity [74]. Although the development of CAD colonography is well advanced, more work is needed to refine existing technology, and large-scale clinical trials are needed to establish performance characteristics [73].

Whether 3-D reconstructions, reformatted views, or endoluminal images should supplement or replace 2-D views is still under evaluation. Which of these imaging display methods will prove to be the best

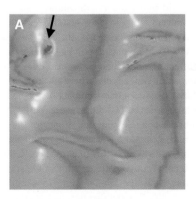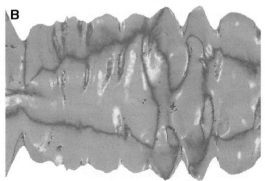

Fig. 6. A novel method of display (*A, B*) provides a colon unwrapping while preserving the local geometry and original surface area. The green areas (*arrow*) represent elevated mucosa that may be possible sites of polypoid lesions.

in terms of speed and accuracy is not yet clear. Although a review of axial views alone can be performed quickly and is often sufficient for interpretation, as computer processing techniques advance, complex image analysis software and computer-aided diagnosis may change the accepted viewing method, and post-processed views may assume a more central role in image interpretation [75]. As workstations continue to improve, it is almost certain that the debate concerning primary 2-D versus primary 3-D interpretation will become moot, and interpretation will consist of the seamless integration of both types of images. In addition, the development of CAD will greatly influence reading strategies and visualization methods.

Screening with CT colonography

Screening

Cancer screening has been shown to reduce mortality by detecting disease at an early asymptomatic stage with a better prognosis. The goal of screening is to identify individuals who are more likely to have unrecognized disease from among the healthy population so that those identified can undergo the more invasive, expensive, but definitive diagnostic procedure [76]. Because traditional methods of colorectal cancer screening are ineffective, colonoscopy has come to be used for screening; however, colonoscopy is not a true screening tool because it is invasive and expensive. The correct use of screening should identify patients who are more likely to have cancer or polyps so that this subgroup can undergo colonoscopy. Colonoscopy should be reserved as a second-line definitive diagnostic and therapeutic test. Virtual colonoscopy or CTC is a true screening tool with minimal invasiveness and acceptable cost. Multiple studies have shown that it has similar accuracy to conventional colonoscopy in high-risk groups [51,67,68] and, more recently, in a low-prevalence screening population [22]. Published reports have shown that virtual colonoscopy is more accurate than alternative methods of colorectal cancer detection such as the barium enema or sigmoidoscopy. In fact, sigmoidoscopy is incapable of detecting more than 50% of lesions because no more than half of the colon is examined [76]. Although several studies have found accuracy approaching that of conventional colonoscopy, conventional video-guided colonoscopy is still considered the gold standard for polyp detection, albeit, a flawed one [77,78]. It is also the only test that combines a complete review of the

colon with the removal of detected polyps. For that reason, CTC is not recommended as a routine substitute for conventional colonoscopy; however, contraindications to sedation, strictures in the colon, and other factors may preclude conventional colonoscopy, and, in many cases, patients may be reluctant to experience the discomfort associated with colonoscopy. CTC should be evaluated seriously for all patients who are unwilling or unable to undergo conventional colonoscopy.

As CTC changes from a research technique to a generally accepted screening test, issues relating to the clinical implementation of a CTC screening program remain. Transitioning a new technology into clinical practice is facilitated by developing a set of standards and practice guidelines. Traditionally, the development of such guidelines follows from an accumulation of clinical data, literature reviews, and consensus opinions from knowledgeable experts in the field [14].

Screening performance of CT colonography

Perhaps the most important measure of CTC as a colorectal screening test is its accuracy in detecting adenomatous polyps and other precursor lesions. CTC does not need to be the equal of endoscopic colonoscopy, because it is only a tool to screen for those persons at higher risk who should undergo a more invasive and definitive endoscopic colonoscopy [76]. From the perspective of preventing colorectal cancer, it is most important to consider only lesions of sufficient size to have a significant likelihood of becoming cancerous, that is, lesions with a diameter of 10 mm. Lesions of this size are recommended for immediate removal because they pose the greatest risk of becoming cancerous (Fig. 7) [79,80]. Nevertheless, controversy still exists as to the exact size that should be used for a threshold. The results of a recent survey suggest that lesions less than 4 mm should not be reported [14]. In addition, one should not consider hyperplastic polyps because they are not premalignant, and their presence does not predict adenomas or cancers elsewhere in the colon [76].

Polyp size has a major impact on the accuracy and performance of CTC. Diagnostic performance and interobserver agreement are high for large polyps (>10 mm) but more variable for smaller ones [81]. Hara and coworkers [82] of the Mayo Clinic evaluated 70 consecutive patients with single slice CT. The sensitivity and specificity were 75% and 90% for patients with adenomatous polyps larger than 10 mm, 66% and 63% for patients with adenomatous polyps larger than 5 mm, and 45% and 80% for patients with

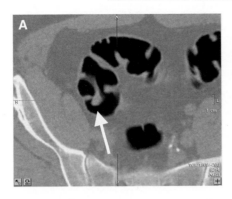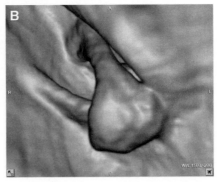

Fig. 7. Pedunculated adenoma. (*A*) Axial CTC image and (*B*) 3-D endoluminal image show a pedunculated 16-mm polyp on a 26-mm stalk in the sigmoid colon (*arrow*).

adenomatous polyps smaller than 5 mm. Hara conducted a subsequent study with MSCT and reported significant improvement of colonic distention and fewer respiratory artifacts. No significant difference in the depiction of polyps larger than 10 mm was demonstrated between single- and multidetector-row CT [83].

Several large studies have found high sensitivity and specificity for lesions and cancers over 1 cm (Fig. 8) [22,64,68,84–87]. On the other hand, Cotton and coworkers [65] and Johnson and coworkers [66] found the results of CTC to be well below those of optical colonoscopy, in contrast to many other studies. The evolving nature of the CTC technique makes direct comparison of reported data difficult, and statistically reliable information is not available. Preliminary results suggest that the accuracy of CTC for polyp detection exceeds that of barium enema and approaches or equals that of conventional colonoscopy [22].

Limitations of CT colonography for colorectal screening

Although CTC has numerous advantages when compared with other leading screening tests (high patient acceptance, lack of sedation, extracolonic review during polyp screening), it has several significant limitations as well [48,88]. Advances in CTC may surmount some of these limitations, whereas others may be more difficult to overcome. As is true for any CT examination, CTC exposes the patient to radiation. Although the dose is below that for a typical abdominal CT or barium enema, it still contributes to the patient's lifetime accumulated radiation exposure.

Unlike conventional colonoscopy, CTC provides no means to remove polyps detected during the examination. Patients with polyps of sufficient size to require removal must schedule a follow-up colonoscopy for polypectomy. In certain cases, the discovery of polyps of intermediate size may present the patient and the physician with a difficult choice as to whether they should be removed. Only conventional colonoscopy combines a full structural review of the entire colon with the option of immediate polypectomy.

Although several studies suggest that it has a higher accuracy than any colorectal screening test other than conventional colonoscopy, the accuracy of CTC is still under study. In particular, some studies have found its sensitivity to be under 65% for polyps smaller than 10 mm but larger than 5 mm [65,66,89]. Although the removal of polyps of this size is of questionable clinical necessity, the inability to detect them is a concern. Moreover, there are conflicting data establishing the accuracy of CTC in a true screening population [22,24,64,66,89]. A large multicenter trial (ACRIN) is now underway, and results in this asymptomatic cohort could prove disappointing. If so, the risk/benefit balance will need reevaluation. In comparison with conventional colonoscopy and barium enema, CTC is safe and highly accepted by patients. Nevertheless, the attendant radiation, rigorous preparation, colonic insufflation, and other demands compare unfavorably with alternative screening methods such as fecal occult blood tests and genetic testing.

CTC performance is highly dependent on many factors, such as the preparation quality, the method of interpretation, the scanning protocol, and the quality of insufflation. Consequently, the imaging center or institution performing the procedure has a significant impact on its success. The center's recommended preparation regimen, scanning equipment, and experience in interpretation of CTC may lead to varying performance in different instances. As is true for con-

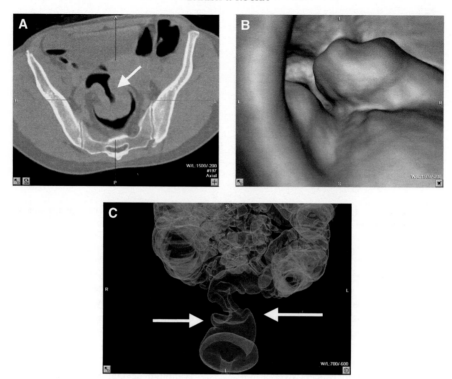

Fig. 8. Sigmoid carcinoma. (*A*) Prone axial CTC image and (*B*) corresponding 3-D endoluminal image show a large circumferential mass in the distal sigmoid colon (*arrow*). (*C*) Volume rendered CT image simulating a double-contrast barium enema shows the "apple core" sigmoid carcinoma (*arrow*).

ventional colonoscopy, CTC interpretation has a substantial learning curve. Several major institutions offer training fellowships or Internet-based tutorials (available at http://www.virtualcolonoscopy.org). The existence of formal training programs is an important step in the widespread adoption of the procedure. At the same time, it reflects the high variability in reader experience, ranging from experts with years of experience to other individuals with only recent training in CTC interpretation.

Other indications for CT colonography

Occlusive carcinoma

Another application of CTC is the preoperative assessment of the colon proximal to an occlusive cancer (defined as a tumor that cannot be traversed endoscopically) (Fig. 8) [90]. In 29 patients with occlusive carcinomas, CTC identified all 29 occlusive cancers and demonstrated 2 cancers and 24 polyps in the proximal colon. Both of the synchronous cancers were confirmed intraoperatively and resected. CTC

successfully demonstrated the proximal colon in 26 of 29 patients studied, whereas a preoperative barium enema failed to demonstrate adequately the proximal colon in any patient studied [90]. Morrin and workers [91] found similar results and reported that CTC was superior to barium enema in assessing the colon proximal to an occlusive tumor. A total of 97% (87 of 90) of all colonic segments were visualized adequately during CTC in patients with obstructing colorectal lesions (15 patients were referred after incomplete colonoscopy) compared with 60% (26 of 42) of segments at barium enema.

Extracolonic findings

Because the entire abdomen and pelvis are scanned, the extracolonic organs can be assessed. CTC commonly detects extracolonic findings that may be considered clinically important when applied to an asymptomatic screening population. In one study, these findings were categorized as being of high clinical importance in 71 individuals (10%), of medium importance in 183 individuals (27%), and of low importance in 341 individuals (50%) [92].

Subsequent medical or surgical interventions resulted from these findings in 9 of the 681 patients (1.3%). Hara and coworkers [93] reported similar findings. No other colorectal screening examination has this advantage of detecting potentially life-threatening conditions in an age group in which those conditions have a higher prevalence.

Summary

In the past few years, many obstacles to the clinical implementation of CTC have been eliminated. The results of CTC published in the recent literature are extremely encouraging for the detection of lesions sized 1 cm or larger with few false-positive findings. The study by Pickhardt and coworkers [22] strongly suggests that CTC can compete favorably against endoscopic colonoscopy in a true screening population. MSCT techniques continue to improve the speed, accuracy, and reproducibility of CTC. This examination will continue to improve with the development of automated (computer) detection programs and 3-D rendering algorithms. In addition, cathartic bowel preparation, one of the biggest obstacles to patient compliance with colorectal cancer screening, may be eliminated if successful fecal tagging can be developed. The major issue remaining is the confident reproducibility of the accuracy of CTC in a purely screening population. When CTC proves to be an accurate, reliable, and cost-effective method for detecting polyps and early cancers in this population, it may dramatically improve population participation in screening programs and have a major role in minimizing the impact of colorectal cancer.

References

[1] Jemal A, Murray T, Ward E, et al. Cancer statistics, 2005. CA Cancer J Clin 2005;55(1):10–30.
[2] Bond JH. Clinical evidence for the adenoma-carcinoma sequence, and the management of patients with colorectal adenomas. Semin Gastrointest Dis 2000;11(4):176–84.
[3] Leslie A, Carey FA, Pratt NR, et al. The colorectal adenoma-carcinoma sequence. Br J Surg 2002;89(7):845–60.
[4] Mandel JS, Bond JH, Church TR, et al. Reducing mortality from colorectal cancer by screening for fecal occult blood: Minnesota Colon Cancer Control Study. N Engl J Med 1993;328(19):1365–71 [erratum in: N Engl J Med 1993;329(9):672].
[5] Winawer SJ, Zauber AG, Ho MN, et al. Prevention of colorectal cancer by colonoscopic polypectomy. N Engl J Med 1993;329:1977–81.
[6] Smith RA, Cokkinides V, Eyre HJ. American Cancer Society Guidelines for the Early Detection of Cancer, 2005. CA Cancer J Clin 2005;55:31–44.
[7] Rex DK, Johnson DA, Lieberman DA, et al. Colorectal cancer prevention 2000: screening recommendations of the American College of Gastroenterology. Am J Gastroenterol 2000;95(4):868–77.
[8] US Preventive Services Task Force. Screening for colorectal cancer: recommendations and rationale. Ann Intern Med 2002;137:129–31.
[9] Winawer S, Fletcher R, Rex D, et al. Colorectal cancer screening: clinical guidelines and rationale—update based on new evidence. Gastroenterology 2003;124:544–60.
[10] Seeff LC, Nadel MR, Klabunde CN, et al. Patterns and predictors of colorectal cancer test use in the adult US population. Cancer 2004;100(10):2093–103.
[11] Nadel MR, Blackman DK, Shapiro JA, et al. Are people being screened for colorectal cancer as recommended? Results from the National Health Interview Survey. Prev Med 2002;35:199–206.
[12] Johnson CD, Hara AK, Reed JE. Computed tomographic colonography (virtual colonoscopy): a new method for detecting colorectal neoplasms. Endoscopy 1997;29(6):454–61.
[13] Fenlon HM, Barish MA, Ferrucci JT. Virtual colonoscopy—technique and applications. Ital J Gastroenterol Hepatol 1999;31(8):713–20.
[14] Barish MA, Soto JA, Ferrucci JT. Consensus on current clinical practice of virtual colonoscopy. AJR Am J Roentgenol 2005;184:786–92.
[15] Fletcher JG, Johnson CD, MacCarty RL, et al. CT colonography: potential pitfalls and problem-solving techniques. AJR Am J Roentgenol 1999;172(5):1271–8.
[16] Macari M, Lavelle M, Pedrosa I, et al. Effect of different bowel preparations on residual fluid at CT colonography. Radiology 2001;218:274–7.
[17] Ji H, Rolnick JA, Haker S, et al. Multislice CT colonography: current status and limitations. Eur J Radiol 2003;47:123–34.
[18] Fletcher JG, Johnson CD, Welch TJ, et al. Optimization of CT colonography technique: prospective trial in 180 patients. Radiology 2000;216:704–11.
[19] Lefere PA, Gryspeerdt SS, Dewyspelaere J, et al. Dietary fecal tagging as a cleansing method before CT colonography: initial results—polyp detection and patient acceptance. Radiology 2002;224:393–403.
[20] Pickhardt PJ, Choi JR. Electronic cleansing and stool tagging in CT colonography: advantages and pitfalls with primary three-dimensional evaluation. AJR Am J Roentgenol 2003;181:799–805.
[21] Ferrucci JT. Colonoscopy: virtual and optical—another look, another view. Radiology 2005;235:13–6.
[22] Pickhardt PJ, Choi JR, Hwang I, et al. Computed tomographic virtual colonoscopy to screen for colo-

rectal neoplasia in asymptomatic adults. N Engl J Med 2003;349(23):2191–200.

[23] Gluecker TM, Johnson CD, Harmsen WS, et al. Colorectal cancer screening with CT colonography, colonoscopy, and double-contrast barium enema examination: prospective assessment of patient perceptions and preferences. Radiology 2003;227:378–84.

[24] Edwards JT, Mendelson RM, Fritschi L, et al. Colorectal neoplasia screening with CT colonography in average-risk asymptomatic subjects: community-based study. Radiology 2004;230:459–64.

[25] Lefere P, Gryspeerdt S, Marrannes J, et al. CT colonography after fecal tagging with a reduced cathartic cleansing and a reduced volume of barium. AJR Am J Roentgenol 2005;184(6):1836–42.

[26] Zalis ME, Perumpillichira J, Del Frate C, et al. CT colonography: digital subtraction bowel cleansing with mucosal reconstruction—initial observations. Radiology 2003;226:911–7.

[27] Zalis ME, Hahn PF. Digital subtraction bowel cleansing in CT colonography. AJR Am J Roentgenol 2001; 176:646–8.

[28] Callstrom MR, Johnson CD, Fletcher JG, et al. CT colonography without cathartic preparation: feasibility study. Radiology 2001;219:693–8.

[29] Iannaccone R, Laghi A, Catalano C, et al. Computed tomographic colonography without cathartic preparation for the detection of colorectal polyps. Gastroenterology 2004;127:1300–11.

[30] Lefere PA, Gryspeerdt S, Baekelandt M, et al. Laxative-free CT colonography. AJR Am J Roentgenol 2004;183:945–8.

[31] Bielen D, Thomeer M, Vanbeckevoort D, et al. Dry preparation for virtual CT colonography with fecal tagging using water-soluble contrast medium: initial results. Eur Radiol 2003;13:453–8.

[32] Yee J, Hung RK, Akerkar GA, et al. The usefulness of glucagon hydrochloride for colonic distention in CT colonography. AJR Am J Roentgenol 1999;173: 169–72.

[33] Morrin MM, Farrell RJ, Keogan MT, et al. CT colonography: colonic distention improved by dual positioning but not intravenous glucagon. Eur Radiol 2002;12:525–30.

[34] Taylor SA, Halligan S, Goh V, et al. Optimizing colonic distention for multi-detector row CT colonography: effect of hyoscine butylbromide and rectal balloon catheter. Radiology 2003;229(1):99–108.

[35] Bruzzi JF, Moss AC, Brennan DD, et al. Efficacy of IV Buscopan as a muscle relaxant in CT colonography. Eur Radiol 2003;13(10):2264–70 [erratum in: Eur Radiol 2004;14(4):756].

[36] Laghi A, Lannaccone R, Panebianco V, et al. Multislice CT colonography: technical developments. Semin Ultrasound CT MR 2001;22(5):425–31.

[37] Schoepf UJ, Becker CR, Obuchowski NA, et al. Multislice computed tomography as a screening tool for colon cancer, lung cancer and coronary artery disease. Eur Radiol 2001;11(10):1975–85.

[38] Iannaccone R, Laghi A, Passariello R. Colorectal carcinoma: detection and staging with multislice CT (MSCT) colonography. Abdom Imaging 2005;30:13–9.

[39] Laghi A, Iannaccone R, Mangiapane F, et al. Experimental colonic phantom for the evaluation of the optimal scanning technique for CT colonography using a multidetector spiral CT equipment. Eur Radiol 2003; 13(3):459–66.

[40] Chen SC, Lu DS, Hecht JR, et al. CT colonography: value of scanning in both the supine and prone positions. AJR Am J Roentgenol 1999;172(3):595–9.

[41] Pescatore P, Glucker T, Delarive J, et al. Diagnostic accuracy and interobserver agreement of CT colonography (virtual colonoscopy). Gut 2000;47: 126–30.

[42] Laks S, Macari M, Bibi EJ. Positional changes in colon polyps at CT colonography. Radiology 2004;231: 761–6.

[43] Morrin MM, Farrell RJ, Kruskal JB, et al. Utility of intravenously administered contrast material at CT colonography. Radiology 2000;217:765–71.

[44] Fletcher JG, Johnson CD, Krueger WR, et al. Contrast-enhanced CT colonography in recurrent colorectal carcinoma: feasibility of simultaneous evaluation for metastatic disease, local recurrence, and metachronous neoplasia in colorectal carcinoma. AJR Am J Roentgenol 2002;178:283–90.

[45] Sosna J, Morrin MM, Kruskal JB, et al. Colorectal neoplasm: role of intravenous contrast-enhanced CT colonography. Radiology 2003;228:152–6.

[46] Iannaccone R, Laghi A, Catalano C, et al. Feasibility of ultra-low-dose multislice CT colonography for the detection of colorectal lesions: preliminary experience. Eur Radiol 2003;13(6):1297–302.

[47] Hara AK, Johnson CD, Reed JE, et al. Reducing data size and radiation dose for CT colonography. AJR Am J Roentgenol 1997;168(5):1181–4.

[48] Mendelson RM, Forbes GM. Virtually viewing the large bowel: the future of colorectal cancer screening? Med J Aust 2000;172:416–7.

[49] Cohnen M, Vogt C, Beck A, et al. Feasibility of MDCT colonography in ultra-low-dose technique in the detection of colorectal lesions: comparison with high-resolution video colonoscopy. AJR Am J Roentgenol 2004;183:1355–9.

[50] Iannaccone R, Laghi A, Catalano C, et al. Detection of colorectal lesions: lower-dose multi-detector row helical CT colonography compared with conventional colonoscopy. Radiology 2003;229:775–81.

[51] Macari M, Bini EJ, Xue X, et al. Colorectal neoplasms: prospective comparison of thin-section low-dose multi-detector row CT colonography and conventional colonoscopy for detection. Radiology 2002;224:383–92.

[52] van Gelder RE, Venema HW, Serlie IW, et al. CT colonography at different radiation dose levels: feasibility of dose reduction. Radiology 2002;224:25–33.

[53] Wessling J, Fischbach R, Meier N, et al. CT colonography: protocol optimization with multi-

detector row CT—study in an anthropomorphic colon phantom. Radiology 2003;228:753–9.

[54] Paik DS, Beaulieu CF, Jeffrey Jr RB, et al. Visualization modes for CT colonography using cylindrical and planar map projections. J Comput Assist Tomogr 2000;24(2):179–88.

[55] Fletcher JG, Johnson CD, Reed JE, et al. Feasibility of planar virtual pathology: a new paradigm in volume-rendered CT colonography. J Comput Assist Tomogr 2001;25(6):864–9.

[56] Ji H, Haker SJ, Barish MA, et al. Area preserving colon unfolding: a novel display for CT colonography. Radiology 2002;225:746 [p].

[57] Sheppard DG, Iyer RB, Herron D, et al. Subtraction CT colonography: feasibility in an animal model. Clin Radiol 1999;54(2):126–32.

[58] Hopper KD, Iyriboz AT, Wise SW, et al. Mucosal detail at CT virtual reality: surface versus volume rendering. Radiology 2000;214(2):517–22.

[59] Samara Y, Fiebich M, Dachman AH, et al. Automated calculation of the centerline of the human colon on CT images. Acad Radiol 1999;6(6):352–9.

[60] Rottgen R, Fischbach F, Plotkin M, et al. CT colonography using different reconstruction modi. Clin Imaging 2005;29(3):195–9.

[61] Sorantin E, Werkgartner G, Balogh E, et al. Virtual dissection and automated polyp detection of the colon based on spiral CT: techniques and preliminary experience on a cadaveric phantom. Eur Surg 2002;34(2):143–9.

[62] Dachman AH, Kuniyoshi JK, Boyle CM, et al. CT colonography with three-dimensional problem solving for detection of colonic polyps. AJR Am J Roentgenol 1998;171:989–95.

[63] Macari M, Milano A, Lavelle M, et al. Comparison of time-efficient CT colonography with two- and three-dimensional colonic evaluation for detecting colorectal polyps. AJR Am J Roentgenol 2000;174:1543–9.

[64] Macari M, Bini EJ, Jacobs SL, et al. Colorectal polyps and cancers in asymptomatic average-risk patients: evaluation with CT colonography. Radiology 2004;230:629–36.

[65] Cotton PB, Durkalski VL, Pineau BC, et al. Computed tomographic colonography (virtual colonoscopy): a multicenter comparison with standard colonoscopy for detection of colorectal neoplasia. JAMA 2004;291(14):1713–9.

[66] Johnson CD, Harmsen WS, Wilson LA, et al. Prospective blinded evaluation of computed tomographic colonography for screen detection of colorectal polyps. Gastroenterology 2003;125:311–9.

[67] Fenlon HM, Nunes DP, Schroy III PC, et al. A comparison of virtual and conventional colonoscopy for the detection of colorectal polyps. N Engl J Med 1999;341:1496–503.

[68] Yee J, Akerkar GA, Hung RK, et al. Colorectal neoplasia: performance characteristics of CT colonography for detection in 300 patients. Radiology 2001;219:685–92.

[69] Vos FM, van Gelder RE, Serlie IWO, et al. Three-dimensional display modes for CT colonography: conventional 3D virtual colonoscopy versus unfolded cube projection. Radiology 2003;228:878–85.

[70] McFarland EG. Reader strategies for CT colonography. Abdom Imaging 2002;27:275–83.

[71] Pickhardt PJ. Translucency rendering in 3D endoluminal CT colonography: a useful tool for increasing polyp specificity and decreasing interpretation time. AJR Am J Roentgenol 2004;183(2):429–36.

[72] Yoshida H, Dachman AH. CAD techniques, challenges, and controversies in computed tomographic colonography. Abdom Imaging 2005;30(1):26–41.

[73] Nicholson FB, Taylor S, Halligan S, et al. Recent developments in CT colonography. Clin Radiol 2005;60:1–7.

[74] Summers RM, Yao J, Johnson CD. CT colonography with computer-aided detection: automated recognition of ileocecal valve to reduce number of false-positive detections. Radiology 2004;233(1):266–72.

[75] Summers RM, Jerebko AK, Franaszek M, et al. Colonic polyps: complementary role of computer-aided detection in CT colonography. Radiology 2002;225:391–9.

[76] Helm J, Choi J, Sutphen R, et al. Current and evolving strategies for colorectal cancer screening. Cancer Control 2003;10(3):193–204.

[77] Hixson LJ, Fennerty MB, Sampliner RE, et al. Prospective blinded trial of the colonoscopic miss-rate of large colorectal polyps. Gastrointest Endosc 1991;37(2):125–7.

[78] Rex DK, Cutler CS, Lemmel GT, et al. Colonoscopic miss rates of adenomas determined by back-to-back colonoscopies. Gastroenterology 1997;112(1):24–8.

[79] Dachman AH. Diagnostic performance of virtual colonoscopy. Abdom Imaging 2002;27:260–7.

[80] Gluecker TM, Fletcher JG. CT colonography (virtual colonoscopy) for the detection of colorectal polyps and neoplasms: current status and future developments. Eur J Cancer 2002;38:2070–8.

[81] McFarland EG, Pilgram TK, Brink JA, et al. CT colonography: multiobserver diagnostic performance. Radiology 2002;225:380–90.

[82] Hara AK, Johnson CD, Reed JE, et al. Colorectal polyp detection with CT colography: two- versus three-dimensional techniques. Work in progress. Radiology 1996;200(1):49–54.

[83] Hara AK, Johnson CD, MacCarty RL, et al. CT colonography: single- versus multi-detector row imaging. Radiology 2001;219:461–5.

[84] Laghi A, Iannaccone R, Carbone I, et al. Detection of colorectal lesions with virtual computed tomographic colonography. Am J Surg 2002;183:124–31.

[85] Wong BC, Wong W, Chan JK, et al. Virtual colonoscopy for the detection of colorectal polyps and cancers in a Chinese population. J Gastroenterol Hepatol 2002;17:1323–7.

[86] Spinzi G, Belloni G, Martegani A, et al. Computed tomographic colonography and conventional colonos-

copy for colon diseases: a prospective, blinded study. Am J Gastroenterol 2001;96(2):394–400.

[87] Miao YM, Amin Z, Healy J, et al. A prospective single centre study comparing computed tomography pneumocolon against colonoscopy in the detection of colorectal neoplasms. Gut 2000;47:832–7.

[88] Rockey DC. Virtual colonoscopy to screen for colorectal cancer. N Engl J Med 2004;350(11):1148–50.

[89] Rockey DC, Paulson E, Niedzwiecki D, et al. Analysis of air contrast barium enema, computed tomographic colonography, and colonoscopy: prospective comparison. Lancet 2005;365:305–11.

[90] Fenlon HM, McAneny DB, Nunes DP, et al. Occlusive colon carcinoma: virtual colonoscopy in the preopera-

tive evaluation of the proximal colon. Radiology 1999; 210:423–8.

[91] Morrin MM, Farrell RJ, Raptopoulos V, et al. Role of virtual computed tomographic colonography in patients with colorectal cancers and obstructing colorectal lesions. Dis Colon Rectum 2000;43(3):303–11.

[92] Gluecker TM, Johnson CD, Wilson LA, et al. Extracolonic findings at CT colonography: evaluation of prevalence and cost in a screening population. Gastroenterology 2003;124(4):911–6.

[93] Hara AK, Johnson CD, MacCarty RL, et al. Incidental extracolonic findings at CT colonography. Radiology 2000;215:353–7.

ELSEVIER
SAUNDERS

Radiol Clin N Am 43 (2005) 1063 – 1077

**RADIOLOGIC
CLINICS**
of North America

Multidetector Row CT of the Small Bowel

Michael A. Patak, MD*, Koenraad J. Mortele, MD, Pablo R. Ros, MD, MPH

Department of Radiology, Brigham and Women's Hospital, Harvard Medical School, Boston, MA, USA

Several factors continue to make multidetector row CT (MDCT) of the small bowel difficult: inherent anatomic limitations, specific challenges because of the pathology sought, and technical constraints. The small bowel is an organ several meters long with a tortuous and variable course prone to change with breathing and peristalsis, and a thin wall difficult to display with imaging. The small bowel method of fixation to the rest of the body (the mesentery) and its blood supply are both complex. In addition, because small bowel diseases have a low incidence, their appearance is less well known and there is an increased risk of missing them. Even for most of the common diseases in the small bowel, early changes are subtle making their diagnoses difficult.

Imaging the small bowel is challenging technically. Because the organ is long and serpentine, a large field of view and a large volume are needed to display it in its entirety. Another problem for imaging is motion, both the intrinsic motion of peristalsis and the positional changes caused by breathing. These two motion patterns can be additive and lead to a complex movement of individual bowel loops, making their tracing very difficult.

The ideal diagnostic imaging tool for the small bowel displays its bowel wall, with detailed information of its mucosal layer; depicts the entire small bowel tube; and provides information about adjacent structures, such as mesenteric and omental fat. To diagnose changes in the mucosa, sufficient and reliable bowel distention has to be obtained. These prerequisites can only be partly fulfilled by most standard methods. Endoscopy and capsule endoscopy can provide a detailed view of the mucosal layer but deeper layers of the bowel wall and the adjacent tissues are out of its diagnostic reach. Conventional small bowel fluoroscopy with enteroclysis provides reliable diagnosis of mucosal changes and can depict indirect findings of deep bowel wall and surrounding tissues, but still has clear limitations in these areas [1].

The development of MDCT allows high-resolution imaging of the whole abdomen in one breathhold obviating motion artifacts. With this acquisition method, a whole abdominal volume can be obtained instead of only single slices as with earlier CT units. Using this volume data set for reconstructions allows concise display of the small bowel [2]. New developments in patient preparation provide stable distention of the small bowel.

For years, the standard of reference for small bowel imaging was fluoroscopic small bowel follow-through (SBFT) and enteroclysis. With the fast and widely available MDCT at hand, however, attention has shifted toward this technique to diagnose small bowel pathology [3]. This article discusses the current status of MDCT for small bowel imaging, gives an overview of the technique and the different oral preparation methods possible, and discusses the normal anatomy and the most common small bowel diseases as detected and characterized with MDCT.

Dr. Patak is funded by the Swiss Research Foundation.

* Corresponding author. Department of Radiology, Brigham and Women's Hospital, Harvard Medical School, 75 Francis Street, Boston, MA 02115.

E-mail address: mpatak@partners.org (M.A. Patak).

Technique

There are several challenges in imaging the small bowel. Ideally, CT of the small bowel should include optimal image acquisition, oral contrast and intra-

doi:10.1016/j.rcl.2005.07.009

venous (IV) contrast administration, and multiplanar reconstruction in the postprocessing phase.

Technical CT considerations

With MDCT, with one breathhold the whole abdomen can be covered. Suspended respiration is an essential aspect for successful imaging of the small bowel. Even with fast MDCT it is not possible to obtain artifact-free images if there is free breathing. The length of the apnea phase is a limiting factor for adequate imaging. The acquisition time must be limited to a maximum of 25 seconds. The newest MDCT units have no time constraints and with 64-row models to scan multiple contrast phases within a breathhold representing a challenge to optimize IV contrast administration. For a good-quality image, a voxel size below 2 mm is recommended.

The current CT protocol the authors use for small bowel evaluation is as follows: oral contrast administration with 1350 mL of VoLumen (EZEM, Lake Success, New York) taken continuously over a period of 45 minutes before imaging. The patient is imaged in supine position at 40 and 70 seconds after IV administration of 100 mL iopromide (Ultravist 300; Berlex, Montville, New Jersey). For 16-row images the authors use a 0.75-mm collimation and for 64-row a 0.6-mm collimation. All image data are reconstructed in axial, coronal, and saggital planes (Table 1).

Reconstruction methods

With standard MDCT scans of the abdomen using slice thickness of less than 2 mm and an approximate coverage in the z-axis of 90 cm, several hundred slices are acquired. The resulting mass of data requires special technical capacities to handle these several hundred images. This is why all abdominal MDCT scans use reconstruction methods image

interpretation. Reconstruction is not only done in coronal and saggital planes but also in the axial plane, resetting the slice thickness (usually 3–5 mm) to a thicker size than the one scanned. The technique of reconstruction should be implemented on all workstations for immediate availability of the needed views. With modern MDCT technique, the in-plane and through-plane resolution is the same, leading to isotropic voxel resolution in the volume, which makes reconstruction in all planes possible without loss of information.

Coronal reconstruction seems to be especially important for small bowel imaging because of the anatomic arrangement of the loops [4]. The possibility of having all three planes available also helps to follow the bowel loops throughout the abdomen. Complex reconstruction techniques, such as surface rendering or virtual fly-through, do not seem to offer any improvement over the diagnostic accuracy of two-dimensional viewing of MDCT images. Thick-slab rendering seems a promising technique for the diagnostic display of the small bowel (Fig. 1). With this technique, a thicker slab of the initially acquired volume is extracted. This display method has the advantage of high-resolution imaging (which is lost in other methods of displaying radiologic information of the abdomen) and the physical possibilities of volumetric information. This technique is very helpful in giving information about complex structures in a limited space, such as the mesenteric artery, the vasa recta to the bowel, and duodenum and proximal jejunum folds.

Intravenous contrast

The peroral contrast must be combined with IV contrast. Specifically, the combination of neutral oral contrast and IV contrast gives a very good display of the bowel wall [5]. Inflammatory bowel disease and neoplasm are optimally displayed with the use of IV contrast [6]. Nonionic iodinated contrast is most

Table 1
Parameter list for multidetector row CT of the small bowel

CT type	Oral	IV	Delay (s)	kV/Ma	Collimation	Recon	MPR
16-row	300 mL VoLumen given at 1 h, 45 min, and 30 min before scan. Add another 300 mL on the table prior examination.	100 mL iopromide 300 at 3–5 mL/s	40 and 70	120/180	0.75	5/5	3 cor; 1.5 sag
64-row	As above.	100 mL iopromide 300 at 3–5 mL/s	40 and 70	120/200	0.6	5/5	3 cor; 1.5 sag

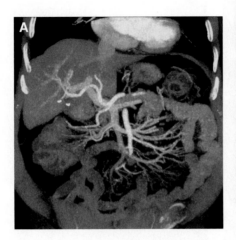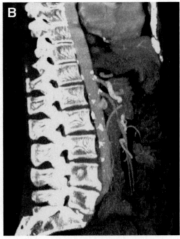

Fig. 1. The combination of submillimeter slices and volume acquisition provides the option for multiplanar recon-structions. Working directly on workstations one can easily reconstruct the mesenteric vessels in both coronal (*A*) and saggital (*B*) planes. The use of thin slab maximum intensity projections can be helpful in getting an overview of complex bowel structures. (Courtesy of Ralph Berther, MD, Winterthur, Switzerland.)

widely used today. The ideal volume and injection rate are 125 mL and 3 to 4 mL/s, respectively. For detailed display of the mesenteric vasculature, a higher volume (150 mL) and a higher flow rate (4–5 mL/s) are chosen. The peak contrast enhance-ment of the bowel wall has a different timing than the liver [5]. A 60-second scan delay is ideal to acquire the small bowel wall in its best enhancement phase, whereas 70 to 90 seconds is best for liver imaging. If there are additional questions about the liver, add the upper abdomen to the liver phase of the scan protocol.

Oral contrast and distention

For an optimal display of the bowel, two things are essential in imaging: intraluminal contrast and dis-tention. Intraluminal contrast is needed to delineate bowel loops in the abdominal cavity, to tell different loops apart, and to depict the bowel wall. There are three ways to contrast the bowel: (1) positively, giv-ing the contents an increased density compared with their surroundings; (2) neutral, using an intermediate density contrast; and (3) negatively, with a contrast of low density. Distention in small bowel imaging is essential to unfold the bowel tube and separate out the bowel wall. It is nearly impossible to find subtle pathology in collapsed bowel loops [7–9]. With stan-dard oral contrast administration for abdominal CT, the distention of the small bowel is not sufficiently achieved and different methods of oral contrast have been developed.

In imaging the small bowel these intraluminal contrast and distention are inseparable. Many authors speak of oral contrast when they actually mean the combination of contrast and distention.

Several techniques are available to combine optimal contrast and distension (Fig. 2). Two differ-ent application methods carry the contrast to its required site: peroral (noninvasive) or CT enter-ography and administration of contrast by a nasogas-tric tube or CT enteroclysis. The next sections explain the different contrast and application techniques.

CT enterography

Positive intraluminal contrast

Positive oral contrast produces a high density to the bowel content and clearly delineates the bowel. Barium sulfate or iodinated solutions are used. Barium should only be used in very low doses to prevent artifacts, commercially available in concen-trations of 2.1% (Readi-CAT; EZEM, Lake Suc-cess, New York) [10]. The iodinated contrast agent meglumine diatrizoate (Gastrographin) is the most widely used agent for CT. Both barium and iodated bowel contrast have wide acceptance and a low adverse-event rate [11]. The use of positive oral contrast leads to a diminished display of the bowel wall because of the high density of the lumen and the consequently decreased contrast between bowel lu-men and wall. Additionally, multiplanar reconstruc-tions (eg, of vascular structures) are hampered by the positive contrast [3]. Another problem with these

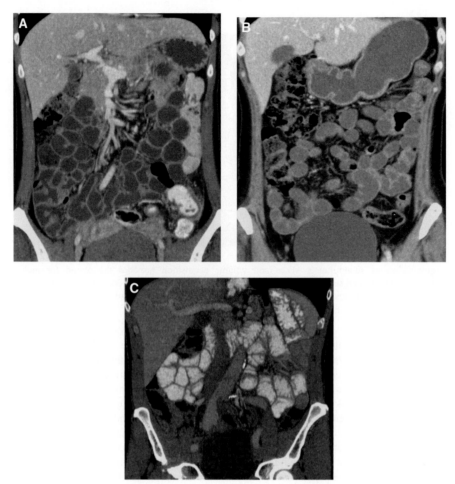

Fig. 2. Coronal reconstructions of different contrast agents for CT enterography. Mannitol (A; courtesy of Ralph Berther, MD, Winterthur, Switzerland) and VoLumen (B) are neutral contrast agents with water-like densities. Meglumine diatrizoate (C) is a positive contrast agent giving the content of the small bowel a higher density. Mannitol and VoLumen provide good distention of small bowel loops, whereas meglumine diatrizoate has a tendency to be absorbed and of showing collapsed bowel segments, especially in the proximal segments.

agents is their relatively low distending capability. The risk with high intraluminal signal is to obscure the bowel wall and to miss an enhancing tumor [2].

Neutral intraluminal contrast

Contrast agents that have an intermediate density (10–30 HU) in MDCT are called neutral. These oral contrast agents are used with increasing frequency [12]. In combination with IV contrast, they provide very good display of the bowel wall. The most widely used neutral oral contrast agent is water. It is inexpensive and universally available, but water alone is not an ideal contrast agent, because it is absorbed early in the gastrointestinal system and is not available in the mid and distal section of the small bowel

[5]. To overcome early absorption, additives that increase the osmolarity of the water are used without changing the contrast characteristics. Mannitol [13,14] or other long-chain sugars can be used. The adverse effects of these additives are nausea and diarrhea.

A newly introduced neutral oral contrast agent is VoLumen. It is based in oral barium sulfate solutions containing all the additives but with only 0.1% of barium sulfate. With such a low concentration of barium it has no possible contrast effect in MDCT and even though containing barium, it is considered a neutral contrast agent. Compared with water or meglumine diatrizoate, VoLumen creates far better distention and the display of the bowel wall is very clear compared with these intraluminal contrast agents [15].

Negative intraluminal contrast

Negative contrast agents display a density below 0 HU in MDCT and are normally fat based. Although they provide a good distention and can result in a good visualization of the small bowel wall they are not so widely used [16–18]. There are some studies showing that carbon dioxide could work as a negative contrast but it is very difficult to apply and patient tolerance is low [19].

CT enteroclysis

A fundamentally different approach to small bowel imaging is CT enteroclysis [20]. Because the peroral administration of contrast is not controllable and needs good patient compliance, some centers use enteroclysis in combination with MDCT for small bowel imaging.

In enteroclysis, a nasojejunal tube is placed under fluoroscopy. With the tube in place, the patient is transported to the CT suite, and there the contrast is applied under direct CT fluoroscopic control. With this technique the distention is closely monitored dynamically. The advantage of this method is the

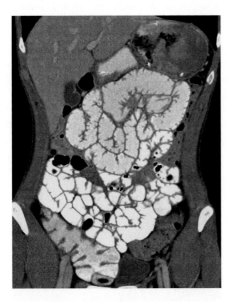

Fig. 3. Enteroclysis. A nasoduodenal tube is placed under fluoroscopy. With the tube in place the bowel is filled with a positive contrast agent, and then the patient is transported to the CT suite and images are acquired. Administration of contrast with a nasoduodenal tube allows the radiologist to have a well-controlled distention of the small bowel; usually a better distention than with orally administered contrast media. The placement of the tube is cumbersome and perceived as unpleasant by patients. (Courtesy of Simon Wildermuth, MD, Zurich, Switzerland.)

close control of the distention and the dynamic filling of the bowel loops under CT fluoroscopy (Fig. 3). The placement of the nasoduodenal tube, however, is unpleasant for patients [21]. It is also invasive, with all the accompanying risks, and needs additional ionizing radiation for tube placement, which is an issue for female patients of childbearing age.

With intensive research on peroral contrast agents, there is an ongoing discussion about the benefit of enteroclysis, but there is evidence that CT enteroclysis is the choice imaging method for diagnosing low-grade small bowel obstruction (SBO) [22,23]. It increases its detection rate and can reveal the cause of obstruction. CT enteroclysis can also be used as a next-step diagnosis in Crohn's disease (CD) after standard technique MDCT, instead of SBFT [6]. Larger studies are needed to confirm the higher diagnostic value of CT enteroclysis versus CT enterography.

Normal anatomy

The small bowel is an intraperitoneal structure, except for the duodenum, which is retroperitoneal. The total length of the small bowel measures 4 to 5 m in autopsy samples; in vivo its length is approximately 2.5 to 3 m. Its course is complex and has been referred to as "a pond of withering snakes" [24], extending roughly from the left to the right upper quadrant, down to the left lower, and then to the right lower quadrant. It is not possible on MDCT images to distinguish exactly between jejunum and ileum, but one can guess by their location in the abdominal cavity. The normal bowel wall thickness by MDCT seems 4 mm or less and can enhance brightly [5]. The thickness may vary depending on distention, but thickness of >5 mm is deemed always pathologic, independent of its distention [25]. The small bowel folds should be visible in the duodenum and the jejunum but are not visible in the ileum. The mesentery is the fixation point of the bowel loops and also provides the vasculature and the lymphatics of the small bowel. Between two thin layers of peritoneum, the mesentery contains mostly fat. The entire small bowel is supplied by the superior mesenteric artery and drains to the superior mesenteric vein and then to the portal vein.

Disease

Small bowel diseases are rare. This article discusses the diseases that most commonly affect the small bowel, such as inflammatory bowel disease, obstruction, ischemia, and neoplasm. A recently published single-center study represents the distribution of disease in 107 patients, which were referred for small bowel MDCT in an 18-month period. The distribution of the diseases in this study was as follows: small bowel masses (18%), CD (10%), obstruction (10%), and normal findings in the rest. The overall sensitivity was 100% for detecting small bowel disease with MDCT, specificity was 95%, and accuracy was 97% [6].

Crohn's disease

CD is an idiopathic inflammatory condition that may include all segments of the gastrointestinal tract. Approximately half a million patients in the United States suffer from this disease [26]. Large reviews have found that two thirds of these patients have some involvement of the small bowel, with 10% to 30% of them in the small bowel alone [27,28]. Symptomatic patients may have active inflammatory disease, chronic changes, or conditions not related to CD. The aim of imaging should be to establish the following: (1) presence, severity, and extent of the disease; (2) its activity; and (3) extraintestinal complications [29].

The classic imaging method to study CD is fluoroscopic SBFT, but the use of MDCT as the primary imaging technique for CD is gaining acceptance, especially because the use of neutral oral contrast media allows depiction of subtle bowel wall changes not possible with positive intraluminal contrast. Another emerging technique to diagnose CD is wireless capsule endoscopy, which is highly sensitive for early disease manifestations, such as small mucosal changes [30]. It is only applicable in patients without strictures, however, because it carries the risk of obstruction [31,32]. For safety reasons, every CD patient should have imaging before wireless capsule endoscopy, ideally by MDCT.

Large studies have evaluated the sensitivity and specificity of MDCT for detection of CD using SBFT as gold standard [25,33,34]. MDCT has a sensitivity and specificity of 95% and 96%, respectively, for advanced disease, but with only 70% sensitivity and specificity for early stage CD. Adding multiplanar image reconstruction to the axial data significantly increases the diagnostic confidence, even if it does not help identify additional lesions [9].

A classification of subtypes of CD was introduced as a guide for medical and surgical therapy: (1) active inflammatory, (2) fistulizing-perforating, (3) fibrostenosing, and (4) reparative or regenerative subtypes

[35]. The characteristics of the active inflammatory subtype include focal inflammation; ulceration (superficial or deep); and activation of the lymphoid tissue with granuloma formation (Fig. 4). This subtype shows only subtle imaging changes in its mild form and can be difficult to determine with MDCT. Administration of IV contrast in combination with a neutral intraluminal contrast agent can increase its detection. Radiologists should be aware of the slight mucosal hyperenhancement and subtle wall thickening as signs of an early form of the active inflammatory subtype. The advanced inflammatory form is readily recognized on MDCT. The signs indicating activity are discussed later.

The active inflammatory type can transform into the fistulating-perforating type by progression of inflammatory activity through the bowel wall. This subtype clinically presents itself with recurrent sinus tracts, fistulae, and abscess formation (Fig. 5). MDCT gives information about fissuring ulcers, sinus tracts, and fistula, including course and organs involved [36].

The dominant feature of the fibrostenosing type is SBO. Narrowing and thickening of the involved bowel segment are seen on MDCT scans. The affected segment typically enhances after IV contrast administration but only moderately because of the fibrous nature of the tissue. In addition, there is no sign of active disease, such as bowel wall edema or mesenteric fat stranding. The stenosis can vary from mild to severe.

The regenerative or reparative subtype is histologically consistent with inactive CD. MDCT find-

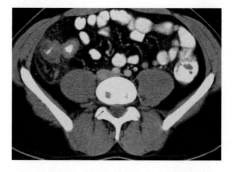

Fig. 4. Axial image of a 28-year-old woman presenting with fever, diarrhea, and right lower quadrant pain. This image is typical for an active inflammatory process in the ileocolic region. There is a marked thickening of the terminal ileum and cecum, stranding of the adjacent mesenteric fat, and enlarged lymph nodes. The wall of the terminal ileum shows multiple layers indicating active inflammation (*high attenuation*) and edema (*low attenuation*). Endoscopy proved active Crohn's disease.

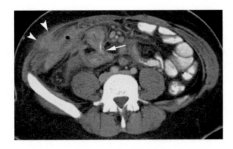

Fig. 5. Crohn's disease can lead to fistulae and abscesses such as seen in this 32-year-old man with known Crohn's disease. In this image there is a bowel-to-bowel fistula (*arrow*) and an abscess in the abdominal wall (*arrowheads*).

ings in this form of CD are submucosal fat replacement and bowel wall thickening with minimal IV contrast enhancement. Findings of active disease, such as mesenteric fat stranding and abscess formation, are not typically seen. Because the course of the illness is recurrent and presents with unpredictable relapses and phases of inactivity, these subtypes can change during the course of a patients' disease.

Besides detection of CD and subtype determination, MDCT can evaluate its activity [37]. Findings include thickening of the bowel wall with marked contrast enhancement; display of layering within the bowel wall [33,38]; local mesenteric hypervascularization (comb sign) (Fig. 6) [39,40]; mesenteric fat stranding; and detection of extraluminal findings, such as adenopathy, mesenteric abscess, and free intraperitoneal fluid [37].

These signs, either alone or in combination, have been correlated to clinical disease activity and symptoms. According to these studies the strongest signs for predicting high activity are mesenteric changes,

such as fat stranding and abscess [37]. The comb sign, a sign of dilated and tortuous course of vessels in the inflamed segment, is also strongly correlated with activity [39,40]. The combination of lymph nodes and fibrofatty proliferation was studied in another trial and this proliferation was found to be significantly increased in patients with active disease [36]. Thickening of the bowel wall alone does not seem to be a sign of active disease, but the combination of thickening, hyperenhancement, and layering shows a significant correlation to disease activity (Fig. 7) [40].

For the detection of extraintestinal findings, MDCT is the method of choice [41]. Such methods as SBFT or endoscopy, which may be better in distinguishing mucosal changes, can only determine extraluminal disease in a very limited way. They may even fail to detect changes in the deep bowel wall that do not involve the mucosal surface. Compared with intraoperative correlation, MDCT is the most accurate imaging method in detecting abscess (91.8%), whereas for the detection of fistula, the sensitivity of MDCT is slightly lower (68%) than that of SBFT (73%), but both have the same specificity [25].

For imaging CD, MDCT is the modality of choice in the acute setting. It can provide the necessary information about the location, subtype, and activity of the disease and extraluminal findings, such as sinus, fistula, or abscess. For subtle mucosal changes,

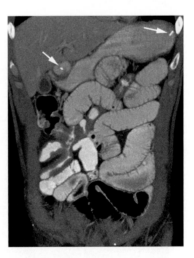

Fig. 7. This 43-year-old woman with known Crohn's disease underwent CT enteroclysis. The nasoduodenal tube is depicted in the stomach and duodenum (*arrows*). The entire small bowel has contrast and is well distended. The coronal reconstruction allows one to observe the thickening of the bowel wall in the distal small bowel. (Courtesy of Simon Wildermuth, MD, Zurich, Switzerland.)

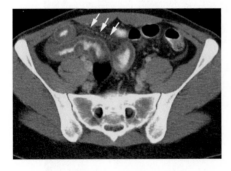

Fig. 6. Comb sign in Crohn's disease in 26-year-old woman. Adjacent to the thickened bowel loops there are small dots seen in the mesentery (*arrows*). These dots represent dilated vasa recta secondary to inflammation. This finding is known as the "comb sign."

SBFT is still better than MDCT and wireless capsule endoscopy may be the diagnostic method of choice for even earlier detection of disease.

Obstruction

One of the leading causes for emergency admission in patients with acute abdomen is intestinal obstruction, accounting for about 20% of admissions for abdominal pain. Most intestinal obstructions are in the small bowel (~80%) and are related to postoperative adhesions (~60%), internal or external hernias (15%), or neoplasms (15%). Less common causes are inflammatory bowel disease, trauma, intussusception, gallstones, foreign bodies, and endometriosis, which account for about 10% of obstruction cases [42].

CT has a significant role in the diagnosis of SBO. The primary diagnostic tool remains the plain film (Fig. 8) [43]. For cost-effectiveness, plain film is the first imaging method of choice to diagnose SBO.

MDCT can provide additional information not possible with plain films and answer questions about the management of disease. Beyond "Is the bowel obstructed," however, the questions are (1) Where is the site? (2) What are the cause and severity of obstruction? (3) Is there a closed-loop obstruction or an obstruction complicated by ischemia (ie, strangulation)? [42], and so forth.

For the detection of SBO, the standard MDCT protocol includes IV contrast administration in the portal-venous phase. One variable to consider is oral contrast administration. In the standard diagnostic work-up, if an abdominal plain film has already diagnosed SBO, then the subsequent use of oral contrast for MDCT can be omitted because the contrast does not progress through an obstructed small bowel system.

The imaging features for the diagnosis of SBO by MDCT scans are thin-walled, dilated, and fluid-filled bowel loops [42]. The most important task after diagnosing SBO is to localize the point of obstruction or the so-called "transition zone" (Fig. 9) [44]. This zone is defined by dilated and air- or fluid-filled bowel loops proximal and collapsed loops distal to the site of obstruction. These findings are the most reliable to diagnose SBO by MDCT and to differentiate it from nonobstructive or paralytic ileus. The bigger the difference between dilated and collapsed bowel loops the easier it is to diagnose SBO by MDCT. The sensitivity and specificity of MDCT in depicting the transition zone varies in different studies [44,45]. In a series of patients with high-grade or complete SBO, the sensitivity and specificity were both reported as 96%. For diagnosing low or partial SBO, the sensitivity was only 63% [43]. The use of multiplanar reconstructions helps to determine the point of transition and to increase the diagnostic confidence.

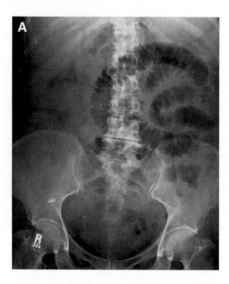 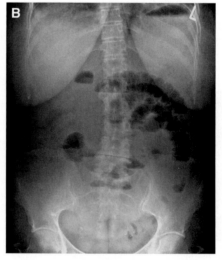

Fig. 8. Abdominal plain film findings of proximal bowel obstruction. Supine (*A*) and erect (*B*) plain film of the abdomen with dilated and air-filled segments. These findings indicate an obstruction with high positive predictive value. In patients with plain film findings suggesting obstruction, CT can help to localize the transition zone, the degree of distention, and the underlying reason for the obstruction.

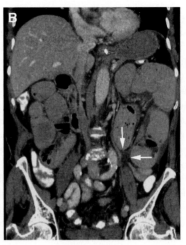

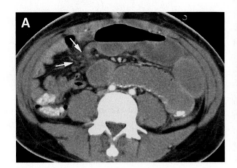

Fig. 9. Axial MDCT (*A*) and coronal reconstruction (*B*) show dilated proximal small bowel loops and collapsed distal bowel in the pelvis indicating a proximal obstruction. The distal small bowel segments, even collapsed, show dense oral contrast, suggesting an incomplete occlusion. The site of obstruction is the region where the bowel loops change from dilated to collapsed, called the transition zone (*arrows*).

MDCT is helpful in grading the severity of SBO and even in diagnosing its underlying cause (Fig. 10) [46,47]. The most common cause in SBO is adhesion. MDCT typically cannot display the actual adhesional band; however, a beaklike distortion of the transition zone without a defined lesion at the site of obstruction suggests this diagnosis. To differentiate complete versus partial SBO clinical evaluation and abdominal plain film findings provide most clues for diagnosis; MDCT can be of help in determining the degree of collapse in the distal segments and the amount of air or fluid and dilation in the proximal loops [48–50].

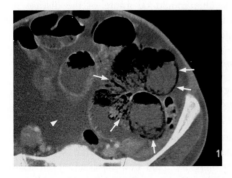

Fig. 10. There are markedly dilated bowel loops caused by obstruction. This obstruction led to underperfusion of bowel loops and to ischemia. The combination of obstruction and ischemia is known as "strangulation." The pneumatosis (*arrows*) and the ascites (*arrowhead*) indicate an advanced stage of ischemia with poor prognosis. (Courtesy of Walter Wiesner, MD, St. Gallen, Switzerland.)

It is important to diagnose closed-loop obstruction (incarceration) by CT and determine whether it is complicated by ischemia. Strangulation is suggested when there is bowel wall edema and mesenteric fat stranding caused by venous outflow obstruction (see Fig. 10) [51,52]. There is still debate about the capability of MDCT to detect vascular compromise in the case of closed-loop obstruction. A study found a 100% positive predictive value of MDCT for the detection of ischemic complications [53].

MDCT can effectively diagnose SBO and its underlying causes, particularly when multiplanar reconstruction is added to the axial images. Nevertheless, plain film radiology remains the method of choice to demonstrate SBO, with MDCT as the next step in diagnosing the obstruction, locating the transition zone, grading the severity of disease, and finding the underlying disease.

Ischemia

Especially for older patients, small bowel ischemia is a rare but often underestimated reason for acute abdomen in daily practice. According to a recently published prospective study, about 8.2% of a nonselected study population presenting with acute abdomen had acute bowel ischemia, 48% of which were small bowel ischemia [54]. The key issue with mesenteric ischemia is its high mortality of more than 50% if not diagnosed and treated in a timely fashion [55–58].

The etiology of acute intestinal ischemia is diverse with most cases caused by either arterial or venous occlusion [59]. In a minority of cases bowel ischemia has a nonocclusive nature caused by low flow rates and hypo-oxygenation of the tissue, such as in cases of hypovolemic shock.

Acute occlusion of the superior mesenteric artery occurs in about 60% to 70% of cases because of thrombosis or embolization. Mesenteric venous thromboses are responsible only for 5% to 10% and non-occlusive conditions for 20% to 30% of cases [60].

Angiography is still the imaging method with highest detection rates for an acute vascular occlusion diagnosis and most of cases of bowel ischemia [61]. Angiography is highly invasive, however, and cannot display other reasons for acute abdomen, which is problematic especially in older and unstable patients. Because acute intestinal ischemia is a rare disease, invasive procedures are performed late in the diagnostic process, leading to a potentially fatal delay in diagnosis and therapy. MDCT has the advantage of depicting a large range of diagnoses in the setting of acute abdomen by covering not only the vascular system (Fig. 11). It also has a similar accuracy than angiography to detect ischemia but because of its noninvasiveness it is performed much earlier in the diagnostic process. Angiography has a sensitivity of 87% in diagnosing bowel ischemia [61], whereas the sensitivity with MDCT for acute ischemia was of 80%, the specificity was 98.51%, positive predictive value was 90.48%, and negative predictive value was 98.15% [54].

Ideally, the MDCT protocol for acute abdomen should be changed to include an arterial phase in

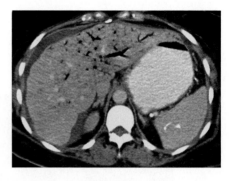

Fig. 12. Contrast-enhanced axial CT slices of the liver in a patient with acute transmural mesenteric ischemia shows intrahepatic portal venous gas.

combination with the use of neutral peroral contrast. Such an altered protocol for bowel ischemia could increase the ability to detect it in the first diagnostic test and facilitate the work-up for these patients. Because it is a rare disease, an arterial phase is normally not included in the routine emergency setting in the acute abdomen MDCT protocol.

Image findings for patients with acute ischemia are wall thickening, mesenteric stranding, and mesenteric fluid. Pneumatosis of the bowel wall and portal venous gas are seen in more severe cases (Fig. 12) [54,62,63]. Given the appropriate protocol, the occlusion itself can be seen and can either be atherosclerotic, thrombotic, or iatrogenic following vascular intervention or operation. Multiplanar reconstructions in the coronal and saggital plane can help tremendously to diagnose occlusion of the mesenteric vascular system. MDCT can detect bowel ischemia with a sensitivity of 80% and a specificity of 98%. One should be aware of the disease in the emergency setting and include it in the differential diagnosis of the acute abdomen.

Neoplasms

Small bowel neoplasms are uncommon, representing fewer than 25% of all gastrointestinal neoplasms and fewer than 2% of all malignant tumors. The annual incidence of small bowel tumors is only 0.5 to 1 per 100,000 population in the Western world, accounting for 5260 new cases and 1130 deaths in the United States in 2004. There is a slight male predominance, and patients are mostly in their fifth decade [64].

Early diagnosis of small bowel tumors poses a significant challenge to clinicians and radiologists. Patients often present with nonspecific symptoms, such as abdominal pain or intestinal bleeding. Fur-

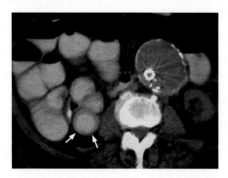

Fig. 11. This 78-year-old man presented with acute abdominal pain 4 days after aortic aneurysm repair. The MDCT scan without intravenous contrast shows slightly thickened small bowel loops in the right lower quadrant (*arrows*). These findings indicate early ischemic changes in the small bowel caused by the postoperative occlusion of the superior mesenteric artery. (Courtesy of Walter Wiesner, MD, St. Gallen, Switzerland.)

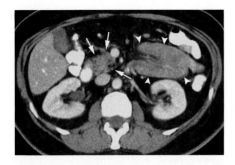

Fig. 13. Contrast-enhanced axial images of a patient with adenocarcinoma of the small bowel. The mass is located in the bowel wall and extends in the surrounding fat in an exophytic manner (*arrows*). Longer segments of the small bowel are affected in this patient showing a loop with diffuse wall thickening (*arrowheads*).

thermore, small bowel tumors tend to be small in early stage and difficult to diagnose.

In patients with suspected neoplasm, the administration of IV contrast has to be modified for imaging in all phases. The use of neutral oral contrast should be considered. Distention is crucial for the detection of small lesions in the bowel wall. Although no hard evidence exists, CT enteroclysis could well be the method of choice at this time because of its capacity for absolute control of distention [20]. If new non-invasive distention methods, such as mannitol, Locust beam gum, or the commercially available VoLumen, prove to produce sufficient distention, these would be the choice methods because of its noninvasiveness and patients' comfort and safety.

Adenocarcinoma is the most common primary tumor of the small intestine accounting for 40% of small bowel neoplasms [65,66]. Most of these tumors are located in the duodenum. MDCT findings for adenocarcinoma are typically a focal area of wall thickening encasing the lumen (Fig. 13). Because these tumors have a fibrotic and rigid consistency, an early sign can be obstruction. CT can localize the tumor and stage it by determining local extension, adenopathy, and metastasis [67]. The liver is the organ most commonly affected by distant metastasis in small bowel adenocarcinoma. Typically, metastases of small bowel adenocarcinoma appear as low-attenuation masses in the liver, which are visualized best during the portal venous phase of enhancement [68].

The second most common primary small bowel neoplasm is carcinoid, representing approximately 25% of all primary small bowel tumors [64]. These tumors are more common in the ileum than in the jejunum and duodenum. About 30% of carcinoid tumors are multicentric, which makes its correct diagnosis and staging difficult with MDCT [69]. In advanced stages, carcinoid tumors grow into the mesentery, with a fairly characteristic appearance on MDCT (Fig. 14) [70]. Calcifications are seen in up to 70% of cases [71,72]. Carcinoid tumors typically metastasize to the liver and normally present as multiple small liver lesions enhancing strongly in the arterial phase.

The third most common malignancy is non-Hodgkin's lymphoma, representing approximately 10% to 15% of all small bowel neoplasms [64].

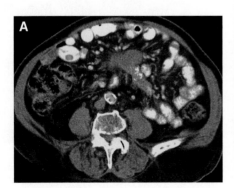
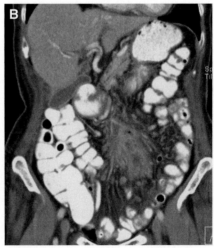

Fig. 14. Contrast-enhanced axial image (*A*) and coronal reconstruction (*B*) of a patient with carcinoid demonstrate a tumor arising in the bowel wall and spreading through the mesentery producing a large mass with central necrosis.

The most common location is in the stomach, but it can occur in any part of the gastrointestinal tract [73]. Several patterns can be seen by imaging [69]. Non-Hodgkin's lymphoma can appear as either multiple small nodules, best seen on small bowel series, or as a single mass of variable size (Fig. 15). This mass can lead to intussusception but rarely causes obstruction because lesions are typically soft and smooth. Infiltrating lymphoma produces a different type of pattern with diffuse wall thickening and destruction of the normal small bowel folds without obstruction. This type of lymphoma commonly infiltrates the muscular layer and disrupts the myoenteric plexus, causing aneurismal dilation of the affected segment in up to 50% of cases [74]. The fourth pattern of lymphoma is an exophytic mass, which can ulcerate. This appearance is very similar to adenocarcinoma or gastrointestinal stromal tumor.

Lymphoma can also be manifested in mesenteric adenopathy and, as the tumor grows, can encase small bowel loops and mesenteric vessels. After IV contrast administration the vascular encasement (bright) of the normal vessels going through the enlarged lymph nodes (lower density on top and at base) is called the "sandwich sign" [2].

The fourth most common primary small bowel tumor is gastrointestinal stromal cell tumor [64], which arises from smooth muscle cells within the bowel wall. It commonly involves the jejunum and the ileum. Gastrointestinal stromal cell tumors are rare, representing only 9% of small bowel tumors; they are slightly more common in males and typically occur in the fifth to the sixth decade of life [75]. Typically, gastrointestinal stromal cell tumors appear as large, bulky, masses (Fig. 16). Central necrosis and ulcerations are common. Tumor spread is through

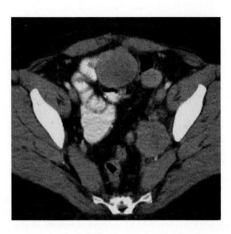

Fig. 16. Contrast-enhanced axial CT image of a patient with metastatic gastrointestinal stromal tumor. The metastatic masses are round-shaped and arise from distal ileal loops.

local extension into adjacent organs and hematogenously to the liver. Liver metastasis can appear either as hypovascular or cystic masses. Peritoneal metastasis may also be seen [76–79].

In a 10-year review of small bowel cancers in a large United States teaching hospital, 50% were primary tumors and 50% were metastatic masses; 43% of the metastases were from colonic cancer, 11% were each of pancreatic and ovarian cancer origin, 9% were from lung cancer, and 6% were melanoma (Fig. 17). The remaining was metastasis from gastric lymphoma and adenocarcinoma, breast, bladder, ureteral, and testicular cancer [66].

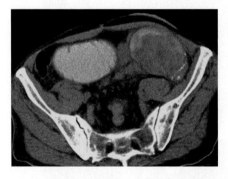

Fig. 15. Axial CT image of a 68-year-old man with abdominal pain. On the CT there is a large mass in the small bowel wall obliterating the lumen and producing an obstruction. Surgery revealed a large small bowel lymphoma.

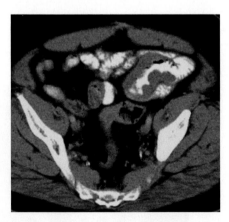

Fig. 17. Contrast-enhanced axial CT image of a patient with known melanoma and lower abdominal pain. The CT shows a thickened bowel wall of the distal ileum. The findings are consistent with melanoma metastasis, which was surgically proved.

Summary

MDCT is a technique that can be applied routinely to evaluate the small bowel. Thin collimation and fast scanning allow coverage of the whole abdomen within one suspended respiration phase with the use of multiphasic IV contrast administration. These technical options provide source images for multiplanar reconstruction.

Bowel distention is a key element for accurately diagnosing small bowel pathology. CT enterography or CT enteroclysis are currently used but larger studies have to determine the best application of these small bowel tailored CT protocols for different indications.

MDCT of the small bowel helps to identify and stage most of the common diseases of the small bowel, such as CD, ischemia, obstruction, and neoplasms. This technique will change the paradigm for diagnosing small bowel disease by setting MDCT in the first line of diagnostic tools for almost all small bowel diseases. It has the needed sensitivity and specificity and the availability and safety for a frontline diagnostic method.

References

[1] Maglinte DD, Lappas JC, Kelvin FM, et al. Small bowel radiography: how, when, and why? Radiology 1987;163:297–305.

[2] Horton KM, Fishman EK. Multidetector-row computed tomography and 3-dimensional computed tomography imaging of small bowel neoplasms: current concept in diagnosis. J Comput Assist Tomogr 2004;28:106–16.

[3] Horton KM, Fishman EK. The current status of multidetector row CT and three-dimensional imaging of the small bowel. Radiol Clin North Am 2003;41:199–212.

[4] Paulson EK, Harris JP, Jaffe TA, et al. Acute appendicitis: added diagnostic value of coronal reformations from isotropic voxels at multi-detector row CT. Radiology 2005;235:879–85.

[5] Horton KM, Eng J, Fishman EK. Normal enhancement of the small bowel: evaluation with spiral CT. J Comput Assist Tomogr 2000;24:67–71.

[6] Boudiaf M, Jaff A, Soyer P, et al. Small-bowel diseases: prospective evaluation of multi-detector row helical CT enteroclysis in 107 consecutive patients. Radiology 2004;233:338–44.

[7] Bender GN, Timmons JH, Williard WC, et al. Computed tomographic enteroclysis: one methodology. Invest Radiol 1996;31:43–9.

[8] Bender GN, Maglinte DD, Kloppel VR, et al. CT enteroclysis: a superfluous diagnostic procedure or valuable when investigating small-bowel disease? AJR Am J Roentgenol 1999;172:373–8.

[9] Raptopoulos V, Schwartz RK, McNicholas MM, et al. Multiplanar helical CT enterography in patients with Crohn's disease. AJR Am J Roentgenol 1997;169:1545–50.

[10] Megibow AJ, Bosniak MA. Dilute barium as a contrast agent for abdominal CT. AJR Am J Roentgenol 1980;134:1273–4.

[11] Raptopoulos V. Technical principles in CT evaluation of the gut. Radiol Clin North Am 1989;27:631–51.

[12] Winter TC, Ager JD, Nghiem HV, et al. Upper gastrointestinal tract and abdomen: water as an orally administered contrast agent for helical CT. Radiology 1996;201:365–70.

[13] Zhang LH, Zhang SZ, Hu HJ, et al. Multi-detector CT enterography with iso-osmotic mannitol as oral contrast for detecting small bowel disease. World J Gastroenterol 2005;11:2324–9.

[14] Antoch G, Kuehl H, Kanja J, et al. Dual-modality PET/CT scanning with negative oral contrast agent to avoid artifacts: introduction and evaluation. Radiology 2004;230:879–85.

[15] Oliva MR, Erturk SM, Ichikawa T, et al. Effectiveness of low attenuation oral contrast medium in abdominal MDCT: comparison with positive oral contrast media and water. Presented at the 16th annual and postgraduate course of the European Society of Gastrointestinal and Abdominal Radiology (ESGAR). Florence, Italy, May 28–31, 2005.

[16] Thompson SE, Raptopoulos V, Sheiman RL, et al. Abdominal helical CT: milk as a low-attenuation oral contrast agent. Radiology 1999;211:870–5.

[17] Ramsay DW, Markham DH, Morgan B, et al. The use of dilute Calogen as a fat density oral contrast medium in upper abdominal computed tomography, compared with the use of water and positive oral contrast media. Clin Radiol 2001;56:670–3.

[18] Raptopoulos V, Davis MA, Davidoff A, et al. Fat-density oral contrast agent for abdominal CT. Radiology 1987;164:653–6.

[19] Pochaczevsky R. Carbon dioxide as a low-attenuation oral contrast agent. Radiology 2000;214:918.

[20] Maglinte DD, Bender GN, Heitkamp DE, et al. Multidetector-row helical CT enteroclysis. Radiol Clin North Am 2003;41:249–62.

[21] Singer AJ, Richman PB, Kowalska A, et al. Comparison of patient and practitioner assessments of pain from commonly performed emergency department procedures. Ann Emerg Med 1999;33:652–8.

[22] Fukuya T, Hawes DR, Lu CC, et al. CT diagnosis of small-bowel obstruction: efficacy in 60 patients. AJR Am J Roentgenol 1992;158:765–9 [discussion: 71–2].

[23] Gollub MJ. Multidetector computed tomography enteroclysis of patients with small bowel obstruction: a volume-rendered "surgical perspective". J Comput Assist Tomogr 2005;29:401–7.

[24] Umschaden HW, Szolar D, Gasser J, et al. Small-bowel disease: comparison of MR enteroclysis images with conventional enteroclysis and surgical findings. Radiology 2000;215:717–25.

[25] Turetschek K, Schober E, Wunderbaldinger P, et al. Findings at helical CT-enteroclysis in symptomatic patients with Crohn disease: correlation with endoscopic and surgical findings. J Comput Assist Tomogr 2002;26:488–92.

[26] Loftus Jr EV, Kane SV, Bjorkman D. Systematic review: short-term adverse effects of 5-aminosalicylic acid agents in the treatment of ulcerative colitis. Aliment Pharmacol Ther 2004;19:179–89.

[27] Mekhjian HS, Switz DM, Melnyk CS, et al. Clinical features and natural history of Crohn's disease. Gastroenterology 1979;77(4 Pt 2):898–906.

[28] Steinhardt HJ, Loeschke K, Kasper H, et al. European Cooperative Crohn's Disease Study (ECCDS): clinical features and natural history. Digestion 1985;31:97–108.

[29] Furukawa A, Saotome T, Yamasaki M, et al. Cross-sectional imaging in Crohn disease. Radiographics 2004;24:689–702.

[30] Hara AK, Leighton JA, Sharma VK, et al. Imaging of small bowel disease: comparison of capsule endoscopy, standard endoscopy, barium examination and CT. Radiographics 2005;25:697–711 [discussion: 11–8].

[31] Enns R, Go K, Chang H, et al. Capsule endoscopy: a single-centre experience with the first 226 capsules. Can J Gastroenterol 2004;18:555–8.

[32] Voderholzer WA, Beinhoelzl J, Rogalla P, et al. Small bowel involvement in Crohn's disease: a prospective comparison of wireless capsule endoscopy and computed tomography enteroclysis. Gut 2005;54:369–73.

[33] Hassan C, Cerro P, Zullo A, et al. Computed tomography enteroclysis in comparison with ileoscopy in patients with Crohn's disease. Int J Colorectal Dis 2003;18:121–5.

[34] Wold PB, Fletcher JG, Johnson CD, et al. Assessment of small bowel Crohn disease: noninvasive peroral CT enterography compared with other imaging methods and endoscopy–feasibility study. Radiology 2003;229:275–81.

[35] Maglinte DD, Gourtsoyiannis N, Rex D, et al. Classification of small bowel Crohn's subtypes based on multimodality imaging. Radiol Clin North Am 2003;41:285–303.

[36] Maconi G, Sampietro GM, Parente F, et al. Contrast radiology, computed tomography and ultrasonography in detecting internal fistulas and intra-abdominal abscesses in Crohn's disease: a prospective comparative study. Am J Gastroenterol 2003;98:1545–55.

[37] Del Campo L, Arribas I, Valbuena M, et al. Spiral CT findings in active and remission phases in patients with Crohn disease. J Comput Assist Tomogr 2001;25:792–7.

[38] Choi D, Jin Lee S, Ah Cho Y, et al. Bowel wall thickening in patients with Crohn's disease: CT patterns and correlation with inflammatory activity. Clin Radiol 2003;58:68–74.

[39] Meyers MA, McGuire PV. Spiral CT demonstration of hypervascularity in Crohn disease: "vascular jejunization of the ileum" or the "comb sign". Abdom Imaging 1995;20:327–32.

[40] Lee SS, Ha HK, Yang SK, et al. CT of prominent pericolic or perienteric vasculature in patients with Crohn's disease: correlation with clinical disease activity and findings on barium studies. AJR Am J Roentgenol 2002;179:1029–36.

[41] Gore RM, Balthazar EJ, Ghahremani GG, et al. CT features of ulcerative colitis and Crohn's disease. AJR Am J Roentgenol 1996;167:3–15.

[42] Scaglione M, Romano S, Pinto F, et al. Helical CT diagnosis of small bowel obstruction in the acute clinical setting. Eur J Radiol 2004;50:15–22.

[43] Maglinte DD, Gage SN, Harmon BH, et al. Obstruction of the small intestine: accuracy and role of CT in diagnosis. Radiology 1993;188:61–4.

[44] Megibow AJ, Balthazar EJ, Cho KC, et al. Bowel obstruction: evaluation with CT. Radiology 1991;180:313–8.

[45] Rubesin SE, Herlinger H. CT evaluation of bowel obstruction: a landmark article–implications for the future. Radiology 1991;180:307–8.

[46] Frager D, Medwid SW, Baer JW, et al. CT of small-bowel obstruction: value in establishing the diagnosis and determining the degree and cause. AJR Am J Roentgenol 1994;162:37–41.

[47] Megibow AJ. Bowel obstruction: evaluation with CT. Radiol Clin North Am 1994;32:861–70.

[48] Taourel PG, Fabre JM, Pradel JA, et al. Value of CT in the diagnosis and management of patients with suspected acute small-bowel obstruction. AJR Am J Roentgenol 1995;165:1187–92.

[49] Donckier V, Closset J, Van Gansbeke D, et al. Contribution of computed tomography to decision making in the management of adhesive small bowel obstruction. Br J Surg 1998;85:1071–4.

[50] Daneshmand S, Hedley CG, Stain SC. The utility and reliability of computed tomography scan in the diagnosis of small bowel obstruction. Am Surg 1999;65:922–6.

[51] Ha HK, Kim JS, Lee MS, et al. Differentiation of simple and strangulated small-bowel obstructions: usefulness of known CT criteria. Radiology 1997;204:507–12.

[52] Khurana B, Ledbetter S, McTavish J, et al. Bowel obstruction revealed by multidetector CT. AJR Am J Roentgenol 2002;178:1139–44.

[53] Scaglione M, Grassi R, Pinto A, et al. Positive predictive value and negative predictive value of spiral CT in the diagnosis of closed loop obstruction complicated by intestinal ischemia. Radiol Med (Torino) 2004;107:69–77.

[54] Wiesner W, Hauser A, Steinbrich W. Accuracy of multidetector row computed tomography for the diagnosis of acute bowel ischemia in a non-selected study population. Eur Radiol 2004;14:2347–56.

[55] Jrvinen O, Laurikka J, Salenius JP, et al. Acute intestinal ischaemia: a review of 214 cases. Ann Chir Gynaecol 1994;83:22–5.

[56] Ruotolo RA, Evans SR. Mesenteric ischemia in the elderly. Clin Geriatr Med 1999;15:527–57.

[57] Martinez JP, Hogan GJ. Mesenteric ischemia. Emerg Med Clin North Am 2004;22:909–28.

[58] Kaminsky O, Yampolski I, Aranovich D, et al. Does a second-look operation improve survival in patients with peritonitis due to acute mesenteric ischemia? A five-year retrospective experience. World J Surg 2005;29(5):645–8.

[59] Segatto E, Mortele KJ, Ji H, et al. Acute small bowel ischemia: CT imaging findings. Semin Ultrasound CT MR 2003;24:364–76.

[60] Wiesner W, Khurana B, Ji H, et al. CT of acute bowel ischemia. Radiology 2003;226:635–50.

[61] Klein HM, Lensing R, Klosterhalfen B, et al. Diagnostic imaging of mesenteric infarction. Radiology 1995;197:79–82.

[62] Bartnicke BJ, Balfe DM. CT appearance of intestinal ischemia and intramural hemorrhage. Radiol Clin North Am 1994;32:845–60.

[63] Ha HK, Rha SE, Kim AY, et al. CT and MR diagnoses of intestinal ischemia. Semin Ultrasound CT MR 2000; 21:40–55.

[64] Chow JS, Chen CC, Ahsan H, et al. A population-based study of the incidence of malignant small bowel tumours: SEER, 1973–1990. Int J Epidemiol 1996;25:722–8.

[65] Brookes VS, Waterhouse JA, Powell DJ. Malignant lesions of the small intestine: a ten-year survey. Br J Surg 1968;55:405–10.

[66] Minardi Jr AJ, Zibari GB, Aultman DF, et al. Small-bowel tumors. J Am Coll Surg 1998;186:664–8.

[67] Merine D, Fishman EK, Jones B. CT of the small bowel and mesentery. Radiol Clin North Am 1989; 27:707–15.

[68] Kuszyk BS, Bluemke DA, Urban BA, et al. Portal-phase contrast-enhanced helical CT for the detection of malignant hepatic tumors: sensitivity based on comparison with intraoperative and pathologic findings. AJR Am J Roentgenol 1996;166:91–5.

[69] Buckley JA, Jones B, Fishman EK. Small bowel cancer. Imaging features and staging. Radiol Clin North Am 1997;35:381–402.

[70] Horton KM, Kamel I, Hofmann L, et al. Carcinoid tumors of the small bowel: a multitechnique imaging approach. AJR Am J Roentgenol 2004;182:559–67.

[71] Seigel RS, Kuhns LR, Borlaza GS, et al. Computed tomography and angiography in ileal carcinoid tumor and retractile mesenteritis. Radiology 1980;134: 437–40.

[72] Pantongrag-Brown L, Buetow PC, Carr NJ, et al. Calcification and fibrosis in mesenteric carcinoid tumor: CT findings and pathologic correlation. AJR Am J Roentgenol 1995;164:387–91.

[73] Crump M, Gospodarowicz M, Shepherd FA. Lymphoma of the gastrointestinal tract. Semin Oncol 1999;26:324–37.

[74] Dudiak KM, Johnson CD, Stephens DH. Primary tumors of the small intestine: CT evaluation. AJR Am J Roentgenol 1989;152:995–8.

[75] Shiu MH, Farr GH, Egeli RA, et al. Myosarcomas of the small and large intestine: a clinicopathologic study. J Surg Oncol 1983;24:67–72.

[76] Horton KM, Juluru K, Montogomery E, et al. Computed tomography imaging of gastrointestinal stromal tumors with pathology correlation. J Comput Assist Tomogr 2004;28:811–7.

[77] Kim HC, Lee JM, Choi SH, et al. Imaging of gastrointestinal stromal tumors. J Comput Assist Tomogr 2004;28:596–604.

[78] Sandrasegaran K, Rajesh A, Rushing DA, et al. Gastrointestinal stromal tumors: CT and MRI findings. Eur Radiol 2005;15(7):1407–14.

[79] Sandrasegaran K, Rajesh A, Rydberg J, et al. Gastrointestinal stromal tumors: clinical, radiologic, and pathologic features. AJR Am J Roentgenol 2005; 184:803–11.

ELSEVIER
SAUNDERS

Radiol Clin N Am 43 (2005) 1079–1095

RADIOLOGIC
CLINICS
of North America

Multidetector CT Evaluation of Abdominal Trauma

Lisa A. Miller, MD*, K. Shanmuganathan, MD

Department of Radiology, University of Maryland Medical Center, Baltimore, MD, USA

Since the 1980s, CT has emerged as the imaging modality of choice to evaluate the hemodynamically stable patient with blunt trauma [1–3]. Many patients admitted to a trauma center have multisystem injuries sustained from high velocity trauma, most commonly a motor vehicle collision. As many as 68% of blunt trauma patients have neurologic impairment owing to injury, drugs, or alcohol, or have a distracting injury, factors that limit the reliability of clinical examination [4]. The speed and accuracy of CT in detecting multisystem injury has proven to be invaluable in the prompt diagnosis and triage of trauma patients. With the advent of multidetector CT (MDCT), scanning times have progressively decreased while image resolution has increased owing to thinner collimation and reduced partial volume and motion artifacts. This high quality image data can be processed further into multiplanar reformatted (MPR) or maximum intensity projection (MIP) images and three-dimensional volumetric (3-D) images, which often aid in the diagnosis of complex injuries in the trauma patient.

Multidetector CT technique

A significant number of patients admitted to the University of Maryland Shock Trauma Center (UMSTC) have multisystem injuries. MDCT evaluation of the abdomen and pelvis is often obtained as part of total body CT in which scans are obtained from the circle of Willis to the symphysis pubis and include the head, cervical spine and neck, chest,

abdomen, and pelvis. Trauma MDCT studies are performed on a 16-slice scanner (MX 8000-IDT; Phillips Medical Systems, Best, Netherlands) using the parameters shown in Table 1. A total of 600 mL of oral contrast (2% sodium diatrizoate [hypaque sodium]) is given before scanning, either orally or via a nasogastric tube. Despite controversy over its use, numerous studies have shown an extremely low risk of aspiration [5–7], and the authors' experience over the past 20 years supports these findings.

Total body CT scan

During a total body scan, a noncontrast MDCT of the head is initially performed. Unless the patient has a known major allergic reaction to contrast material or renal insufficiency, nonionic intravenous contrast material (150 mL of 300 mg I^2/mL, Omnipaque 300) is administered using a biphasic power injector (90 mL at 6 mL/s followed by 60 mL at 4 mL/s). A bolus pro technique is used to initiate scanning at the circle of Willis. The region of interest is placed over the ascending aorta, with the threshold to initiate the scan set at 90 Hu. Delayed images through the abdomen are routinely obtained at 2 to 3 minutes after the initial contrast injection during the renal excretory phase. Delayed images are used to assess the symmetry of renal function and renal collecting system injury, and to differentiate between arterial contrast extravasation and vascular injuries including pseudoaneurysms or traumatic arteriovenous fistulas.

At the authors' center, 3-mm axial soft copy images of the abdomen and pelvis are viewed by the emergency radiologist. In patients who have abdominal or pelvic organ or bony injuries, high resolution MPR images are routinely obtained in the coronal and sagittal planes through the abdomen and pelvis. MIP and color 3-D images are selectively obtained in

---

* Corresponding author. Department of Radiology, University of Maryland Medical Center, 22 South Greene Street, Baltimore, MD 21201.

E-mail address: lmiller1@umm.edu (L.A. Miller).

Table 1
Helical and multidetector CT protocols

Method	Volume of IV contrast (mL)	Delay[a]	Injection rate	Collimation (mm)	Table speed (mm)	Pitch
Single-slice helical CT	150	60 s	3 mL/s	8	8	1
4-slice MDCT	150	Bolus pro	6 mL/s for 90 mL then 4 mL/s for 60 mL	2.5	10	1
16-slice MDCT	150	Bolus pro	6 mL/s for 90 mL then 4 mL/s for 60 mL	1.2	10	1.1

Abbreviation: IV, intravenous.

[a] Delay in initiation of scan from beginning of intravenous contrast bolus.

patients with vascular or bony injuries. The large image data sets that are generated from the total body scan can be processed quickly using a separate work station (TeraRecon, San Mateo, California). These volume images are more than just esthetically pleasing and help the radiologist with the diagnosis and decision-making process. One can better comprehend the exact anatomic location and relationship of the injury to major vessels on volume images when compared with axial images.

Intraperitoneal fluid and hemoperitoneum

The dependent portions of the abdomen and pelvis should be scrutinized thoroughly in the trauma patient to detect small quantities of fluid that may indicate a subtle intraperitoneal injury [8]. These areas include Morison's pouch, the paracolic gutters, and the region directly posterior to the urinary bladder. Free fluid is also commonly seen in the perihepatic and perisplenic spaces in patients with liver or splenic injuries. Density measurements of intraperitoneal fluid are easily obtained and can help to differentiate simple ascites, urine, blood, active bleeding, and bile. Bile may be below zero in Hounsfield units because of its high cholesterol content. Simple ascites and urine will measure between 0 and 15 Hu. The CT attenuation of free intraperitoneal blood measures between 20 and 40 Hu, whereas clotted blood or hematoma measures between 40 and 70 Hu. Active bleeding measures within 10 Hu of the density of the vascular contrast material seen within an adjacent major vessel [8,9].

Isolated free intraperitoneal fluid

Free intraperitoneal fluid in the blunt abdominal trauma patient without evidence of organ injury may represent an occult solid organ, bowel, or mesenteric injury [10–12]. A small amount of pelvic free fluid

can normally be seen in women of childbearing age, and careful correlation with the physical examination and menstrual history is needed to determine the significance of this finding. Occult bowel or mesenteric injury should be suspected when free fluid is seen in males who do not have pelvic fractures, in females with a moderate to large amount of free fluid, or in any patient in whom free fluid is seen interdigitating between the leaves of the mesentery. Several options exist to evaluate the cause of the free fluid:

- Observation with serial physical examinations to detect early peritonitis
- Follow-up MDCT in 4 to 6 hours to demonstrate resolution of free fluid
- Diagnostic peritoneal lavage and determination of the white blood cell count in lavage fluid
- Laparoscopy to detect occult injuries
- Exploratory laparotomy in patients with abdominal pain and a moderate to large amount of free fluid

Splenic trauma

The spleen is the most commonly injured intraperitoneal organ in blunt trauma [13]. Since the 1970s, the major immunologic role of the spleen and the high mortality associated with overwhelming sepsis from encapsulated bacteria in postsplenectomy patients have been well recognized, leading to non-operative management of splenic injuries in the pediatric population. The high success rate of splenic conservation in this group of patients has initiated similar management in the adult trauma population, frequently in conjunction with transcatheter splenic artery embolization. Pachter and coworkers [14] studied the impact of nonoperative management on the changing pattern of management of adult splenic injuries. In their study, 13% of the surgeons used nonoperative management between 1984 and 1990. This rate increased significantly to 54% between 1990 and 1996.

Nonoperative management has now become the standard of care for splenic injury in the majority of patients who are hemodynamically stable with no other injuries requiring laparotomy [15–17]. Splenic arteriography and transcatheter embolization have increased the number of patients with blunt splenic injury who can be managed nonoperatively [15,17]. A recent study by Haan and coworkers [15] evaluated the 5-year experience with nonoperative management at the authors' center using splenic arteriography and MDCT. Of the 648 patients admitted with blunt splenic injury, 280 underwent immediate laparotomy, whereas the remaining 368 underwent planned nonoperative management. Based on the MDCT findings, 70 patients (19%) were treated conservatively with serial physical examinations and a follow-up MDCT scan. The splenic salvage rate in this group was 100%. Among the 132 patients who were treated with splenic artery embolization, the salvage rate was 90%.

MDCT has a vital role in the selection of patients for nonoperative management of splenic injury. Contrast-enhanced MDCT has a 98% accuracy rate in detecting significant splenic injury [18] and is useful in determining the presence of splenic vascular injuries or a site of active bleeding. Preliminary data from ongoing studies at the authors' center suggest that MDCT can better demonstrate these lesions when compared with single slice helical CT. These two MDCT findings have a high association with failure of nonoperative management and require angiographic embolization or surgery for treatment [9,19].

Splenic injury grading scales

To compare outcomes and to standardize reporting, several splenic injury grading systems have been developed, most notably the American Association for the Surgery of Trauma (AAST) Splenic Injury Grading Scale [20]. This grading system includes parameters such as the length of laceration and the amount of surface area involved by the subcapsular or intraparenchymal hematoma. In this surgically based grading scale, the grade of injury is typically assigned at the time of laparotomy. Several CT-based grading systems have been developed from the AAST scale, including one designed by Mirvis and coworkers [21] that is used by the authors (Box 1). CT-based scales have the advantage of assigning a grade of injury

---

Box 1. CT-based injury severity grades and criteria for blunt splenic trauma

CT grade I: Capsular avulsion, laceration(s), or subcapsular hematoma < 1 cm diameter
CT grade II: Laceration(s) 1–3 cm deep, central/subcapsular hematoma 1–3 cm diameter
CT grade III: Laceration(s) 3–10 cm deep, central/subcapsular hematoma > 3 cm diameter
CT grade IV: Laceration(s) > 10 cm deep, central/subcapsular hematoma > 10 cm diameter, massive lobar maceration or devascularization
CT grade V: Bilobar tissue maceration or devitalization

Modified from Mirvis SE, Whitley NO, Gens DR. Blunt splenic trauma in adults: CT-based classification and correlation with prognosis and treatment. Radiology 1989;171:34; with permission.

---

before laparotomy, at which time they would be useful in guiding the management of splenic injury. Nevertheless, considerable controversy continues over the accuracy of all CT-based splenic injury scales in predicting the successful outcome of nonoperative management of splenic injury [22–25]. Although a high association of failure of nonoperative management with vascular lesions and active extravasation has been reported in prior studies, these two injuries have not been included in the current grading scales. At the UMSTC, the grade of injury is used as one of the parameters to guide the management of blunt splenic trauma.

Multidetector CT appearance of splenic injury

MDCT is highly accurate in diagnosing splenic injury. It is vital to image in the portal venous phase during peak splenic parenchymal enhancement to demonstrate splenic injury optimally. Imaging during the early arterial phase may simulate injury owing to normal transient heterogeneous enhancement of splenic tissue during this period. Delayed imaging during the excretory phase can obscure injury. Splenic laceration "fill-in" with contrast material and vascular lesion "wash out" occur during this phase,

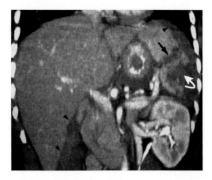

Fig. 1. Splenic lacerations and contusions. MDCT MPR image shows a grade IV splenic injury including a laceration (*arrow*) and an area of contusion (*curved arrow*) more inferiorly. Hemoperitoneum (*arrowheads*) is seen around the liver and spleen.

and the lesions may become isodense with the normal splenic parenchyma, decreasing their conspicuity.

The spectrum of MDCT findings seen in splenic injury includes contusion, laceration, intraparenchymal or subcapsular hematoma, splenic infarction, vascular lesions (traumatic arteriovenous fistula and pseudoaneurysm), and active extravasation. A splenic contusion appears on MDCT as a poorly circumscribed region of hypodensity. A splenic laceration appears as a sharply marginated linear or branching region of hypodensity within enhancing parenchyma (Fig. 1). With healing, the laceration decreases in size, and the margins become less distinct. These changes can be seen within 2 to 3 days of injury but typically take weeks or months for complete resolution of the CT findings. Subcapsular hematomas are more common than intraparenchymal hematomas following trauma. Subcapsular hematomas appear

as a low-density crescentic collection between the splenic capsule and splenic parenchyma, frequently compressing the underlying splenic tissue (Fig. 2). As the subcapsular hematoma matures, it progressively decreases in size and becomes more hypodense as the blood products gradually resorb.

Posttraumatic splenic infarctions are an uncommon manifestation of blunt splenic trauma [26,27]. A splenic infarction appears as a well-defined, wedge-shaped region of hypodensity, with the base of the wedge toward the periphery of the spleen. The mechanism of splenic infarction is thought to be stretching of a splenic blood vessel at the time of trauma, which causes a focal intimal tear and leads to thrombosis. Most splenic infarctions gradually decrease in size and resolve without sequelae. Splenic abscess or delayed rupture is an uncommon complication of infarction that may necessitate angiographic or surgical intervention.

Posttraumatic vascular lesions and active extravasation

Pseudoaneurysms and traumatic arteriovenous fistulas are the two types of vascular lesions seen in splenic trauma. A splenic pseudoaneurysm is formed when there is injury to the wall of branches of the intraparenchymal splenic artery. A small amount of blood tracks into the injured vessel wall but is retained by the adventitia or surrounding tissue, effectively localizing the injury. A traumatic arteriovenous fistula is formed by an abnormal communication between the adjacent artery and vein. Arteriovenous fistulas and pseudoaneurysms have an identical appearance on CT and can only be differentiated by

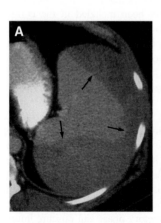
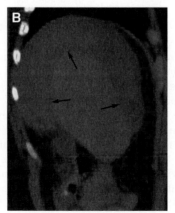
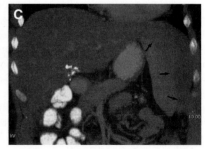

Fig. 2. Subcapsular hematoma of spleen. (*A*) Axial, (*B*) MPR sagittal, and (*C*) MIP coronal reformatted MDCT images show a large subcapsular hematoma (*arrows*) of the spleen compressing and deforming the underlying splenic parenchyma.

splenic angiography. Both of these injuries appear on CT as high-density, well-circumscribed round lesions surrounded by a low-attenuation area. The attenuation of the lesion is typically within 10 Hu of the adjacent contrast-enhanced artery. On images obtained during the renal excretory phase, these lesions will wash out and become slightly hyperdense or isodense when compared with normal splenic tissue (Fig. 3).

Active extravasation indicates bleeding from an injured vessel at the time the CT scan was performed. This injury appears as an irregular or linear high attenuation area of intravenous contrast material extravasation. On excretory phase images, the site of active extravasation remains high in attenuation and increases in size as contrast-enhanced blood continues to extravasate from the injured vessel (Fig. 4). Active bleeding may be seen in the splenic parenchyma, subcapsular space, or within the peritoneum.

Multidetector CT and the management of splenic injuries

Numerous studies indicate improved success of nonoperative management when angiographic embolization is used as an adjunct to treat splenic vascular lesions or active bleeding [17,28–31]. At the UMSTC, hemodynamically stable patients with MDCT evidence of either of these injuries undergo splenic angiography. Other MDCT findings that indicate the need for angiography are high-grade splenic injury (grade III to V) or evidence of progression of splenic injury on follow-up CT [29]. Using these guidelines in 43 hemodynamically stable patients with blunt splenic injury, Haan and coworkers [30] reported a 100% success rate of nonoperative management and a decrease in hospital stay by 3.5 days.

The role of follow-up CT in patients with splenic trauma is not yet defined. Surgical studies have

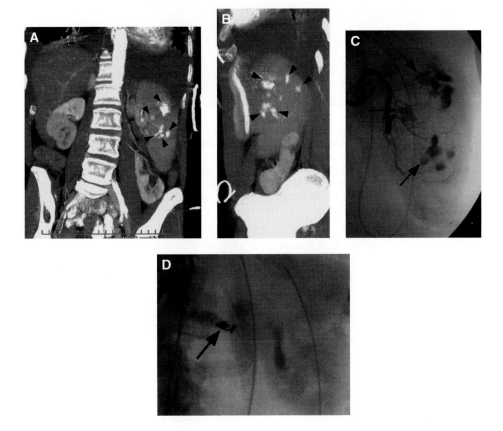

Fig. 3. Splenic pseudoaneurysms in a male admitted following motor vehicle collision. (*A*) Coronal and (*B*) sagittal MPR MDCT images show multiple splenic pseudoaneurysms (*arrowheads*) within splenic parenchyma. (*C*) Splenic arteriogram shows multiple pseudoaneurysms (*arrows*) within splenic parenchyma. (*D*) Completion splenic arteriogram shows main splenic artery embolization (*arrow*) with successful treatment of splenic pseudoaneurysms.

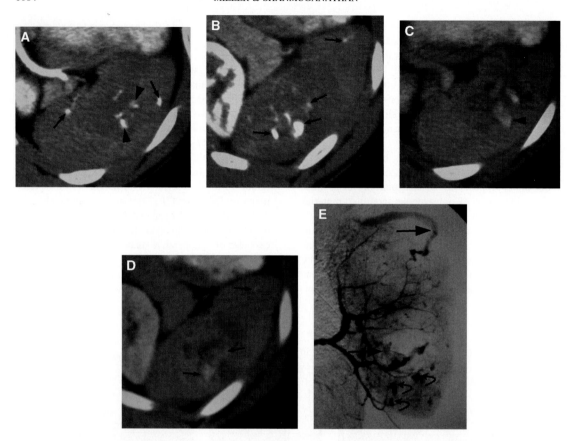

Fig. 4. Splenic active bleeding and pseudoaneurysms. (*A* and *B*) Axial MDCT images obtained in the portal venous phase show multiple rounded pseudoaneurysms (*arrows*) and areas of intraparenchymal active bleeding (*arrowheads*) in the spleen. (*C* and *D*) Delayed axial images obtained in the excretory phase in the same anatomic location show that areas of active bleeding (*arrowheads*) enlarge in size while pseudoaneurysms washout and become isodense or slightly hyperdense (*arrows*) when compared with splenic parenchyma. (*E*) Splenic arteriogram shows active bleeding (*arrows*) and pseudoaneurysms (*curved arrows*). Main splenic artery embolization was performed to treat these lesions.

demonstrated no benefit of repeat CT in clinically stable patients with splenic injury [32,33]. Other studies have shown that as many as 29% of patients with splenic injury have delayed bleeding hours to days following injury [34]. At the UMSTC, a repeat MDCT is performed 48 to 72 hours after the initial scan in all patients with blunt splenic trauma, regardless of the grade of injury. A repeat MDCT is also performed in patients with clinical findings of ongoing bleeding from splenic injury.

Hepatic trauma

The liver is the second most frequently injured intra-abdominal organ in blunt trauma. The right hepatic lobe constitutes 80% of the volume of the liver and is more commonly affected by blunt trauma. Left hepatic lobe injuries are associated with duodenal and pancreatic injuries. Isolated injuries to the liver occur in as many as 50% of patients.

Because as many as 70% of liver injuries have stopped bleeding by the time of surgery [35], and because transfusion requirements and intra-abdominal complications are higher in patients undergoing laparotomy [36,37], nonsurgical management of liver injuries in the hemodynamically stable trauma patient has become more widely accepted. MDCT helps to triage patients with more severe hepatic injuries who may require laparotomy from those who can be managed safely nonoperatively.

Grading systems for hepatic trauma have been devised in an attempt to predict outcome. The most commonly used grading system is the surgically based American AAST Liver Injury Scale [20]. Using the AAST injury scale, Mirvis and coworkers [38] developed a CT-based injury severity grading scale for blunt hepatic trauma (Box 2).

Based on conventional CT findings, investigators found that hepatic injury grading systems were unreliable in predicting the need for surgery [39–41]. Nevertheless, Poletti and coworkers [42] studied 72 patients with blunt hepatic trauma who underwent single slice helical CT and hepatic angiography and demonstrated that the Mirvis CT-based grading system was useful in predicting prognosis and guiding management. In that study, which was biased toward high-grade hepatic injuries (grade III to V) requiring hepatic angiography, grade IV injuries had a higher likelihood of bleeding and delayed complications when compared with grade III injuries. The study also demonstrated that the higher the grade of hepatic injury, the more likely the patient was to fail nonsurgical management.

Multidetector CT appearance of hepatic injuries

MDCT is the preferred imaging modality to diagnose the extent of blunt hepatic injury in hemodynamically stable patients [42,43]. MDCT findings in hepatic trauma include contusion, laceration, subcapsular hematoma, active bleeding, and vascular lesions such as pseudoaneurysms and traumatic arteriovenous fistulas.

Hepatic contusion appears on contrast-enhanced MDCT as a poorly marginated low attenuation area compared with the normal enhancing hepatic parenchyma. Contusions are invariably a minor injury and gradually decrease in size as the injury heals. Hepatic lacerations appear as well-defined, linear, or branching areas of low attenuation within the enhancing liver parenchyma. Perihepatic and intraperitoneal blood are common with liver lacerations and indicate tearing of the hepatic capsule. Lacerations that involve only the "bare area" of the liver rarely have associated hemoperitoneum, because this area of the liver is directly in contact with the retroperitoneum [44]. A bare area laceration is commonly associated with a right adrenal or renal injury and hematoma in the right retroperitoneum [45]. With healing, the margins of a liver laceration will become less distinct and will gradually enlarge into a rounded or oval shape. This rounded lesion may completely resolve or persist as a posttraumatic hepatic cyst.

The location of the hepatic laceration may have ramifications on management and outcome. Poletti and coworkers [42] reported that lacerations extending into the region of hepatic or portal veins were likely to fail nonoperative management and require surgery. Hepatic angiography and transcatheter embolization were helpful in patients with high-grade liver injuries extending into the region of the hepatic or portal veins or in the presence of vascular injury to increase the number of patients managed nonoperatively.

Injuries to the retrohepatic vena cava have a high mortality rate ranging from 90% to 100% owing to hemorrhage and difficulty in obtaining adequate surgical exposure to control hemorrhage [46–48]. These rare but potentially fatal injuries should be suspected on CT when a liver laceration extends into the region of the major hepatic veins or inferior vena cava (Fig. 5). These patients usually have a significant amount of hemorrhage in the lesser sac, adjacent to the right diaphragm, or behind the right hepatic lobe.

Hepatic subcapsular hematomas are seen on contrast-enhanced MDCT as a low-density crescentic collection of blood, typically around the right lateral hepatic margin. A subcapsular hematoma often compresses the underlying hepatic parenchyma, a characteristic that is useful in distinguishing this lesion from perihepatic blood (Fig. 6). Subcapsular hema-

---

Box 2. CT-based injury severity grades and criteria for blunt hepatic trauma

CT grade I: Capsular avulsion, laceration < 1 cm deep, subcapsular hematoma < 1 cm thick

CT grade II: Laceration(s) 1–3 cm deep, intraparenchymal/subcapsular hematoma 1–3 cm in diameter

CT grade III: Laceration > 3 cm deep, intraparenchymal/subcapsular hematoma > 3 cm in diameter

CT grade IV: Intraparenchymal/subcapsular hematoma > 10 cm in diameter, lobar maceration or devascularization

CT grade V: Bilobar maceration or devascularization

Modified from Mirvis SE, Whitley NO, Vainwright JR, et al. Blunt hepatic trauma in adults: CT-based classification and correlation with prognosis and treatment. Radiology 1989;171:30; with permission.

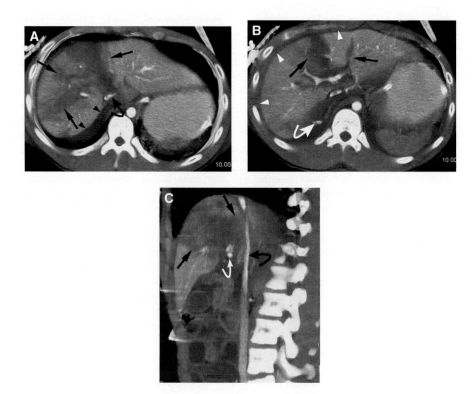

Fig. 5. Retrohepatic caval liver injury in a patient admitted following a high-speed motor vehicle collision. (*A* and *B*) Axial 3-D images show a grade V liver injury involving the right and medial segments of the left lobe of the liver. Lacerations extend into the region of the inferior vena cava (*black curved arrow*) and portal veins. Retroperitoneal active bleeding (*white curved arrow*) and hemorrhage (*black arrowheads*) are seen. Free intraperitoneal blood (*white arrowheads*) is seen around the liver. (*C*) Sagittal 3-D image shows liver lacerations (*arrows*) and the relationship to the inferior vena cava (*black curved arrow*) and portal vein (*white curved arrow*).

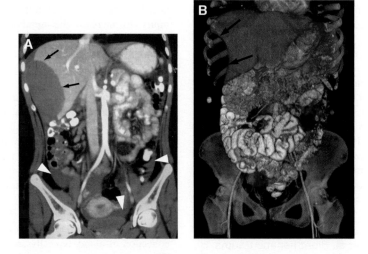

Fig. 6. Hepatic subcapsular hematoma in a patient admitted following blunt trauma. (*A* and *B*) Coronal MPR and 3-D images show a subcapsular hematoma (*arrows*) along the right lobe of the liver compressing the underlying liver parenchyma. Hemoperitoneum (*arrowheads*) is seen in both lower paracolic gutters and the pelvis.

tomas generally become increasingly hypodense and decrease in size until complete resolution in 6 to 8 weeks [49].

Pseudoaneurysms and arteriovenous fistulas are hepatic vascular injuries that have a similar appearance on contrast-enhanced MDCT. Each of these lesions is seen as a well-circumscribed, rounded, high-density focus, usually surrounded by a low-attenuation area. The attenuation of the lesion is typically within 10 Hu of the nearest contrast-enhanced artery. On excretory phase images, the lesions wash out and become slightly hyperdense or isodense with the adjacent normal hepatic parenchyma. Active bleeding within the liver appears as an irregular or linear high-attenuation focus of extravasated intravenous contrast material that remains persistently high in attenuation and typically increases in size on excretory phase images. Active extravasation in the liver may be seen in the hepatic parenchyma, subcapsular space, or peritoneum. Hepatic vascular injuries and active extravasation resulting in bleeding into the peritoneal cavity through a tear in the capsule of liver have been shown to be strong predictors of failure of nonoperative management [50–52]. Helical CT has been shown to have 65% to 100% sensitivity and 76% to 85% specificity for detection of arterial vascular injury [42,53].

Multidetector CT and management of acute hepatic injury

At the UMSTC, MDCT has a key role in management of the hemodynamically stable patient with blunt hepatic trauma. Indications for hepatic angiography include a high-grade (grade III to V) hepatic injury with laceration extending into the region of the hepatic or portal vein or the presence of active hemorrhage or vascular injury (irrespective of the grade of injury). Angiography is also performed if multiple blood transfusions are required because of ongoing hepatic hemorrhage.

Complications of hepatic trauma

The first priority in the treatment of patients with liver trauma is to control hemorrhage. Most hemodynamically stable patients with hepatic injury do not require surgical intervention and heal without any sequelae; however, complications of hepatic trauma can be seen in 10% to 25% of patients [54,55] and may occur weeks to months after the initial injury [56]. MDCT can aid in the diagnosis of complications such as delayed hemorrhage, abscess, and biloma.

Delayed hemorrhage is the most common complication of nonsurgically managed blunt hepatic trauma, occurring in 1.7% to 5.9% of patients treated [36,54,57]. Hemorrhage may occur owing to an increase in size of the laceration at the initial site of injury or from delayed formation of a pseudoaneurysm of the hepatic artery, portal vein, or its branches. Bleeding should be suspected in patients with a decreasing hemoglobin level requiring multiple transfusions or in whom there is new onset of right upper quadrant abdominal pain. Angiographic or surgical intervention may be required to treat patients with delayed hemorrhage.

Hepatic abscesses occur in 0.6% to 4% of patients who have blunt hepatic trauma [41,58] and are most commonly seen in patients managed operatively [59]. A hepatic abscess should be suspected in patients with persistent abdominal pain, tenderness over the liver, fever, and leukocytosis. On CT, a hepatic abscess appears as a well-circumscribed fluid collection within the parenchyma or subcapsular space. Small gas bubbles may be present within the abscess, and the collection may demonstrate an enhancing rim. Percutaneous needle aspiration with drain placement is commonly used for the treatment of post-traumatic hepatic abscess.

Bilomas are an uncommon complication of hepatic trauma. Intrahepatic biliary ducts are invariably injured along with the hepatic parenchyma at time of trauma, but most of these injuries heal without sequelae. Patients with high-grade liver injuries have a higher risk of biloma formation. Bilomas can form weeks to months after the initial trauma as the slow progressive leakage of bile into the traumatized tissue gradually forms a collection [60]. Patients may be asymptomatic or present with right upper quadrant abdominal pain or fullness, fever, or jaundice. On CT, bilomas appear as a round, well-circumscribed collection of low-density fluid. The appearance is similar to that seen with hepatic abscess or resolving hematoma, and differentiating among these three entities on CT is difficult. Percutaneous needle aspiration or Tc-99m IDA scintigraphy can confirm the diagnosis [61]. Symptomatic patients can be treated with a combination of percutaneous drain placement and endoscopic retrograde biliary stent placement [54,62]. Interventional procedures in an asymptomatic patient in whom a biloma is discovered incidentally are generally avoided, because most bilomas will gradually decrease in size with time without any complication. Serial CT scans can document the progressive decrease in size of the biloma, which can take months to years.

Gallbladder trauma

Gallbladder injury resulting from blunt abdominal trauma is rare, with an incidence of 2% to 8% [63]. The gallbladder may be contused, perforated, or avulsed. Although there are no CT signs specific for gallbladder injury, several findings have been described in association with gallbladder trauma [64,65]. A contusion can be suspected on MDCT when there is focal thickening of the gallbladder wall or a high-density intraluminal hematoma. Perforation of the gallbladder results in a full-thickness injury to the gallbladder wall. CT may show a collapsed gallbladder with pericholecystic fluid. A free mucosal flap projecting into the lumen of the gallbladder may also be seen. In avulsion, the gallbladder is torn away from the gallbladder fossa and, in some cases, may only be attached to the cystic artery and duct (Fig. 7). Because of the nonspecific CT findings and rarity of this injury, the final diagnosis of gallbladder injury is often made at the time of laparotomy.

Bowel and mesenteric trauma

Bowel and mesenteric injuries from blunt abdominal trauma are rare. An analysis of more than 275,000 patients with blunt abdominal trauma enrolled in the EAST Multi-Institutional Hollow Viscus Injury Research Group study, the largest retrospective hollow viscus injury study to date, found the incidence of blunt colonic injury to be 0.3% and the incidence of blunt small bowel injury to be 1.1% [66,67]. The most common sites of full-thickness

bowel injury are the jejunum and ilium, with an incidence of 81%, followed by the colon and rectum, duodenum, and stomach [68,69].

Prompt detection of bowel and mesenteric injuries is crucial. A delay in diagnosis may result in peritonitis, ongoing hemorrhage, bowel ischemia, and necrosis. A delay in diagnosis of bowel injury of only 8 hours has been shown to increase morbidity and mortality [67,70]. The accuracy of conventional or single slice helical CT in detecting blunt bowel and mesenteric injuries has been shown in prior studies to range from 84% to 94% [71–73]. Nevertheless, the ability of CT to diagnose bowel injury has been challenged recently by Williams and coworkers, who found CT to have a less than 50% negative predictive value and less than 75% positive predictive value for diagnosing blunt colonic injuries [66]. Several investigators have shown that a normal CT scan can be seen in 10.2% to 17% of patients with surgically proven perforated small bowel injury [67,69,74].

Multidetector CT findings

Bowel trauma can be classified as a partial or full-thickness injury. Partial-thickness bowel injury results in contusion of the bowel wall and can be seen on MDCT as a focal region of bowel wall thickening, usually greater than 3 to 4 mm in thickness [75–79]. Although most cases of bowel wall contusion resolve spontaneously, serial physical examinations or follow-up MDCT in 4 to 6 hours are useful to demonstrate healing of this injury.

Pathognomonic MDCT signs of full-thickness bowel injury are extravasation of oral contrast mate-

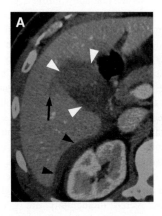
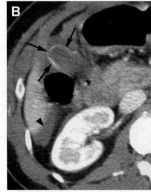
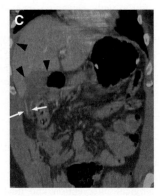

Fig. 7. Gallbladder avulsion following blunt trauma. (*A* and *B*) Axial MDCT images show a liver laceration (*arrow*) extending into gallbladder fossa with hemoperitoneum in the gallbladder (*white arrowheads*) and hepatorenal fossa (*black arrowheads*). The gallbladder (*arrows*) is not seen in the gallbladder fossa but more inferiorly in the peritoneal cavity. (*C*) Coronal MPR image shows the deformed gallbladder in the peritoneal cavity with perihepatic hemoperitoneum (*arrowheads*). At surgery, an avulsed gallbladder (*white arrows*) was seen in the upper right peritoneal cavity.

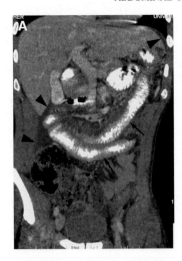
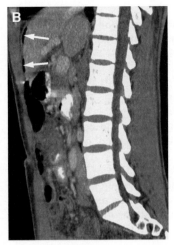

Fig. 8. Full-thickness bowel injury in a male patient admitted following blunt trauma. (*A*) Coronal and (*B*) sagittal 3-D reformatted images show proximal small bowel wall thickening (*black arrows*) with free intraperitoneal fluid (*arrowheads*) in the left upper abdomen and right flank. Free intraperitoneal air (*white arrows*) is seen anterior to the liver in the most nondependent aspect of the abdomen. Enterotomy was performed for full-thickness small bowel injury at laparotomy.

rial, extraluminal intestinal content, and discontinuity of the bowel wall [75,76,79,80]. Pneumoperitoneum may be subtle, and its presence is strongly suggestive of full-thickness bowel injury in the correct clinical setting (Fig. 8). Pneumoperitoneum can also result from air introduced into the peritoneal cavity during diagnostic peritoneal lavage or Foley catheter placement in patients with intraperitoneal bladder rupture. Extra-alveolar air may also decompress from the thorax into the peritoneal cavity, leading to a false-positive diagnosis of full-thickness bowel injury [81,82].

There should be a high index of suspicion for a bowel or mesenteric injury in a patient with blunt abdominal trauma when free intraperitoneal fluid is seen on MDCT without evidence of solid organ injury [10–12]. Unlike hemorrhage due to solid organ injury that is commonly seen in the perisplenic, perihepatic, hepatorenal space, and paracolic gutters, small triangles of free intraperitoneal fluid seen between the folds of the mesentery are especially concerning for occult bowel or mesenteric injury [83,84]. Free fluid without solid organ injury was found by Fakhry and coworkers to be associated with

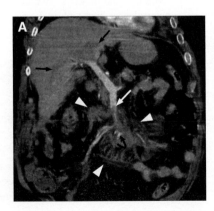
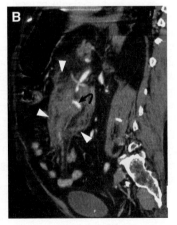

Fig. 9. Mesenteric injury in a 63-year-old man admitted following a motorcycle collision. (*A*) Coronal and (*B*) sagittal MPR images show a large mesenteric hematoma (*arrowheads*) with active bleeding (*curved arrows*) in the midabdomen. A mesenteric hematoma surrounds the superior mesenteric vein. Thrombus (*white arrow*) is also seen within the superior mesenteric vein. A grade III liver laceration (*black arrows*) is seen extending into the porta hepatis.

Box 3. American Association for the
Surgery of Trauma Renal Injury grading
scale and description

AAST grade I[a]: Renal contusion or subcapsular hematoma
AAST grade II[a]: Laceration < 1 cm deep
that does not involve the collecting
system, nonexpanding perinephric
hematoma
AAST grade III: Laceration > 1 cm deep
without collecting system involvement
AAST grade IV: Laceration extending into
the collecting system, main renal artery, or vein injury with contained
hemorrhage
AAST grade V: Shattered kidney, avulsion
of renal hilum with devascularized
kidney

[a] Advance one grade for bilateral injuries
up to grade III.
From Moore EE, Shackford SR, Pachter
HL, et al. Organ injury scaling: spleen,
liver and kidney. J Trauma 1989;29:1664;
with permission.

an 84.2% incidence of small bowel injury [67]. The
combination of free fluid and pneumoperitoneum
increased the sensitivity in detecting perforated small
bowel injury to 97%.

Mesenteric injuries can be divided into surgical or
nonsurgical lesions. The accuracy of CT in predicting
the need for surgical intervention ranges from 54% to
100% [72,78,85]. CT signs of a surgical mesenteric
injury include active bleeding within the mesentery or
bowel wall thickening associated with mesenteric
stranding or hematoma (Fig. 9). Focal mesenteric
stranding or hematoma without bowel wall thickening and isolated free intraperitoneal fluid are nonspecific CT findings of mesenteric injury. In these
patients, serial physical examinations and a repeat CT
scan at 6 to 8 hours are important means of assessing
the progression of injury [78,80,85].

Renal trauma

Renal injury is seen in approximately 10% of all
patients with blunt abdominal trauma [86,87].

Patients with renal trauma may be asymptomatic,
present with flank pain, or have microscopic or gross
hematuria. As many as 85% of patients with gross
hematuria have a major renal injury [88], whereas
microhematuria can be seen in 25% to 35% of patients with grade IV or V injuries [89,90]. The decision to image for evaluation of potential renal injury
rests not only on the presence of hematuria but also
on the mechanism of injury and clinical factors such
as hemodynamic stability, the reliability of physical
examination, a decreasing hematocrit, or evidence of
major flank impact [91].

Traditionally, a one-shot intravenous pyelogram
has been used to exclude a major renal injury in the
hemodynamically stable patient with blunt trauma.
CT has since replaced the intravenous pyelogram
owing to its high diagnostic accuracy and is currently
the test of choice for assessing renal injury.

Types of renal injuries

The spectrum of renal injuries ranges from minor
trauma requiring no treatment to major life-
threatening renal injuries that require surgical intervention. To help predict the outcome and to guide
management of renal trauma, the AAST has created
a renal injury grading scale (Box 3) [92]. The scale
ranges from grades I to V, with severity increasing
with higher grade. Grades I and II represent minor
injuries and account for approximately 85% of all
renal injuries. These injuries do not typically require
treatment. Grades IV and V are severe injuries that
always require treatment, often surgical. A grade III
injury may or may not require intervention.

Minor renal injuries include contusions, small
subcapsular or perinephric hematomas, and super-

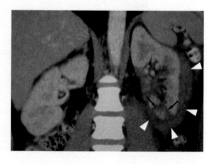

Fig. 10. Minor renal injury in a 42-year-old man. MDCT
coronal MPR image shows a small perinephric hematoma
(*arrowheads*) with lacerations (*arrows*) in the lower pole of
the left kidney that do not involve the calyx.

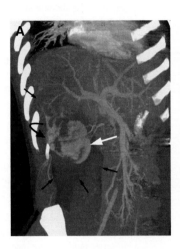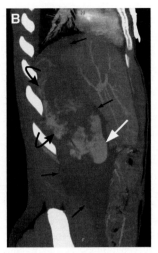

Fig. 11. Catastrophic renal injury in a 16-year-old male involved in a motor vehicle collision. (*A*) MDCT coronal oblique and (*B*) sagittal 3-D images show active bleeding (*curved arrows*) from a shattered kidney (*white arrows*). A large retroperitoneal hematoma (*black arrows*) is seen extending from the diaphragm into the pelvis. This hematoma displaced the liver and small bowel anteriorly. Renal arteriography and embolization were performed to control bleeding.

ficial lacerations. A contusion is seen on CT as an ill-defined region of hypodensity within the renal parenchyma. Subcapsular renal hematomas are infrequently seen owing to the strong attachment of the capsule to the underlying parenchyma. A subcapsular hematoma will usually be crescent shaped and indent the underlying renal tissue. These injuries typically resolve over time without sequelae. Rarely, a Page kidney may result from a subcapsular hematoma. In this entity, there is chronic compression of the underlying renal parenchyma from a nonresolving subcapsular hematoma. Local ischemia causes excess secretion of renin, resulting in hypertension.

A laceration will appear as a linear or branching well-defined hypodensity (Fig. 10). A minor renal laceration will be less than 1 cm deep and will not extend into the medulla or collecting system. Once a laceration extends into the collecting system, it is considered a grade IV injury. Initial CT images are obtained before the excretory phase of the kidney. Delayed images obtained 1 to 2 minutes after initial images are necessary to identify correctly the extravasation of contrast material from the injured collecting system.

Grade V injuries include avulsion of vessels at the renal hilum causing devascularization of the entire kidney and shattered kidney (Fig. 11). These catastrophic injuries require angiographic embolization or surgery to control bleeding.

Two other types of injuries can be seen that are not included on the current AAST renal injury grading scale. The first is subtotal or segmental renal infarction (Fig. 12). CT will show a well-defined, wedge-shaped region of hypodensity within the parenchyma. Segmental renal infarctions are thought to result from abrupt mechanical stretching of a renal arterial branch at the time of impact, causing a focal intimal tear and subsequent thrombosis [93]. If the segmental infarction is an isolated renal injury, no treatment is required [94,95].

The second type of injury not included on the current AAST renal injury grading scale is a renal parenchymal vascular injury, such as active extravasation of contrast. Unlike extravasation from an injured urinary collecting system, active extravasation from an injured renal parenchymal blood vessel will be evident on the initial CT images (Fig. 11).

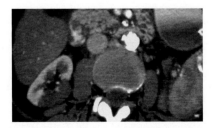

Fig. 12. Segmental renal infarction in a 66-year-old woman. MDCT axial image shows a lower pole segmental infarction of the right kidney (*black arrowhead*). Well-defined margins are seen between the infarct and normal renal parenchyma.

These injuries are considered major renal injuries that require surgery or angiographic embolization.

Summary

MDCT is the imaging modality of choice to evaluate the hemodynamically stable patient who has blunt trauma. Technical advances have made it possible to scan rapidly during vascular, parenchymal, and excretory phases with optimal contrast enhancement. The volumetric data acquired can be used to obtain high-resolution MPR, MIP, and 3-D color images. These views have not only helped to display complex injuries but have also significantly increased the diagnostic capabilities, accuracy, and confidence of the trauma radiologist. MDCT has had a major impact on the number of patients with solid organ injury managed nonoperatively at the authors' center.

References

[1] Fabian TC, Mangiante EC, White TJ, et al. A prospective study of 91 patients undergoing both computed tomography and peritoneal lavage following blunt trauma. J Trauma 1986;26:602–8.

[2] Kearney Jr PA, Vahey T, Burney RE, et al. Computed tomography and diagnostic peritoneal lavage in blunt abdominal trauma: their combined role. Arch Surg 1989;124:344–7.

[3] Federle MP. Computed tomography in blunt abdominal trauma. Radiol Clin North Am 1983;21:461–75.

[4] Malhotra AK, Fabian TC, Katsis SB, et al. Blunt bowel and mesenteric injuries: the role of screening computed tomography. J Trauma 2000;48:991–8.

[5] Nastanski F, Cohen A, Lush SP, et al. The role of oral contrast administration immediately prior to the computed tomographic evaluation of the blunt trauma victim. Injury 2001;32(7):545–9.

[6] Federle MP, Peitzman A, Krugh J. Use of oral contrast material in abdominal trauma CT scans: is it dangerous? J Trauma 1995;38(1):51–3.

[7] Federle MP, Yagan N, Peitzman AB, et al. Abdominal trauma: use of oral contrast material for CT is safe. Radiology 1997;205(1):91–3.

[8] Federle MP, Goldberg HI, Kaiser JA, et al. Evaluation of abdominal trauma by computed tomography. Radiology 1981;138(3):637–44.

[9] Shanmuganathan K, Mirvis SE, Sover ER. Value of contrast-enhanced CT in detecting active hemorrhage in patients with blunt abdominal and pelvic trauma. AJR Am J Roentgenol 1993;161(1):65–9.

[10] Livingston DH, Lavery RF, Passamante MR, et al.

Free fluid on abdominal computed tomography without solid organ injury after blunt abdominal trauma does not mandate celiotomy. Am J Surg 2001;182(1): 6–9.

[11] Harris HW, Morabito DJ, Mackersie RC, et al. Leukocytosis and free fluid are important indicators of isolated intestinal injury after blunt trauma. J Trauma 1999;46(4):656–9.

[12] Brasel KJ, Olson CJ, Stafford RE, et al. Incidence and significance of free fluid on abdominal computed tomographic scan in blunt trauma. J Trauma 1998; 44(5):889–92.

[13] Mirvis SE, Duham CM. Abdominal/pelvic trauma. In: Mirvis SE, Young JW, editors. Imaging in trauma and critical care. 1st edition. Baltimore: Williams and Wilkins; 1992. p. 155–61.

[14] Pachter HL, Guth AA, Hofstetter SR, et al. Changing patterns in the management of splenic trauma: the impact of nonoperative management. Ann Surg 1998; 227(5):708–17.

[15] Haan JM, Bochicchio GV, Kramer N, et al. Nonoperative management of blunt splenic injury: a 5-year experience. J Trauma 2005;58:492–8.

[16] Wasvary H, Howells G, Villalba M, et al. Nonoperative management of adult blunt splenic trauma: a 15-year experience. Am Surg 1997;68(8):694–9.

[17] Sclafani SJA, Shaftan GW, Scalea TM, et al. Nonoperative salvage of computed tomography–diagnosed splenic injuries: utilization of angiography for triage and embolization for hemostasis. J Trauma 1995; 39(5):818–25.

[18] Wing VW, Federle MP, Morris JA, et al. The clinical impact of CT for blunt abdominal trauma. AJR Am J Roentgenol 1985;145:1191–4.

[19] Federle MP, Courcoulas AP, Powell M, et al. Blunt splenic injury in adults: clinical and CT criteria for management, with emphasis on active extravasation. Radiology 1998;206(1):137–42.

[20] Moore EE, Cogbill TH, Jurkovich GJ, et al. Organ injury scaling: spleen and liver (1994 revision). J Trauma 1995;38(3):323–4.

[21] Mirvis SE, Whitley NO, Gens DR. Blunt splenic trauma in adults: CT-based classification and correlation with prognosis and treatment. Radiology 1989; 171:33–9.

[22] Navarrete-Navarro P, Vazquez G, Bosch JM, et al. Computed tomography vs clinical and multidisciplinary procedures for early evaluation of severe abdominal and chest trauma—a cost analysis approach. Intensive Care Med 1996;22:208–12.

[23] Becker CD, Spring P, Glattli A, et al. Blunt splenic trauma in adults: can CT findings be used to determine the need for surgery? AJR Am J Roentgenol 1994;162: 343–7.

[24] Buntain WL, Gould HR, Maull KI. Predictability of splenic salvage by computed tomography. J Trauma 1998;28:24–34.

[25] Peitzman AB, Heil B, Rivera L, et al. Blunt splenic injury in adults: multi-institutional study of the Eastern

Association for the Surgery of Trauma. J Trauma 2000;49(2):177–87.

[26] Miller LA, Mirvis SE, Shanmuganathan K, et al. CT diagnosis of splenic infarction in blunt trauma: imaging features, clinical significance and complications. Clin Radiol 2004;59(4):342–8.

[27] Romano S, Scaglione M, Gatta G, et al. Association of splenic and renal infarctions in acute abdominal emergencies. Eur J Radiol 2004;50(1):48–58.

[28] Davis KA, Fabian TC, Croce MA, et al. Improved success in nonoperative management of blunt splenic injury: embolization of splenic artery pseudoaneurysm. J Trauma 1998;44:1008–13.

[29] Shanmuganathan K, Mirvis SE, Boyd-Kranis R, et al. Nonsurgical management of blunt splenic injury: use of CT criteria to select patients for splenic arteriography and potential endovascular therapy. Radiology 2000;217(1):75–82.

[30] Haan J, Ilahi ON, Kramer M, et al. Protocol-driven nonoperative management in patients with blunt splenic trauma and minimal associated injury decreases length of stay. J Trauma 2003;55(2):317–21.

[31] Hagiwara A, Fukushima H, Murata A, et al. Blunt splenic injury: usefulness of transcatheter arterial embolization in patients with a transient response to fluid resuscitation. Radiology 2005;235(1):57–64.

[32] Uecker J, Pickett C, Dunn E. The role of follow-up radiographic studies in nonoperative management of spleen trauma. Am Surg 2001;67(1):22–5.

[33] Thaemert BC, Cogbill TH, Lambert PJ. Nonoperative management of splenic injury: are follow-up computed tomographic scans of any value? J Trauma 1997;43(5): 748–51.

[34] Federle MP. Splenic trauma: is follow-up CT of value? Radiology 1995;194(1):23–4.

[35] Carmona RH, Lim Jr RC, Clark GC. Morbidity and mortality in hepatic trauma: a 5-year study. Am J Surg 1982;144(1):88–94.

[36] Croce MA, Fabian TC, Menke PG, et al. Nonoperative management of blunt hepatic trauma is the treatment of choice for hemodynamically stable patients: results of a prospective trial. Ann Surg 1995;221(6):744–53.

[37] Sherman HF, Savage BA, Jones LM, et al. Nonoperative management of blunt hepatic injuries: safe at any grade? J Trauma 1994;37(4):616–21.

[38] Mirvis SE, Whitley NO, Vainwright JR, et al. Blunt hepatic trauma in adults: CT-based classification and correlation with prognosis and treatment. Radiology 1989;171(1):27–32.

[39] Becker CD, Gal I, Baer HU, et al. Blunt hepatic trauma in adults: correlation of CT injury grading with outcome. Radiology 1996;201(1):215–20.

[40] Meredith JW, Young JS, Bowling J, et al. Nonoperative management of blunt hepatic trauma: the exception or the rule? J Trauma 1994;36(4):529–34.

[41] Pachter HL, Knudson MM, Esrig B, et al. Status of nonoperative management of blunt hepatic injuries in 1995: a multicenter experience with 404 patients. J Trauma 1996;40:31–8.

[42] Poletti PA, Mirvis SE, Shanmuganathan K, et al. CT criteria for management of blunt liver trauma: correlation with angiographic and surgical findings. Radiology 2000;216:418–27.

[43] Shanmuganathan K, Mirvis SE. CT scan evaluation of blunt hepatic trauma. Radiol Clin North Am 1998; 36:399–411.

[44] Patten RM, Spear RP, Vincent LM, et al. Traumatic lacerations of the liver limited to the bare area: CT findings in 25 patients. AJR Am J Roentgenol 1993; 160:1019–22.

[45] Shanmuganathan K. Multidetector row CT imaging of blunt abdominal trauma. Semin Ultrasound CT MRI 2004;25:180–204.

[46] Beal SL. Fatal hepatic hemorrhage: an unresolved problem in the management of complex liver injuries. J Trauma 1990;30:163–9.

[47] Ochsner MG, Jaffin JH, Golocovsky M, et al. Major hepatic trauma. Surg Clin North Am 1993;73:337–52.

[48] Ciresi KF, Lim Jr RC. Hepatic vein and retrohepatic vena caval injury. World J Surg 1990;14:472–7.

[49] Savolaine ER, Grecos GP, Howard J, et al. Evolution of CT findings in hepatic hematoma. J Comput Assist Tomogr 1985;9:1090–6.

[50] Fang JF, Chen RJ, Wong YC, et al. Classification and treatment of pooling of contrast material on computed tomographic scan of blunt hepatic trauma. J Trauma 2000;49:1083–8.

[51] Fang JF, Chen RJ, Wong YC, et al. Pooling of contrast material on computed tomography mandates aggressive management of blunt hepatic injury. Am J Surg 1998;176:315–9.

[52] Wong YC, Wang LJ, See LC, et al. Contrast material extravasation on contrast-enhanced helical computed tomographic scan of blunt abdominal trauma: its significance on the choice, time, and outcome of treatment. J Trauma 2003;54:164–70.

[53] Hagiwara A, Murata A, Matsuda T, et al. The efficacy and limitations of transarterial embolization for severe hepatic injury. J Trauma 2002;52(6):1091–6.

[54] Carillo EH, Spain DA, Wohltmann CD, et al. Interventional techniques are useful adjuncts in nonoperative management of hepatic injuries. J Trauma 1999;46: 619–22.

[55] Goldman R, Zilkowski M, Mullins R, et al. Delayed celiotomy for the treatment of bile leak, compartment syndrome, and other hazards of nonoperative management of blunt liver injury. Am J Surg 2003; 185:492–7.

[56] Goffette PP, Laterre PF. Traumatic injuries: imaging and intervention in post-traumatic complications (delayed intervention). Eur Radiol 2002;12:994–1021.

[57] Allins A, Ho T, Nguyen TH, et al. Limited value of routine follow-up CT scans in nonoperative management of blunt liver and splenic injuries. Am Surg 1996; 62(1):883–6.

[58] Hsieh CH, Chen RJ, Fang JF, et al. Liver abscess after nonoperative management of blunt liver injury. Langenbecks Arch Surg 2003;387:343–7.

[59] Knudson MM, Lim Jr RC, Oakes DD, et al. Non-operative management of blunt liver injuries in adults: the need for continued surveillance. J Trauma 1990; 30(12):1494–500.

[60] Esensten M, Ralls PW, Colletti P, et al. Posttraumatic intrahepatic biloma: sonographic diagnosis. AJR Am J Roentgenol 1983;140(2):303–5.

[61] Weissmann HS, Byun KJ, Freeman LM. Role of Tc-99m IDA scintigraphy in the evaluation of hepato-biliary trauma. Semin Nucl Med 1983;13(3):199–222.

[62] D'Amours SK, Simons RK, Scudamore CH, et al. Major intrahepatic bile duct injuries detected after laparotomy: selective nonoperative management. J Trauma 2001;50:480–4.

[63] Ball DS, Friedman AC, Radecki PD, et al. Avulsed gallbladder: CT appearance. J Comput Assist Tomogr 1988;12(3):538–9.

[64] Erb RE, Mirvis SE, Shanmuganathan K. Gallbladder injury secondary to blunt trauma: CT findings. J Comput Assist Tomogr 1994;18(5):778–84.

[65] Soderstrom CA, Maekawa K, Dupriest Jr RW, et al. Gallbladder injuries resulting from blunt abdominal trauma: an experience and review. Ann Surg 1981; 193(1):60–6.

[66] Williams MD, Watts D, Fakhry S. Colon injury after blunt abdominal trauma: results of the EAST Multi-Institutional Hollow Viscus Injury study. J Trauma 2003;55:906–12.

[67] Fakhry S, Watts D, Luchette FA for the EAST Multi-Institutional HVI Research Group. Current diagnostic approaches lack sensitivity in the diagnosis of perforated blunt small bowel injury: analysis from 275,557 trauma admissions from the EAST Multi-Institutional HVI Trial. J Trauma 2003;54:295–306.

[68] Watts DD, Fakhry SM for the EAST Multi-Institutional HVI Research Group. Incidence of hollow viscus injury in blunt trauma: an analysis from 275,557 trauma admissions from the EAST Multi-Institutional Trial. J Trauma 2003;54:289–94.

[69] Sharma OP, Oswanski MF, Singer D, et al. The role of computed tomography in diagnosis of blunt intestinal and mesenteric trauma (BIMT). J Emerg Med 2004; 27(1):55–67.

[70] Fakhry SM, Browstein M, Watts DD, et al. Relatively short diagnostic delays (<8 hours) produce morbidity and mortality in blunt small bowel injury: an analysis of time to operative intervention in 198 patients from a multicenter experience. J Trauma 2000; 48:408–14.

[71] Malhotra AK, Fabian TC, Katsis SB, et al. Blunt bowel and mesenteric injuries: the role of screening computed tomography. J Trauma 2000;48(6):991–8.

[72] Killeen KL, Shanmuganathan K, Poletti PA, et al. Helical computed tomography of bowel and mesenteric injuries. J Trauma 2001;51(1):26–36.

[73] Janzen DL, Zwirewich CV, Breen DJ, et al. Diagnostic accuracy of helical CT for detection of blunt bowel and mesenteric injuries. Clin Radiol 1998;53(3): 193–7.

[74] Fang JF, Chen RJ, Lin BC, et al. Small bowel perforation: is urgent surgery necessary? J Trauma 1999; 47:515–20.

[75] Mirvis SE, Gens DR, Shanmuganathan K. Rupture of bowel after blunt abdominal trauma: diagnosis with CT. AJR Am J Roentgenol 1992;159(6):1217–21.

[76] Rizzo MJ, Federle MP, Griffiths BG. Bowel and mesenteric injury following blunt abdominal trauma: evaluation with CT. Radiology 1989;173(1):143–8.

[77] Breen DJ, Janzen DL, Zwirewich CV, et al. Blunt bowel and mesenteric injury: diagnostic performance of CT signs. J Comput Assist Tomgr 1997;21: 706–12.

[78] Dowe MF, Shanmuganathan K, Mirvis SE, et al. CT findings of mesenteric injury after blunt trauma: implications for surgical intervention. AJR Am J Roentgenol 1997;168:425–8.

[79] Brody JM, Leighton DB, Murphy BL, et al. CT of blunt trauma bowel and mesenteric injury: typical findings and pitfalls in diagnosis. Radiographics 2000; 20:1525–36.

[80] Donahue JH, Federle MP, Griffiths BG, et al. Computed tomography in the diagnosis of blunt intestinal and mesenteric injuries. J Trauma 1987;27(1):11–7.

[81] Cook DE, Walsh JW, Vick CW, et al. Upper abdominal trauma: pitfalls in CT diagnosis. Radiology 1986;159: 65–9.

[82] Kane NM, Francis IR, Burney RE, et al. Traumatic pneumoperitoneum: implications of computed tomography diagnosis. Invest Radiol 1991;26:574–8.

[83] Nghiem HV, Jeffrey RB, Mindelzun RE. CT of blunt trauma to the bowel and mesentery. Semin Ultrasound CT MR 1995;16:82–90.

[84] Levine CD, Gonzales RN, Wachsberg RH, et al. CT findings of bowel and mesenteric injury. J Comput Assist Tomogr 1997;21:974–9.

[85] Scaglione M, Pinto F, Lassandro F, et al. Value of contrast-enhanced CT for managing mesenteric injuries after blunt trauma: review of a five year experience. Emerg Radiol 2002;9:26–31.

[86] Bretan PN, McAninch JW, Federle MP, et al. Computerized tomographic staging of renal trauma: 85 consecutive cases. J Urol 1986;136:561–5.

[87] Brower P, Paul J, Brosman SA. Urinary tract abnormalities presenting as a result of blunt abdominal trauma. J Trauma 1978;18:719–22.

[88] Hardeman SW, Husmann DA, Chinn HKW, et al. Blunt urinary tract trauma: identifying those patients who require radiologic diagnostic studies. J Urol 1987; 138:99–101.

[89] Santucci RA, McAninch JM. Grade IV renal injuries: evaluation, treatment and outcome. World J Surg 2001;12:1565–72.

[90] Guerriero WG, Carlton CE, Scott R, et al. Renal pedicle injuries. J Trauma 1971;11:53–62.

[91] Mirvis SE. Injuries to the urinary system and retroperitoneum. In: Mirvis SE, Shanmuganathan K, editors. Imaging in trauma and critical care. 2nd edition. Philadelphia: Saunders; 2003. p. 483–517.

[92] Moore EE, Shackford SR, Pachter HL, et al. Organ injury scaling: spleen, liver and kidney. J Trauma 1989;29:1664–6.

[93] Clark DE, Georgitis JW, Ray FS. Renal arterial injuries caused by blunt trauma. Surgery 1981;90: 87–96.

[94] Mirvis SE. Trauma. Radiol Clin North Am 1996; 34:1225–57.

[95] Lewis DR, Mirvis SE. Segmental renal artery infarction following blunt abdominal trauma: clinical appearance and appropriate management. Emerg Radiol 1996;3:236–40.

ELSEVIER
SAUNDERS

Radiol Clin N Am 43 (2005) 1097 – 1118

RADIOLOGIC
CLINICS
of North America

Multidetector CT of the Female Pelvis

Kristina A. Siddall, MD*, Deborah J. Rubens, MD

Department of Imaging Sciences, University of Rochester Medical Center, Rochester, NY, USA

During the past 10 years, single-slice helical CT has been steadily replaced by multidetector row CT (MDCT). Multislice MDCT has allowed the acquisition of images of larger volumes in a single breathhold. Similar to high-resolution CT of the chest in the evaluation of interstitial lung disease, MDCT provides thinly collimated images with less volume averaging and much greater detail. Some images achieve resolution close to that of a gross pathology specimen.

Like single-slice CT, MDCT is the modality of choice for patients who cannot undergo MR imaging because of the presence of a pacemaker or a metallic foreign body, such as an aneurysm clip, and for patients who are claustrophobic. MDCT is becoming more widely available and less expensive than MR imaging and allows acquisition of an image series in a fraction of the time needed to obtain the multiple sequences of images in a single MR study.

Trauma centers in the United States are replacing single-slice helical CT scanners with MDCT scanners adjacent to patient-care areas. MDCT is now more accessible and is used in the setting of trauma and for excluding comorbid conditions in a patient who has vague symptoms. On newer picture archiving and communications systems, instantaneous reconstructions in any plane can be generated at the radiologist's workstation.

Staging of malignancy and screening for recurrent tumor are other uses of MDCT that have gained popularity recently. Current clinical applications of multislice CT of the abdomen include MDCT angiography of the liver for evaluation before liver transplantation in patients who have end-stage liver disease and of pancreatic tumors to determine resectability [1]. CT angiography of the abdomen is also used for evaluation of suspected mesenteric ischemia [1].

Multidetector CT of the pelvis

CT of the pelvis, in either males or females, usually is obtained in conjunction with CT of the abdomen. Incidental gynecologic findings are visualized more frequently now, because the adnexa, for example, are better seen with MDCT than on single-slice CT (Fig. 1). This improvement results largely from the decrease in partial-volume averaging. Suspected local or systemic disease in the pelvis that prompts CT evaluation can affect the adnexa or uterus, and these abnormalities now can be seen better with MDCT (Fig. 2). CT also plays a leading role in the aspiration or drainage of fluid collections such as pus or blood [2].

MDCT has been used successfully for staging and treatment planning of cervical and ovarian malignancy. CT has an advantage over clinical examination for staging, particularly for detecting ascites, metastases to the liver, and pelvic and para-aortic lymph node involvement [3]. In the past, inability to resolve abnormalities smaller than 1 cm has been cited as a disadvantage of CT, but resolution is much improved with new MDCT technology, and partial-volume averaging is significantly decreased. Ultrasound had been claimed to be superior to CT for staging ovarian cancer, because scanning occurs in both transverse

* Corresponding author. Department of Imaging Sciences, University of Rochester Medical Center, 601 Elmwood Avenue, Rochester, NY 14642.

E-mail address: kristina_siddall@urmc.rochester.edu (K.A. Siddall).

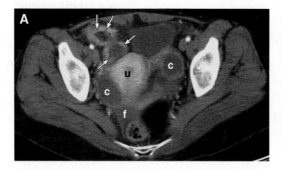
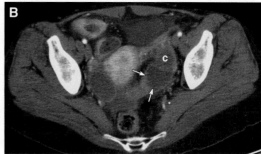

Fig. 1. A 33-year-old woman who had a Crohn's disease exacerbation. (*A*) The anterior loops of bowel, fluid-filled ileum (*arrows*) have thickened, enhancing walls. Incidental bilateral, physiologic adnexal cysts (c) are noted. u, uterus; f, free fluid. (*B*) The normal left ovarian cyst (c) is difficult to distinguish from the adjacent fluid-filled small bowel loop (*arrows*); in this case, the images must be interpreted sequentially.

and longitudinal planes; however, two-dimensional and three-dimensional reconstructions are now available with new MDCT technology. Coronal, sagittal, and oblique multiplanar reconstructions (MPRs) are performed using the source data obtained in the axial plane and can be used to evaluate the complex female pelvic anatomy. In addition to its capability of multiplanar imaging, CT is superior to ultrasound in detecting tumor adherence to bowel, retroperitoneal lymphadenopathy, and peritoneal implants. Furthermore, gynecologic oncologists may be more familiar with cross-sectional anatomy as seen with CT as opposed to ultrasound.

Evaluation of female pelvic vasculature has included MDCT of fibroids after uterine artery embolization and of pelvic arteriovenous malformations after embolization.

In addition to providing a multidimensional survey of pathology, the speed of MDCT reduces motion artifact that complicates interpretation. In fact,

CT boasts a more rapid acquisition of images and fewer contraindications and less motion artifact than MR imaging. Speed of scanning also allows the injection of a smaller bolus of intravenous (IV) contrast media to obtain optimal enhancement of anatomy and pathology while maintaining the diagnostic value of the study and preserving kidney function.

Protocols

At the University of Rochester Medical Center, there are single-slice, two-slice, six-slice, 16-slice, and 40-slice scanners. Standard protocols for evaluating the abdomen and pelvis and the pelvis alone do not vary significantly among these scanners (Table 1). Offline reconstructions are taken from the raw data acquired at 5-mm collimation, and coronal and sagittal reformats are then produced at 3-mm intervals.

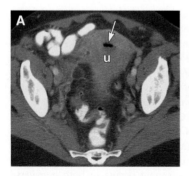
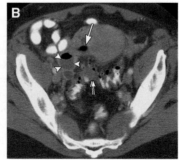
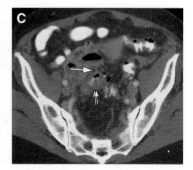

Fig. 2. Axial images from MDCT of the pelvis of a 68-year-old woman who had a perforated diverticular abscess. The abscess communicates with the uterus (u) and fallopian tube (*arrowheads*), both containing air (*arrows*). Note the inflamed, thickened sigmoid colon (*double arrows*) and fistula to the right adnexa in the third image (*arrow*).

Table 1
CT protocol

Area	Oral contrast	IV contrast injection rate (cm^3/s)	Delay before image acquisition (s)
Abdomen and pelvis	2 h when concern for colon or pelvic pathology	2	65–75
Pelvis	2 h	2	80–90

Pannu and colleagues [4] developed a multidetector scanner protocol for evaluation of peritoneal carcinomatosis, using a fast injection of 3 cm^3/second with a 30-second scan delay for the arterial phase and a 60-second scan delay for venous phase of the lower abdomen and pelvis. They developed a similar protocol for cervical cancer staging. Images were acquired in the opposite direction, from the symphysis pubis to the diaphragm, to image the cervix during maximal enhancement [5].

Other strategies have been used for optimal evaluation of the pelvis. Water has been used as an oral contrast agent to facilitate differentiation of calcified tumor implants from bowel loops. Cystic ovarian tumor can be easily confused with unopacified small bowel or unenhanced bladder. Delaying imaging until 1 hour after oral contrast administration has been completed and obtaining delayed images of contrast-filled bladder, respectively, can clarify these findings [6]. A scan delay after routine injection to image the pelvis optimizes venous enhancement for distinguishing between tumor and lymph nodes [6].

Normal anatomy

Familiarity with the normal radiologic anatomy of a female pelvis is necessary for assessing pathology on MDCT.

The true (lesser) pelvis is separated from the more superior false (greater) pelvis by an oblique plane extending across the pelvic brim from the sacral promontory to the symphysis pubis. The true pelvis of a woman contains the rectum, bladder, pelvic ureters, vagina, uterus, and ovaries. The broad ligament, a two-layer structure continuous with the peritoneum, contains the paired fallopian tubes, ovaries, uterine/ovarian vessels, and the parametrium and connects the uterus to the pelvic sidewall.

The uterus is a pear-shaped organ that is about the size of an adult fist, approximately 8 cm × 5 cm ×

2.5 cm or 9 cm × 6 cm × 4 cm in length, width, and thickness for nulliparous and multiparous women, respectively [7]. During menstruation, the uterus enlarges, is more vascular, and takes on a more globular shape.

The fundus or dome of the uterus is superior to the insertion of the fallopian tubes and is covered by peritoneum. The endometrial cavity of the uterus is central, flat, and triangular and can contain low-attenuation fluid. The amount of endometrial fluid is dependent upon the time of the menstrual cycle. The upper limit of the short-axis endometrial thickness in an asymptomatic postmenopausal female is about 12 mm, slightly higher than the 8-mm parameter used for ultrasound, probably because of the difference in imaging plane [8].

The uterine artery supplies the uterus and gives off superior and inferior branches to the cervix, fallopian tubes, and upper vagina. Anatomically, the uterine artery arises from the anterior branch of the internal iliac artery and crosses the ureter as it enters the bladder. The uterine veins drain into the internal iliac veins.

The cervix is the lower one third of the uterus, a cylindrical tube about 2 to 3 cm in length. The inferior aspect of the cervix is surrounded by the vaginal fornix. The vagina can be H-shaped in the axial plane, whereas the cervix is the elliptical or circular in cross-section, but distinguishing the two on CT can be difficult. If needed, placement of a tampon will provide contrast between the vagina and the cervix by adding air to the vaginal canal. The vagina lies anterior to the rectum and posterior to the bladder and is approximately 7 to 9 cm in length. The ureter passes lateral to the lateral vaginal fornix. The posterior fornix is a surgical landmark, providing direct access to the cul-de-sac [9].

The cul-de-sac, or rectouterine pouch of Douglas, is a virtual space that is outlined anteriorly by the posterior wall of the uterus, the supravaginal cervix, and the upper one fourth of the vagina; posteriorly by the rectum and sacrum; superiorly by the small bowel and the rectouterine ligament; and laterally by the sacrouterine ligaments (Fig. 3). A small amount of physiologic low-attenuation free fluid may be seen in the cul-de-sac dependent on the day of the patient's menstrual cycle. On ultrasound, free fluid in the cul-de-sac is observed over the whole length of the cycle in asymptomatic women of reproductive age but is seen most frequently during the 5 days before menses [10].

The oviduct is 1 to 5 mm in diameter at the isthmus and up to 1 cm in diameter at the ampulla [11]. The normal fallopian tubes or oviducts are not

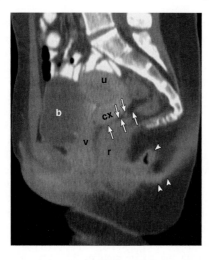

Fig. 3. Sagittal reformat of MDCT in a young female with Crohn's disease and concern for fistula formation. The cul-de-sac (*arrows*) is preserved without evidence of abnormal communication. A rectocutaneous fistula (*arrowheads*) is present. b, bladder; u, uterus; cx, cervix; r, rectum; v, vagina.

the external iliac vessels to its origin in the superolateral broad ligament.

The ovaries are paired, oval or almond-shaped, and seen on either side of the uterus. In a woman of childbearing age, the ovaries have a variable appearance of fluid attenuation, soft tissue attenuation, or physiologic cysts [12]. A normal ovary does not enhance significantly (Fig. 5) [13]. The position of the ovaries within the pelvis is variable and is affected by uterine size and orientation, bladder or distal colon distention, the presence of pelvic fluid or a pelvic mass, and by ovarian shape and size. In a woman of reproductive age, the average volume of the ovary is 11 cm^3 and is up to 4 cm on the long axis [9,14]. An important caveat is that sometimes, in the presence of a physiologic ovarian cyst in a premenopausal patient, the overall ovarian size will appear increased, perhaps 7 cm in length, even if the amount of ovarian tissue is normal.

In a normal premenarchal girl, the ovary is one third its adult size, and visualization on conventional CT is infrequent. Occasionally microcysts less than 9 mm in diameter can be seen [12]. Adolescent girls can have macrocysts larger than 9 mm and smaller than 3 cm in diameter. With MDCT, visualization of the ovaries in pediatric patients may become more commonplace. Ovaries in postmenopausal women are also small and are typically featureless with homogenous soft tissue attenuation [12].

The suspensory or infundibulopelvic ligament is a peritoneal fold that extends from the superolateral aspect of the ovary to the pelvic sidewall and carries the ovarian vessels. The suspensory ligament is contiguous with the peritoneum covering external iliac vessels and psoas muscle and posterolateral pelvic sidewall. The ovary is suspended by the mesovarium, a double peritoneal fold, which attaches to the upper and posterior broad ligament and carries the

visualized easily on routine CT; with the high resolution of MDCT, visualization may improve.

The ovaries can be difficult structures to identify on CT; however, with the new MDCT technique, reconstructions and thinly collimated images can be obtained, and unenlarged ovaries are seen more easily. Two different methods have been used in the past to locate the ovary on CT [12]. The course of the ovarian vein anterior to the psoas muscle leads directly to the ovary (Fig. 4). A second method for locating the normal ovary involves tracing the suspensory ligament from the peritoneum overlying

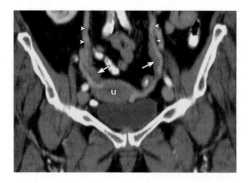

Fig. 4. Coronal reconstruction of a normal pelvis of a 75-year-old woman. Note that the ovarian veins (*arrowheads*) lead directly to the bilateral adnexal tissue (*arrows*). There is a faintly enhancing, small, postmenopausal uterus (u).

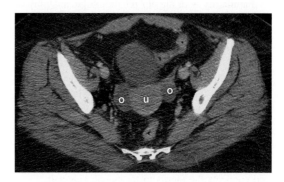

Fig. 5. An adolescent girl with a normal uterus (u) and ovaries (o) on contrast-enhanced MDCT.

ovarian vessels from the suspensory ligament to the ovarian hilum. The ovarian ligament connects the lower pole of the ovary to the uterus and carries the ovarian branches of the uterine artery.

The ovarian arteries arise from either side of the aorta inferior to the takeoff of the renal arteries. Each ovarian artery courses medial to the ureter at level of lower renal poles, crosses anterior to the ureter at the mid-lower lumbar level, and then courses lateral to the ureter in the pelvis.

Acute conditions

Ovarian cysts and rupture

Ovarian cysts are common incidental findings on MDCT of the female pelvis. On both unenhanced and contrast-enhanced CT, functional ovarian cysts are well circumscribed, usually less than 5 cm in diameter, demonstrating homogeneous, low-attenuation contents and an absence of internal architecture [15,16]. These physiologic cysts can be categorized further as follicular or corpus luteal cysts. On contrast-enhanced CT, corpus luteal cysts have thickened, crenulated, hyperdense or enhancing walls, which correspond to the collapsed, vascularized follicular walls formed after ovulation (Fig. 6) [17]. Distinction between follicular and corpus luteal cysts on CT is difficult because they are similar in size and composition, but differentiation is important because hypervascular corpus luteal cysts are more likely to be hemorrhagic. The presence of high-attenuation contents and an enhancing rim are suggestive of a hemorrhagic corpus luteal cyst (Fig. 7) [18].

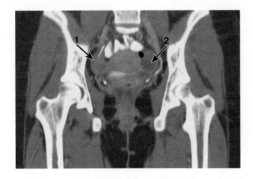

Fig. 6. Coronal multiplanar reformatting view in an adolescent girl with pelvic pain. The right corpus luteal cyst has a thicker wall and higher attenuation of its contents (*arrow 1*) compared with the functional cyst of the left ovary (*arrow 2*).

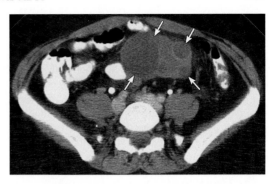

Fig. 7. A 45-year-old woman who had a multiloculated cystic mass (*arrows*) in the expected location of the left adnexa. Differential diagnosis would include a hemorrhagic cyst, paraovarian cyst, or adnexal torsion. Pathology confirmed hemorrhagic corpus luteal cyst.

Ruptured ovarian cysts are a common cause of an acute abdomen in women of reproductive age [19]. A ruptured hemorrhagic ovarian cyst is also a frequent cause of hemoperitoneum in young women [20]. Discontinuity or irregularity of the cyst wall and the presence of blood or contrast medium in the pelvis are CT findings indicative of cyst rupture [18,20].

Adnexal torsion

Ovarian or adnexal torsion is defined as partial or complete rotation of the ovarian pedicle, which carries the ovarian vessels. Torsion can occur in normal-sized or pathologically enlarged ovaries and can cause an acute abdomen in adolescent or older women [19]. The nonspecific presentation of adnexal torsion frequently prevents prompt diagnosis and treatment. Although ultrasound is the accepted first-line imaging modality for suspected torsion, it is important to be familiar with CT findings of ovarian torsion, because MDCT is being used more frequently for emergency department patients who have unclear clinical presentations. For example, if a torsed right adnexa rotates out of the pelvis and into the right lower quadrant, symptoms may mimic those seen in appendicitis [21]. Moreover, in a patient who has right lower pain suspected of being caused by appendicitis, early diagnosis of right adnexal torsion on CT could prevent irreversible damage.

Unenhanced CT findings of adnexal torsion include the presence of an adnexal mass that is relatively hyperdense to normal contralateral ovary. The mass may contain peripheral, small, hypodense, cystlike lesions and a small amount of pelvic free fluid [22]. Contrast-enhanced CT findings of adnexal torsion include (1) a peripheral, thickened, edematous ovarian cortex; (2) ipsilateral fallopian tube thickening; (3) ascites; and (4) uterine deviation to the side of the twisted adnexa [23,24]. In a case report of a 10-year-old prepubertal girl with torsion of a large ovarian cyst, contrast-enhanced CT revealed an enlarged ovary with small peripheral cystic structures, probably follicles [25]. Another marker of ovarian torsion is rotation of the adnexal mass to the contralateral side of the pelvis [26].

In addition to an adnexal cyst, a benign cystic teratoma (BCT), a benign ovarian tumor, is prone to torsion. Imaging findings of a torsed BCT include (1) wall thickness greater than 1 cm; (2) peritumoral infiltration; and (3) the presence of an enlarged, solid mass adjacent to uterus [27].

Initially, adnexal torsion disrupts the lymphatic and venous drainage of the ovary, and the arterial circulation is relatively preserved. If left untreated, torsion eventually can lead to disruption of the arterial supply and hemorrhagic infarction of the ovary. CT findings of infarction include a torsed mass with internal hemorrhage, mass wall thickness greater than 10 mm, and lack of enhancement of the solid component of the mass (Fig. 8) [24].

Pelvic inflammatory disease and tubo-ovarian abscess

Each year in the United States, more than 1 million women experience an episode of acute pelvic inflammatory disease (PID), with the rate of infection

highest among teenagers. PID is an ascending, polymicrobial cervical infection with *Chlamydia trachomatis*, *Neisseria gonorrhoeae,* or other organisms. Each year, more than 100,000 women become infertile because of scarring related to PID [28]. Eight percent of affected women develop tubal occlusion after one episode, 20% do so after two episodes, and 40% do so after three episodes [29].

Because many patients who have PID present with vague symptoms, treating physicians usually order MDCT through the emergency department. Although ultrasound and laparoscopy are regularly used for evaluating PID, early identification with MDCT could be helpful in preventing infertility, especially in the younger population affected by PID. CT is also useful when ultrasound results are equivocal or in assessing patients for whom routine antibiotic therapy has failed [26].

Early changes of PID detected on CT are an enlarged cervix with an enhancing canal, enlarged ovaries, dilated and enhancing fallopian tubes, periovarian stranding, and peritoneal enhancement [15,29]. In addition to these features, as PID progresses, CT demonstrates loculated or complex fluid collections associated with pyosalpinx, abnormal endometrial fluid and enhancement, loss of normal pelvic fat planes, and free fluid in the pelvis [29]. CT can also identify ileus, mechanical bowel obstruction, hydronephrosis or hydroureter, and rectosigmoid and other adjacent organ involvement (Fig. 9) [15,29]. Late findings of PID are peritonitis, tubo-ovarian or pelvic abscess, adhesions, or mesenteric infiltrates [21]. A tubo-ovarian abscess can be a thick-walled, fluid-density mass in the adnexal region

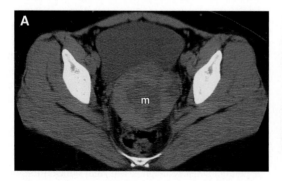 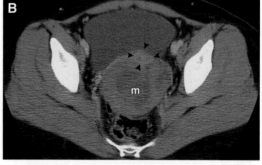

Fig. 8. A 31-year-old woman who had pelvic pain. (*A*) Axial image (without contrast) shows hyperdense, heterogeneous mass (m) in the cul-de-sac measuring 50 to 55 Houndsfield units (HU) peripherally and 10 to 20 HU centrally with peripheral low-attenuation cystic areas. The mass was attributed to adnexal pathology or a fibroid uterus. Nonvisualization of the left ovary, however, was concerning for torsion. (*B*) After IV contrast, a second axial image revealed no significant enhancement of the large mass (m), measuring 50 to 60 HU peripherally and 10 to 20 HU centrally. The mass displaces and compresses the normally enhancing uterus (*arrowheads*) anteriorly. Laparotomy revealed infarction of the left ovary.

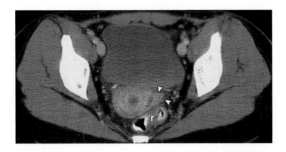

Fig. 9. A 28-year-old woman who had pelvic pain. Axial image shows an enlarged, enhancing cervix and adjacent inflammatory changes (*arrowheads*) consistent with cervicitis. Wall thickening and enhancement of the rectum (r) suggests extension of infection.

with internal septation and associated para-aortic lymphadenopathy (Fig. 10) [30]. Gas bubbles within this abnormal mass are specific for tubo-ovarian abscess and are rarely seen in PID [2].

Multidetector CT of the uterus

On unenhanced CT of the female pelvis, the uterus has a homogeneous, soft tissue density and a central low-density region that represents the endometrial cavity [8]. Kaur and colleagues [31] categorize the appearance of the uterus on contrast-enhanced CT into three patterns. Type 1 uterine enhancement is seen in the young, premenopausal patient who has a very vascular uterus. The enhancement is early in the subendometrial region then later appears in the subserosal tissue. The type 2 pattern, seen in both pre- and postmenopausal women, differs from type 1 in that there is no early subendometrial enhancement. Rather, early diffuse myometrial enhancement increases from the outer to inner myometrium over time. Type 3 enhancement, seen exclusively in postmenopausal patients, is faint or minimal within the myometrium [31]. Understanding these patterns of enhancement can be helpful in identifying uterine pathology such as fibroids or tumor.

Uterine myomas or fibroids

With MDCT, uterine myomas, also called leiomyomata or fibroids, are more frequent incidental findings. Fibroids are the most common benign tumors of the uterus and, except for pregnancy, are the most common cause of uterine enlargement. They are composed of smooth muscle and fibrous tissue and occur in 20% to 40% of women of reproductive age. Fibroids are asymptomatic in most cases but can present with bleeding, pelvic pain or pressure, urinary incontinence, or constipation. They also can contribute to infertility.

Fibroids typically are classified on MR imaging and are identified incidentally on CT or ultrasound [32]. Ninety percent of fibroids occur in the corpus and can be seen in a submucosal, intramural, or subserosal location [33,34]. The most common CT appearance of fibroids is enlargement of the uterus with lobulation of the outer contour [35]. Irregular areas of low attenuation, which can simulate tumor, are seen if the fibroid is undergoing hyaline degeneration or necrosis and hemorrhage [13,15]. On contrast-enhanced CT, uterine myomas can be

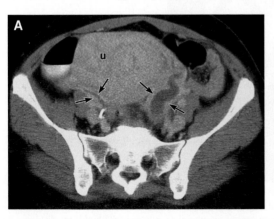

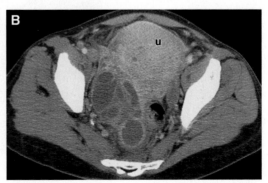

Fig. 10. (*A*) A 42-year-old woman who had abdominal pain. Bilateral tubular structures (*arrows*) with enhancing, thickened walls (left greater than right in caliber), consistent with hydrosalpinx or pyosalpinx in acute PID. Incidental note is made of enlarged fibroid uterus (u). (*B*) A 45-year-old woman who had fever and pelvic pain. A large, loculated, cystic mass with thickened, enhancing walls is located posterior to the uterus and cervix, consistent with tubo-ovarian abscess. Incidental note is made of enlarged fibroid uterus (u).

either homogeneous or heterogeneous and hypodense, isodense, or hyperdense relative to normal contrast-enhanced myometrium. Sometimes, a
whorled enhancement pattern is seen (Fig. 11).
Coarse calcifications are specific but are seen in only
10% of fibroids [15].

Very infrequently (<1% of cases), leiomyomata
degenerate into uterine sarcoma, and these two
entities are indistinguishable on CT [33]. A clue to
malignancy is the growth of a fibroid in a postmenopausal woman or the sudden growth in a
previously stable fibroid in a premenopausal woman
[15,35]. Of note, because fibroids are estrogen-
dependent, rapid enlargement can occur under estro-
gen stimulation.

Endometriosis

Endometriosis and adenomyosis are rarely identified on CT. Endometriosis, or functioning endometrium outside the uterus, can be found throughout the
body, most commonly in the ovary, and is evaluated
at laparoscopy. Ectopic endometrium in the ovary is
also referred to as a chocolate cyst or endometrioma.
A hyperdense focus inside an ovarian cyst is
suggestive of endometrioma [36]. Endometriosis has
variable attenuation on CT and is difficult to
distinguish from normal ovarian tissue or ovarian
pathology such as a teratoma or hemorrhagic cyst
[32]. For example, a complex cystic mass with high-
density fluid components and surrounding inflamma-

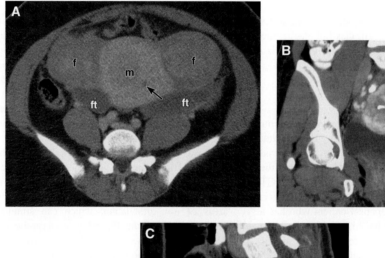

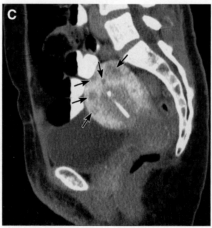

Fig. 11. (*A*) A 37-year-old woman who had pelvic pain. Bilateral large, exophytic, subserosal fibroids (f) demonstrate a whorled
enhancement pattern, secondary to hyaline degeneration. A more central intramural or submucosal fibroid (m) displaces the
endometrial cavity posteriorly and to the left side (*arrow*). Incidental note is made of bilateral fluid-filled dilated fallopian tubes
(ft), posterior to the uterus, consistent with hydrosalpinx. No inflammatory change or intense enhancement is seen to suggest
acute PID. (*B*) Coronal multiplanar reformatting view in a different patient shows the relationship of the fibroids to the
intrauterine device–containing uterine cavity. (*C*) Sagittal multiplanar reformatting view from same study as in B shows multiple
low-attenuation fibroids (*arrows*) in the myometrium.

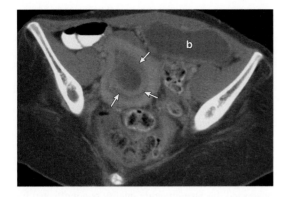

Fig. 12. A 23-year-old woman who had a 6-week pregnancy scheduled for dilation and curettage presenting with pelvic pain. A fluid-filled gestational sac (*arrows*) is seen in the endometrial cavity with wall enhancement similar to the myometrium. The bladder (b) is displaced anteriorly.

tory changes and fibrosis could be consistent with both endometriosis and tubo-ovarian abscess. Overall, CT can provide important information about extensive pelvic involvement (eg, in the cul-de-sac, bowel, bladder, or uterosacral ligaments) and can be particularly helpful in localizing a source of recurrent pain after hysterectomy [15].

Pregnancy

Normal gravid uterus

On CT, the gravid uterus is enlarged (Fig. 12). If contrast is used, placenta should enhance heteroge-

neously. Inhomogeneous enhancement of the placenta after contrast administration, hydronephrosis (in the second and third trimesters), and enlarged ovarian veins (up to 1 cm in diameter) are normal findings on the CT of a pregnant woman [37,38]. The ovaries and fallopian tubes are displaced superiorly and laterally. Periuterine venous varices are physiologic in pregnancy and in the postpartum period [13,39]. Fetal parts are not seen on CT until the late first or early second trimesters, and an appreciable fetal skeleton is not seen until the end of second trimester [37].

The postpartum uterus

On CT, the normal postpartum uterus appears enlarged with an average size of 9 cm × 12 cm × 14 cm [15]. A small amount of intrauterine blood or fluid can be a normal finding within 24 hours of an uncomplicated vaginal delivery [40]. About one fourth of patients also have intrauterine air on CT after vaginal delivery (Fig. 13) [41]. Uterine size returns to normal 6 to 8 weeks after delivery.

Enhanced CT of the pelvis after cesarean section can show transverse or vertical discontinuity at the incision site in the uterine wall, variable attenuation endometrial fluid, and small low-attenuation parametrial seromas or hematomas [39]. About half of patients have intrauterine air on CT after cesarean section [42].

Postpartum complications

CT often is used to evaluate postpartum women who have unexplained pain. Post–cesarean section

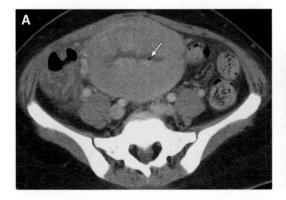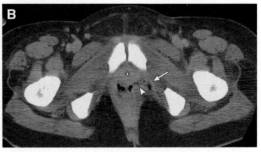

Fig. 13. A 25-year-old woman 4 days after vaginal delivery of twins with subsequent vaginal laceration and repair. (*A*) Contrast-enhanced MDCT demonstrates an enlarged, bulky uterus with homogeneous myometrial enhancement, a small amount of endometrial air (*arrow*), and low-attenuation endometrial fluid. (*B*) More caudal image demonstrates air in the vaginal fornix, a thickened vaginal wall, a vaginal wall defect (*arrowhead*), and adjacent soft tissue stranding and air (*arrow*) indicating infection.

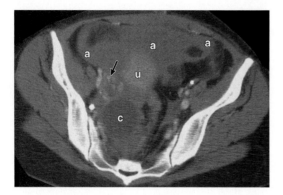

Fig. 14. A 35-year-old woman who had right lower quadrant pain. There is normal enhancement of the uterine fundus (u). A 4-cm low-attenuation cyst (c), probably a functional cyst, is seen in the expected location of the right adnexa. Just anterior to this cyst is a heterogeneous, cystic region with wall enhancement and discontinuity (*arrow*). A large amount of ascites (a) surrounds the uterus and adnexa, measuring 45 to 60 HU, consistent with blood. Findings were suspicious for ruptured ectopic pregnancy, ruptured corpus luteal cyst, or possible ovarian tumor. At surgery, patient had a ruptured right tubal pregnancy.

abscesses can be seen at the incision site, in the subcutaneous tissue, or elsewhere in the pelvis.

Endometritis complicates the postpartum course in 1% to 6% of patients undergoing cesarean section [42]. Uncomplicated endometritis may be undetectable on CT, or minimal endometrial fluid, debris, or gas can be seen. Imaging usually is reserved for patients who have suspected endometritis and persis-

tent fever and symptoms after adequate antibiotic therapy. CT is particularly useful to assess the extent of uterine involvement and to detect extrauterine complications such as abscess formation or septic ovarian vein thrombophlebitis, so that surgical intervention or anticoagulation can be planned [43,44].

Ovarian vein septic thrombophlebitis, or ovarian vein thrombosis, is an uncommon complication of postpartum endometritis or other infections, such as complicated PID. CT, not ultrasound, is the preferred imaging modality when septic thrombophlebitis is suspected, because imaging quality is not affected by bowel gas or free fluid. On contrast-enhanced CT, the affected ovarian vein is larger than 1 cm in diameter, contains a central low-density thrombus, and demonstrates an enhancing wall [39,41]. Eighty percent of ovarian vein thromboses occur on the right side and can extend into the inferior vena cava. Ovarian vein thrombosis is associated with inflammatory changes adjacent to the uterus, endometrial fluid, and ureteral compression and hydronephrosis [15].

Ectopic pregnancy

Most ectopic pregnancies are a consequence of scarring related to PID [28]. With in vitro fertilization and embryo transfer, the rate of ectopic pregnancy has increased [45]. The most common location of ectopic pregnancy is the fallopian tube [9]. Ultrasound detection of ectopic pregnancy is 99% sensitive and 84% specific [21], and MR imaging has been used for complicated cases [45]. On the other hand,

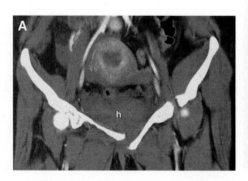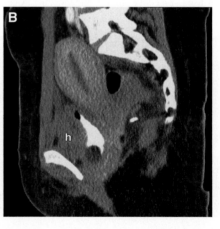

Fig. 15. A 23-year-old woman 3 weeks postpartum injured in a high-speed motor vehicle accident. Coronal (*A*) and sagittal (*B*) multiplanar reformatting views were obtained to evaluate the extent of pelvic fractures. Note the normal coronal and sagittal images of the uterus. Patient sustained bilateral acetabular fractures, pubic dislocation, and right inferior pubic ramus fracture. A large pelvic hematoma (h) displaces the intact bladder superiorly.

little has been written about CT detection of ectopic pregnancy. A patient who has a ruptured ectopic pregnancy and a nonspecific presentation may undergo CT, which may show hemoperitoneum and an abnormal mass (Fig. 14). As with ultrasound, hemoperitoneum seen on CT in a sexually active female can represent a ruptured ectopic pregnancy, even if the pregnancy test is negative.

Trauma

CT is the reference standard for demonstrating the sequelae of blunt injury to solid organs and is the imaging modality of choice to evaluate hemodynamically stable patients suffering blunt abdominal trauma (Fig. 15) [46,47]. MDCT's rapidly obtained high-resolution images and optimal timing of contrast enhancement provide improved detection of vascular injuries [47].

Contrast-enhanced MDCT is ideal for the evaluation of severe maternal trauma because visceral injuries without intraperitoneal hemorrhage are not detected routinely by ultrasound, and because CT is less user-dependent than ultrasound [46]. Despite these advantages, the appearance of the gravid uterus, as described in the prior section, can confound CT interpretation (Fig. 16).

The most common serious cause of blunt maternal trauma is motor vehicle accident, followed by physical abuse, assault, or fall [48]. The most common causes of fetal death associated with maternal trauma are maternal death, placental injury, or maternal hypotension [32,37]. Placental separation from the uterus or placental tear can lead to life-threatening fetal and maternal hemorrhage. If placental or uterine injury is not managed, it may lead to

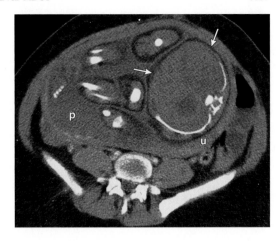

Fig. 17. A 20-year-old pregnant woman at 8 months' gestation ejected from a vehicle during collision. There is no fetal enhancement (*arrows*) and minimal placental (p) enhancement consistent with placental infarction and fetal death. u, uterus.

spontaneous abortion. Ultrasound evaluation after maternal injury alerts the clinician to possible fetal distress but does not consistently identify placental damage. Contrast-enhanced CT can distinguish avascular or infarcted regions of the placenta and identifies high attenuation regions in the nonplacenta uterus that indicate uterine disruption, contusion, or tear [37,47]. Although CT can demonstrate uterine rupture and retroperitoneal hemorrhage, direct detection of fetal injuries is rare (Fig. 17) [37].

Tumors of the female pelvis

Currently, CT, MR imaging, and ultrasound are used to detect and stage gynecologic malignancy. Each modality has its own limitations, and none supplants laparotomy as the reference standard. CT or MR staging is more helpful in advanced gynecologic cancer, when primary treatment is chemotherapy aimed at diffuse disease followed by possible surgery [32]. CT often is used to evaluate a palpable pelvic mass and can help identify the source, nature, and extension of the primary tumor [21].

Both understaging and overstaging of gynecologic malignancies occurs with CT, MR imaging, and ultrasound. In the evaluation of cervical cancer, CT may overstage tumor by identifying normal parametrium as abnormal or understage tumor when there is microscopic invasion of the parametrium or pelvic viscera [3]. Similarly, tumor invasion of lymph nodes smaller than 1.5 cm in diameter cannot be distin-

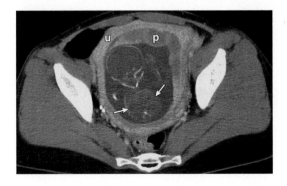

Fig. 16. MDCT of a 23-year-old woman at 20 weeks' gestation after motor vehicle rollover. Note the normal uterine (u), placental (p), and fetal (*arrows*) enhancement. No free fluid is seen.

guished from normal uninvolved lymph nodes on CT [3]. Both CT and MR imaging are limited in the evaluation of lymph node involvement because it is not possible to differentiate metastatic from non-metastatic hyperplastic nodes of similar size and shape [49].

In some cases, MDCT can be used for determining resectability of tumor and predicting surgical outcome. In a study of patients who had recurrent ovarian cancer and secondary cytoreduction, preoperative CT scans using oral and IV contrast agents identified hydronephrosis and pelvic sidewall invasion as significant indicators of tumor nonresectability [50].

Benign ovarian tumors

Seventy-five percent of ovarian tumors are benign [6]. The mature teratoma, otherwise known as the BCT or dermoid cyst, is the most common benign ovarian tumor in patients younger than 20 years old and is bilateral in 25% of cases [16,32]. On CT, an area of fat density within a cystic mass is diagnostic (Fig. 18) [51]. CT may show subtle calcification and an intralesional fat–fat or fat–fluid level [16,32,35]. The Rokitansky nodule, a classic finding of BCT, is a protuberance into the cystic cavity that may contain hair, bone, or teeth [32,51].

Rarely, BCT undergoes malignant degeneration, and CT can show a huge multiloculated, ovarian mass with intra-abdominal findings of ascites, omental infiltration, and retroperitoneal lymphadenopathy [52].

Other benign cystic neoplasms are mostly large (>10 cm in diameter) and thin-walled with central fluid attenuation [3,15]. Serous cystadenoma is the most common and is bilateral in 10% to 20% of cases [15]. The mucinous type of cystadenoma is much less common and demonstrates central fluid density higher than that of water, internal septation, and wall thickening [3].

Detection of smaller ovarian tumors is difficult for several reasons, mainly because the normal ovary itself is difficult to identify. If the ipsilateral suspensory ligament leads to or merges with a mass, this "ovarian suspensory ligament sign" is a "highly reliable" indicator that the suspected mass is ovarian in origin [12]. When the suspensory ligament is not obvious, identification of the ovarian vein joining the suspicious mass indicates that the mass probably arises from the ovary (Fig. 19).

Distinguishing between an ovarian mass and an adjacent lymph node can be also difficult, but in most cases the ovarian mass displaces the ureter postero-laterally and a lymph node displaces the ureter anteromedially [12]. Differentiating an ovarian mass from the uterus is possible by identifying the myometrial enhancement and the triangular endometrial cavity of the uterus [3].

Ovarian cancer

Once the ovarian origin of a mass is determined, identifying more suspicious lesions can lead to early detection and early treatment of malignancy. CT features that favor benign ovarian cyst over tumor are

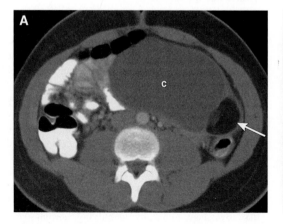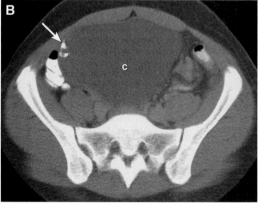

Fig. 18. A 13-year-old girl with crampy, left pelvic pain. (*A*) A large mass of fat and fluid (c) density is seen in the anterior abdomen arising from the left adnexa. The rounded area of fat density (*arrow*) seen laterally contains wispy strands of soft tissue, probably hair. (*B*) The contralateral dermoid cyst (c) in the same patient demonstrates a "toothlike" peripheral calcification (*arrow*).

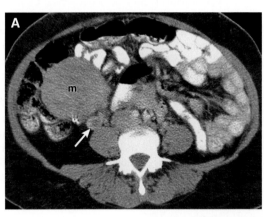

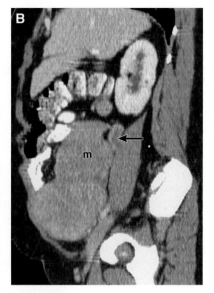

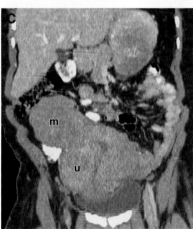

Fig. 19. A 44-year-old woman with abdominal pain. (*A*) Axial and (*B*) sagittal images demonstrate an intraluminal thrombus in the ovarian vein (*arrow*) adjacent to a large mass (m) in the expected location of the right adnexa. (*C*) Coronal image confirms that the right adnexal mass (m) is actually an exophytic fibroid arising from the uterus (u).

thin and smooth walls, homogenous contents, and absence of internal architecture [16]. In contrast, ovarian cancer on CT appears as a thick-walled, cystic or solid mass with irregular margins and with or without soft tissue components [35]. The soft tissue component of a malignant tumor enhances more than the adjacent pelvic musculature and less than myometrium [3].

Kawamoto and colleagues [6] proposed primary and secondary criteria to determine if an ovarian mass is benign or malignant (Box 1). If primary and secondary criteria are used, CT is 92% to 94% accurate in determining whether an ovarian mass is

benign or malignant [6]. For example, a predominantly cystic mass with a nodular enhancing wall and thick enhancing septa would be classified as malignant (Fig. 20).

Ovarian cancer accounts for 3% of new cancer cases in women and carries the worst prognosis of the gynecologic tumors with a 5-year survival rate of 44% [53]. Most ovarian malignancies are diagnosed at advanced stage III or stage IV. No good screening tool exists for ovarian malignancy. Seventy percent to 90% of malignant ovarian tumors are epithelial in origin, most commonly cystadenocarcinoma [3,6,16]. Germ cell tumors, stromal tumors, and metastasis, most commonly from gastrointestinal tract tumor, make up the remaining 30% of ovarian malignancies [3,16].

Ovarian cancer staging typically is done at exploratory laparotomy and resection, but preliminary staging by imaging is important for planning chemo-therapy and radiation and for determining the suitability of surgical resection (Box 2) [54]. Preoperative CT can aid in predicting which patients may not be amenable to primary surgical debulking and which patients may be better served by neoadjuvant chemotherapy [55]. It is important to identify solid implants to use chemotherapy to debulk tumor before surgery [32]. In 1999, Kurtz and colleagues [56] reported 92% sensitivity and 89% specificity for CT staging of ovarian tumors.

Metastases from epithelial-based ovarian tumors spread by direct extension to the uterus, fallopian tubes, colon, small bowel, and bladder. Pelvic lymph nodes often are bypassed in favor of para-aortic lymph nodes at the renal hilum, because the lymphatic drainage follows the ovarian veins. Advanced cystadenocarcinoma of the ovary is associated with ascites, hydronephrosis and urinary tract obstruction, and omental and peritoneal implants. The malignant ascites can be helpful in diagnosis in providing contrast from other pelvic and peritoneal structures. Omental metastases, or "omental cake," are soft tissue masses that replace the anterior intra-abdominal fat and displace the bowel from the anterior abdominal wall (Fig. 21) [3]. Mesenteric metastases appear as enhancing soft tissue masses infiltrating the mesenteric fat.

Peritoneal carcinomatosis, or peritoneal tumor implants, is found most commonly under the right hemidiaphragm, on the liver surface, and in the right paracolic gutter (Fig. 22) [3,4]. In the past, it was thought that CT was ineffective for staging ovarian

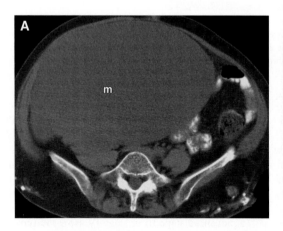
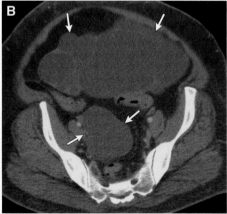

Fig. 20. (*A*) A premenopausal woman who had abdominal pain and increased abdominal girth. MDCT shows a large cystic mass (m) filling the abdomen and arising from the left adnexa. Pathology revealed ovarian cystadenocarcinoma. (*B*) A 52-year-old woman who had increasing abdominal girth and left lower quadrant pain. MDCT showed bilateral large, lobulated, septated, cystic adnexal masses (*arrows*) found to be cystadenocarcinomas.

Box 2. Ovarian cancer ataging

Stage 0: No evidence of primary tumor
Stage I: Tumor confined to the ovaries
  IA: Tumor limited to one ovary with capsule intact; no tumor on ovarian surface and no malignant ascites
  IB: Tumor limited to both ovaries with capsules intact; no tumor on ovarian surfaces and no malignant ascites
Stage II: Tumor of one or both ovaries with pelvic extension
  IIA: Tumor involvement of the uterus and/or fallopian tubes; no malignant ascites
  IIB: Tumor involvement of other pelvic organs; no malignant ascites
  IIC: Stages IIA or B with malignant ascites present
Stage III: Tumor of one or both ovaries with microscopic extrapelvic peritoneal metastasis and/or regional lymph node metastasis[a]
  IIIA: Microscopic extrapelvic peritoneal metastasis
  IIIB: Macroscopic extrapelvic peritoneal metastasis ≤ 2 cm in greatest dimension
  IIIC: Extrapelvic peritoneal metastasis > 2 cm in greatest dimension with or without regional lymph node metastasis
Stage IV: Distant metastasis beyond the peritoneal cavity[b]

[a] Involvement of the liver capsule is stage III disease.
[b] Involvement of the liver parenchyma is stage IV disease.
Adapted from Benedet JL, Pecorelli S. Staging classifications and clinical practice guidelines of gynaecologic cancers. Int J Gynaecol Obstet 2000;70:238; with permission.

cancer because peritoneal implants smaller than 2 cm in size were not adequately visualized [3,56]. Data from conventional and single-detector spiral CT scanners estimated 50% detection of peritoneal metastasis [4]. With thin-section MDCT and multi-

planar reformatting, small-volume primary disease, small metastases, and metastases at sites difficult to explore at surgery, such as the diaphragm, lesser sac, and porta hepatis, can now be identified. The false-negative rate for detection of metastases may be lower with these improvements in CT scanner technology. Reformatted images in the coronal, sagittal, and oblique planes facilitate identification and better characterization of tumor.

After any ovarian cancer therapy, CT is the imaging modality of choice to document residual tumor. It detects postoperative recurrence with an accuracy of 70% to 90% [35]. Postoperative CT scanning after surgical debulking may provide objective confirmation of the surgeon's assessment of residual disease [55]. Optimal resection demonstrates residual tumor less than 1 cm in greatest diameter [50].

Recurrent ovarian cancer is defined as the presence of disease after complete initial response to first-line therapy, negative findings at a second-look operation (if performed), and a disease-free interval longer than 6 months [50]. CT can detect response to therapy, residual tumor, or tumor recurrence with a sensitivity of 59% to 83% and a specificity of 83% to 88% before second-look surgery and may obviate the need for an additional laparotomy [6]. Early recurrent disease often can be detected at the margins of the vaginal cuff after hysterectomy (Fig. 23).

Uterine cancer

Endometrial cancer is the most common gynecologic malignancy, with approximately 40,000 new cases reported in the United States each year [53]. Patients present with postmenopausal bleeding, and therefore uterine cancer can be detected in its early stage. Endometrial cancer has the best prognosis of the gynecologic cancers, with a 5-year relative survival rate of 86% [53,54]. Ninety percent to 95% of endometrial cancers are adenocarcinoma by pathology [3,35]. Most uterine cancers do not require imaging at initial presentation; however, CT is helpful in patients who have equivocal pelvic examinations, obese patients, and patients who have aggressive disease or a large tumor such as uterine sarcoma [3]. Noncontrast CT is ineffective for detecting endometrial cancer, because the tumor typically is isodense to the uterus [35]. The uterus may be enlarged, and, on occasion, the mass may be hypodense to the normal uterine tissue or cause a nonspecific heterogeneous uterine attenuation [16]. Contrast-enhanced CT shows an enhancing lesion in the myometrium [3]. A fluid-filled endometrial

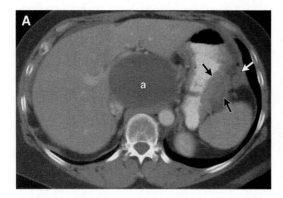

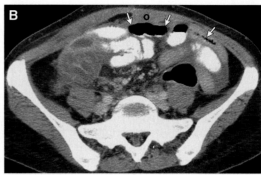

Fig. 21. (*A*) A 55-year-old woman who had a history of stage IIIC ovarian cancer. There is a soft-tissue density mass (*arrows*) between the stomach and spleen, consistent with omental cake. A stable fluid collection in the lesser sac represents loculated ascites (a). (*B*) A 46-year-old woman who had stage IV ovarian cancer. Omental cake (o) displaces bowel loops (*arrows*) posteriorly in the midline.

cavity may signify an obstructing tumor or may be secondary to surgery or radiation (Box 3) [3,16,54].

In the evaluation of endometrial cancer, the preoperative clinical examination understages the disease 22% of the time [57]. Cervical involvement is detected on physical examination or endocervical curettage. In the late 1990s, MR was identified as the only imaging modality to depict cervical invasion accurately [58]. CT now is valuable for staging endometrial cancer. CT detection of uterine disease and extrauterine disease is 83% and 86% accurate, respectively [16].

In the past, difficulties delineating the cervix and uterine corpus in the axial imaging plane limited evaluation of cervical tumor extension by CT [55]. Thin-collimation MDCT provides better detection of the depth of macroscopic cervical invasion. In the evaluation of advanced endometrial cancer, MDCT offers the advantages of screening for lymph node involvement and noninvasive confirmation of local or extrapelvic metastasis [3,32]. The greatest advantage of CT scanning in staging endometrial cancer lies in its ability to confirm pelvic sidewall or parametrial extension, because the presence of parametrial invasion requires irradiation rather than immediate surgery [58].

CT also is useful for diagnosing endometrial cancer recurrence, which appears as pelvic soft tissue

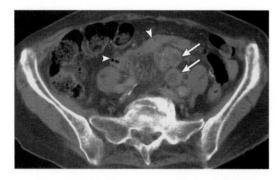

Fig. 22. An 83-year-old woman who had abdominal pain and vomiting. There are multiple mesenteric tumor implants, which demonstrate edge enhancement (*arrows*) and could easily be mistaken for loops of small bowel (*arrowheads*). MDCT multiplanar reformatting views could be useful to demonstrate that these lesions are not contiguous with bowel.

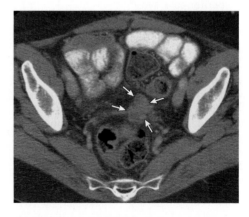

Fig. 23. A 55-year-old woman who had a history of stage IIIC ovarian cancer, status post cytoreduction and bilateral salpingo-oophorectomy 6 years ago. An enhancing cystic and nodular mass (*arrows*) arises from the left vaginal apex, consistent with recurrence.

Box 3. Uterine cancer staging

Stage 0: Carcinoma in situ (preinvasive)
Stage I: Confined to the body of the uterus
  IA: Tumor limited to endometrium
  IB: Tumor invades less than
    50% myometrium
  IC: Tumor invades more than
    50% myometrium
Stage II: Invades cervix but does extend
  beyond uterus
  IIA: Endocervical gland involvement only
  IIB: Cervical stromal invasion
Stage III: Local and/or regional spread
  IIIA: Involvement of the uterine serosa,
    direct extension or metastasis to
    the adnexa, and/or malignant cells
    detected in peritoneal fluid
  IIIB: Direct extension or metastasis
    to vagina
  IIIC: Metastasis to pelvic and/or para-
    aortic lymph nodes
Stage IV
  IVA: Invasion of bladder and/or
    bowel mucosa
  IVB: Distant metastasis

Adapted from Benedet JL, Pecorelli S.
Staging classifications and clinical practice guidelines of gynaecologic cancers.
Int J Gynaecol Obstet 2000;70:260;
with permission.

volume averaging, which can blur the planes between uterus, bladder, and bowel.

MDCT technology has improved CT staging for cervical cancer. The thinner tissue slices, better spatial resolution, and the availability of multiplanar reconstructions allow better detection of parametrial extension, pelvic sidewall disease, local organ involvement, lymphadenopathy, local tumor recurrence, and distant metastatic disease [5]. Sagittal

Box 4. Cervical cancer staging

Stage 0: Carcinoma in situ (preinvasive)
Stage I: Tumor confined to uterus
  IA: Microscopic invasion only
    IA1: Stromal invasion ≤3 mm deep
      or ≤7 mm wide
    IA2: Stromal invasion >3 mm or
      <5 mm deep or ≤7 mm wide
  IB: Clinically visible lesion or lesion
    greater in size than IA2
    IB1: ≤4 cm in greatest dimension
    IB2: >4 cm in greatest dimension
Stage II: Tumor invasion beyond uterus
  but not to pelvic wall or lower third
  of vagina
  IIA: No parametrial invasion
  IIB: Parametrial invasion
Stage III: Tumor extension to pelvic wall
  and/or lower third of vagina and/or
  tumor causing hydronephrosis or
  nonfunctioning kidney
  IIIA: Tumor involvement of the lower
    third of the vagina without pelvic
    sidewall involvement
  IIIB: Tumor involvement of the pelvic
    sidewall and/or hydronephrosis or
    a nonfunctioning kidney
Stage IV
  IVA: Tumor invasion of bladder or
    rectum and/or extension beyond
    true pelvis
  IVB: Distant metastasis

Adapted from Benedet JL, Pecorelli S.
Staging classifications and clinical practice guidelines of gynaecologic cancers. Int J Gynaecol Obstet 2000;70:294;
with permission.

masses or nodal enlargement, most often occurring within 2 years of initial staging and treatment [3,16].

Cervical cancer

Formerly, CT lacked the resolution necessary for primary staging of the low-volume and microscopic cervical cancer and was used only for staging, not for detection, of known cervical carcinoma. MR imaging also was used for staging and demonstrated a higher sensitivity for parametrial invasion and lymph node involvement than CT [49]. CT is, however, more accurate than clinical staging in stage II disease with parametrial involvement and in stage III disease with extension to the pelvic sidewall (Box 4) [16,54]. The major limitation of using axial CT images is partial-

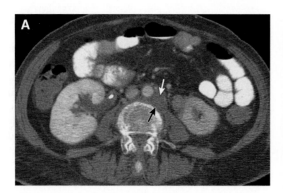
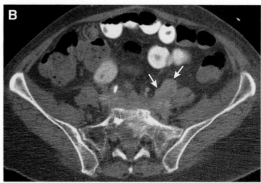

Fig. 24. A 61-year-old woman who had a history of stage IV recurrent squamous cell carcinoma of the cervix. (*A*) MDCT shows enlarged left para-aortic lymph node (*black arrow*) consistent with metastatic disease. (*B*) More caudally, enlarged left common iliac lymph nodes (*arrows*) also denote tumor spread. The left ureter (*white arrow*) is thickened and infiltrated with tumor. Right ureteral stent is seen.

reformatted images can confirm tumor involvement of the vagina and the body of the uterus. Three-dimensional volume rendering can define more accurately the location of tumor relative to surrounding structures and the precise relation of involved lymph nodes to the surrounding vessels [5].

On CT, early cervical cancer may appear as a cervical mass with areas of low attenuation secondary to necrosis, ulceration, or reduced vascularity. IV contrast agent should be administered for cervical cancer staging, because myometrial enhancement is necessary to distinguish normal cervical borders from the irregular hypodense borders of tumor [3]. Up to 50% of stage IB cervical cancers still are described as undetectable because they are isodense to normal cervical parenchyma [5].

CT findings of more advanced cervical cancer include cervical enlargement greater than 4 cm in diameter and an enlarged, fluid-filled endometrial cavity secondary to uterine obstruction by tumor [32,35]. Local spread and parametrial invasion are suspected if the cervical border is effaced and linear soft tissue stranding extends from the cervix into the paracervical fat [3]. Encasement of the ureter and a parametrial soft tissue mass are also specific signs of parametrial invasion on CT [59]. The International Federation of Gynecology and Obstetrics (FIGO) staging does not include evaluation of lymph node involvement; however, the prognosis of cervical cancer "depends heavily" on lymph node involvement [49]. Cervical cancer spreads along the iliac nodal chains and to the para-aortic lymph nodes (Fig. 24) [59]. Metastatic disease may also lead to bladder wall or ureteral invasion and subsequent hydronephrosis (Fig. 25). The advantage of MDCT

over other imaging modalities is the ability to detect extrapelvic metastasis without significant additional scanning time.

Brachytherapy or external beam radiotherapy is used for stage IIB, III, and IV cervical cancer [49]. CT can be used to evaluate tumor extent for radiotherapy, determine radiation therapy portals [3,16], and detect complications of radiation including uterine perforation, rectovesical fistula, sigmoiditis, rectal

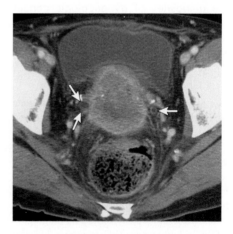

Fig. 25. A 67-year-old woman diagnosed with cervical cancer is seen for staging. An irregular, heterogeneous, bulky mass arises from posterior lip of an enlarged cervix and projects into the parametrial space. The mass encases the distal right ureter (*double arrows*), which is dilated as compared with the left ureter (*arrow*). Marked right hydronephrosis was present. Diagnosis was stage IIIB carcinoma of the cervix.

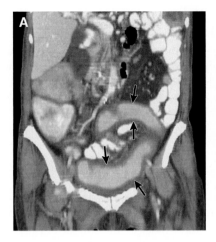
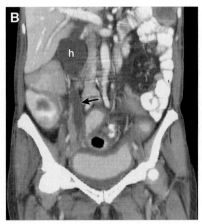

Fig. 26. Treated stage IIIB cervical cancer complicated by radiation proctitis and colitis. (*A*) Coronal reconstruction shows the abnormal wall thickening (*arrows*) of the sigmoid colon. (*B*) More posterior coronal image from the same patient shows marked right hydronephrosis (h) and hydroureter (*arrow*), secondary to extrinsic compression by distal tumor.

stricture, ureteral stricture, and sacral insufficiency fracture (Fig. 26) [16,60]. CT guidance is used for high-dose brachytherapy of cervical cancer. By correlating uterine wall thickness and the proximity of the uterus and cervix to the surrounding viscera on CT, it has been observed that thinner anterior lower uterine walls correlated to an increased late bladder and ureteral toxicity, and that thinner anterior upper uterine walls correlated with increased late small-bowel toxicity [61].

CT is effective for detecting recurrent cervical cancer, but the ability to differentiate postoperative fibrosis, postradiation fibrosis, and tumor recurrence is limited, and biopsy may be necessary [5,60]. Cervical cancer most frequently recurs at the sidewall in the pelvis or as a central soft tissue mass at the fornix after hysterectomy [5,60].

Vascular abnormalities

The ovarian vein arises from the periuterine venous plexus, courses anterior to the psoas muscle, and drains into the left renal vein or into the inferior vena cava on the right side. A dilated ovarian vein is larger than 7 to 8 mm in diameter. Dilated parauterine and ovarian veins are a common finding in multiparous women of childbearing age. On the other hand, pelvic varices may also indicate a serious underlying pathology, such as portal hypertension.

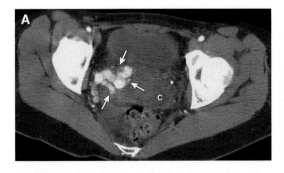
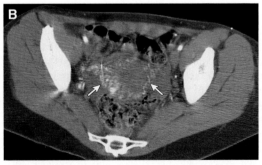

Fig. 27. A 34-year-old woman who had persistent uterine bleeding after embolization of uterine arteriovenous malformation. (*A*) Contrast-enhanced image 30 seconds after injection of contrast shows a tangle of dilated contrast-filled vessels (*arrows*) consistent with the known arteriovenous malformation. Low-density material in expanded vaginal cavity represents clot (c). (*B*) Delayed image obtained 90 seconds after injection shows retention of contrast and the bilateral uterine artery feeders (*arrows*) of the arteriovenous malformation. Patient returned to the interventional radiology suite for further embolization.

Incompetent ovarian veins are associated with the pelvic congestion or pelvic pain syndrome [62]. Retrograde filling of ovarian veins during the arterial phase of CT indicates valvular incompetence and, when associated with prominent pelvic veins, is diagnostic for pelvic congestion syndrome [63]. On imaging, pelvic varicosities are dilated, tortuous, tubular parauterine structures that are isodense to veins after contrast administration. They can extend from the periuterine region laterally into the broad ligament to reach the pelvic sidewall or inferiorly to the paravaginal venous plexus [62].

A pelvic arteriovenous malformation appears masslike, often identical to the appearance of pelvic varices on CT. The pelvic arteriovenous malformation demonstrates brisk enhancement because of the direct communication between the feeding artery and the draining vein [62]. Like fibroids, symptomatic arteriovenous malformations are treated with arterial embolization (Fig. 27).

Uterine artery embolization

Uterine artery embolization (UAE) is used effectively for treatment of symptomatic fibroids. CT is sometimes obtained after UAE to demonstrate adequate embolization and should show retention of contrast in the uterus without washout [64]. One month after UAE, CT of the pelvis may show central necrosis and cavitation with flecks of gas and cyst formation [64]. CT can be used evaluate complications after UAE and may show infection in the endometrium or myometrium or an infarcted fibroid [65].

Summary

In the emergency room setting, MDCT of the female pelvis offers rapid, noninvasive, multiplanar evaluation of patients who have acute pelvic pain. Familiarity with CT findings of ovarian cyst, adnexal torsion, and PID is valuable in the prompt treatment of these entities. MDCT has been integrated into several of the major trauma centers, and its use may surpass the use of ultrasound in the trauma evaluation of the pregnant patient.

In the nonemergent setting, MDCT can be used to stage gynecologic malignancy and to evaluate for tumor recurrence. Multiplanar MDCT has received some acceptance for evaluation of small primary tumor volume and small metastatic implants. MDCT also has a role in the evaluation of pelvic varices and suspected pelvic congestion syndrome.

Acknowledgments

The authors thank Margaret Kowaluk for the preparation of image graphics and Agnieska Flor, Sue Ronzo, Megan Ernst, Angela Holland, Lori Burlaka, Josephine Odey, Casey Russo, Stephen L. Wolak, David McDougall, and Michele Burkle for assistance with image preparation.

References

[1] Maher MM, Kalra MK, Sahani DV, et al. Techniques, clinical applications and limitations of 3D reconstruction in ct of the abdomen. Korean J Radiol 2004;5(1): 55–67.

[2] Ghiatas AA. The spectrum of pelvic inflammatory disease. Eur Radiol 2004;14(Suppl 3):E184–92.

[3] Sawyer RW, Walsh JW. CT in gynecologic pelvic diseases. Semin Ultrasound CT MR 1988;9:122–42.

[4] Pannu HK, Bristow RE, Montz FJ, et al. Multidetector CT of peritoneal carcinomatosis from ovarian cancer. Radiographics 2003;23(3):687–701.

[5] Pannu HK, Fishman EK. Evaluation of cervical cancer by computed tomography: current status. Cancer 2003; 98(9 Suppl):2039–43.

[6] Kawamoto S, Urban BA, Fishman EK. CT of epithelial ovarian tumors. Radiographics 1999;19:S85–102.

[7] Standring S. Uterus. In: Williams PL, Bannister LH, Berry MM, editors. Gray's anatomy: anatomical basis of clinical practice. 39th edition. London: Churchill Livingstone; 2004. p. 1331–8.

[8] Lim PS, Nazarian LN, Wechsler RJ, et al. The endometrium on routine contrast-enhanced CT in asymptomatic postmenopausal women: avoiding errors in interpretation. Clin Imaging 2002;26(5):325–9.

[9] Reproductive anatomy. In: Stenchever MA, Droegemueller W, Herbst AL, et al, editors. Comprehensive gynecology. 4th edition. St. Louis (MO): Mosby; 2001. p. 39–69.

[10] Davis JA, Gosink BB. Fluid in the female pelvis: cyclic patterns. J Ultrasound Med 1986;5(2):75–9.

[11] Standring S. Uterine tubes. In: Williams PL, Bannister LH, Berry MM, editors. Gray's anatomy: anatomical basis of clinical practice. 39th edition. London: Churchill Livingstone; 2004. p. 1327–9.

[12] Saksouk FA, Johnson SC. Recognition of the ovaries and ovarian origin of pelvic masses with CT. Radiographics 2004;24(Suppl 1):S133–46.

[13] Urban BA, Fishman EK. Helical (spiral) CT of the female pelvis. Radiol Clin North Am 1995;33(5): 933–48.

[14] Standring S. Ovaries. In: Williams PL, Bannister LH, Berry MM, editors. Gray's anatomy: anatomical basis of clinical practice. 39th edition. London: Churchill Livingstone; 2004. p. 1321–6.

[15] Langer JE, Dinsmore BJ. Computed tomographic evaluation of benign and inflammatory disorders of

the female pelvis. Radiol Clin North Am 1992;30(4): 831–42.

[16] Gross BH, Moss AA, Mihara K, et al. computed tomography of gynecologic diseases. AJR Am J Roentgenol 1983;141(4):765–73.

[17] Borders RJ, Breiman RS, Yeh BM, et al. Computed tomography of corpus luteal cysts. J Comput Assist Tomogr 2004;28(3):340–2.

[18] Choi HJ, Kim SH, Kim HC, et al. Ruptured corpus luteal cyst: CT findings. Korean J Radiol 2003; 4(1):42–5.

[19] Differential diagnosis of major gynecologic problems by age groups. In: Stenchever MA, Droegemueller W, Herbst AL, et al, editors. Comprehensive gynecology. 4th edition. St. Louis (MO): Mosby; 2001. p. 155–77.

[20] Miele V, Andreoli C, Cortese A, et al. Hemoperitoneum following ovarian cyst rupture: CT usefulness in the diagnosis. Radiol Med (Torino) 2002;104(4): 316–21.

[21] Pinto A, Merola S, De Lutio Di Castelguidone E, et al. Pictorial essay: common and uncommon CT features of acute pelvic pain in women. Radiol Med (Torino) 2004;107:524–32.

[22] Zissin R. Case report: torsion of a normal ovary in a post-pubertal female: unenhanced helical CT appearance. Br J Radiol 2001;74:762–3.

[23] Schlaff WD, Lund KJ, McAleese KA, et al. Diagnosing ovarian torsion with computed tomography. A case report. J Reprod Med 1998;43(9):827–30.

[24] Rha SE, Byun JY, Jung SE, et al. CT and MR imaging features of adnexal torsion. Radiographics 2002;22: 283–94.

[25] Gittleman AM, Price AP, Goffner L, et al. Ovarian torsion: CT findings in a child. J Pediatr Surg 2004; 39:1270–2.

[26] Bennett GL, Slywotzky CM, Giovanniello G. Gynecologic causes of acute pelvic pain: spectrum of CT findings. Radiographics 2002;22(4):785–801.

[27] Kim YH, Cho KS, Ha HK, et al. CT features of torsion of benign cystic teratoma of the ovary. J Comp Assist Tom 1999;23(6):923–8.

[28] Pelvic inflammatory disease. National Institute of Allergy and Infectious Diseases fact sheet. Bethesda (MD): National Institute of Allergy and Infectious Diseases; 1998.

[29] Sam JW, Jacobs JE, Birnbaum BA. Spectrum of CT findings in acute pyogenic inflammatory disease. Radiographics 2002;22:1327–34.

[30] Wilbur AC, Aizenstein RI, Napp TE. CT findings in tuboovarian abscess. AJR Am J Roentgenol 1992;158: 575–9.

[31] Kaur H, Loyer EM, Minami M, et al. Patterns of uterine enhancement with helical CT. Eur J Radiol 1998;28:250–5.

[32] Fielding JR. MR imaging of the female pelvis. Radiol Clin North Am 2003;41:179–92.

[33] Wallach EE, Vlahos NF. Uterine myomas: an overview of development, clinical features, and management. Obstet Gynecol 2004;104(2):393–406.

[34] Hamm B, Kubik-Huch RA, Fleige B. MR imaging and CT of the female pelvis: radiologic-pathologic correlation. Eur Radiol 1999;9:3–15.

[35] Brant WE. Pelvis. In: Webb WR, Brant WE, Helms CA, editors. Fundamentals of body CT. 2nd edition. Philadelphia: WB Saunders; 1998. p. 291–305.

[36] Buy JN, Ghossain MA, Mark AS, et al. Focal hyperdense areas in endometriomas: a characteristic finding on CT. AJR Am J Roentgenol 1992;159(4): 769–71.

[37] Lowdermilk C, Gavant ML, Qaisi W, et al. Screening helical CT for evaluation of blunt traumatic injury in the pregnant patient. Radiographics 1999;19: S243–55.

[38] Standring S. Anatomy of pregnancy and parturition. In: Williams PL, Bannister LH, Berry MM, editors. Gray's anatomy: anatomical basis of clinical practice. 39th edition. London: Churchill Livingstone; 2004. p. 1339–52.

[39] Urban BA, Pankov BL, Fishman EK. Postpartum complications in the abdomen and pelvis: CT evaluation. Crit Rev Diagn Imaging 1999;40(1):1–21.

[40] Garagiola DM, Tarver RD, Gibson L, et al. Anatomic changes in the pelvis after uncomplicated vaginal delivery: a CT study on 14 women. AJR Am J Roentgenol 1989;153(6):1239–41.

[41] Zuckerman J, Levine D, McNicholas MM, et al. Imaging of pelvic postpartum complications. AJR Am J Roentgenol 1997;168:663–8.

[42] Twickler DM, Setiawan AT, Harrell RS, et al. CT appearance of the pelvis after cesarean section. AJR Am J Roentgenol 1991;156:523–6.

[43] Apter S, Shmamann S, Ben-Baruch G, et al. CT of pelvic infection after cesarean section. Clin Exp Obstet Gynecol 1992;19(3):156–60.

[44] Van Hoe L, Gryspeerdt S, Amant F, et al. Abdominal pain in the postpartum: role of imaging. J Belge Radiol 1995;78(3):186–9.

[45] Dialani V, Levine D. Ectopic pregnancy: a review. Ultrasound Q 2004;20(3):105–17.

[46] Weishaupt D, Grozaj AM, Willmann JK, et al. Traumatic injuries: imaging of abdominal and pelvic injuries. Eur Radiol 2002;12:1295–311.

[47] Shanmuganathan K. Multi-detector row CT imaging of blunt abdominal trauma. Semin Ultrasound CT MR 2004;25(2):180–204.

[48] Trauma in pregnancy. In: Cunningham FG, editor. Williams obstetrics. 22nd edition. New York: McGraw-Hill; 2005. p. 997–9.

[49] Bipat S, Glas AS, van der Velden J, et al. Computed tomography and magnetic resonance imaging in staging of uterine cervical carcinoma: a systematic review. Gynecol Oncol 2003;91(1):59–66.

[50] Funt SA, Hricak H, Abu-Rustum N, et al. Role of CT in the management of recurrent ovarian cancer. AJR Am J Roentenol 2004;182:393–8.

[51] Outwater EK, Siegelman ES, Hunt JL. Ovarian teratomas: tumor types and imaging characteristics. Radiographics 2001;21:475–90.

[52] Zissin R. CT Diagnosis of malignant degeneration of an ovarian teratoma. Gynecol Oncol 2000;77: 482–5.

[53] Cancer statistics 2005 presentation. Atlanta (GA): American Cancer Society, Inc; 2005.

[54] Benedet JL, Pecorelli S. Staging classifications and clinical practice guidelines of gynaecologic cancers. Int J Gynaecol Obstet 2000;70:207–312.

[55] Barakat RR, Hricak H. What do we expect from imaging? Radiol Clin North Am 2002;40(3):521–6 [vii.].

[56] Kurtz AB, Tsimikas JV, Tempany CM, et al. Diagnosis and staging of ovarian cancer: comparative values of Doppler and conventional US, CT, and MR imaging correlated with surgery and histopathologic analysis. Radiology 1999;212:19–27.

[57] Hardesty LA, Sumkin JH, Hakim C, et al. The ability of helical CT to preoperatively stage endometrial cancer. AJR Am J Roentgenol 2001;176(3):603–6.

[58] Kinkel K, Kaji Y, Yu KK, et al. Radiologic staging in patients with endometrial cancer: a meta-analysis. Radiology 1999;212(3):711–8.

[59] Pannu HK, Corl FM, Fishman EK. CT evaluation of cervical cancer: spectrum of disease. Radiographics 2001;21(5):1155–68.

[60] Jeong YY, Kang HK, Chung TW, et al. Uterine cervical carcinoma after therapy: CT and MR imaging findings. Radiographics 2003;23:969–81.

[61] Mai J, Rownd J, Erickson B. CT-guided high-dose-rate dose prescription for cervical carcinoma: the importance of uterine wall thickness. Brachytherapy 2002; 1(1):27–35.

[62] Coakley FV, Varghese SL, Hricak H. CT and MRI of pelvic varices in women. J Comput Assist Tomogr 1999;23(3):429–34.

[63] Rozenblit AM, Ricci ZJ, Tuvia J, et al. Incompetent and dilated ovarian veins: a common CT finding in asymptomatic parous women. AJR Am J Roentgenol 2001;176(1):119–22.

[64] Vott S, Bonilla SM, Goodwin SC, et al. CT findings after uterine artery embolization. J Comput Assist Tomogr 2000;24(6):846–8.

[65] Worthington-Kirsch RL, Siskin GP. Uterine artery embolization for symptomatic myomata. J Intensive Care Med 2004;19(1):13–21.

**ELSEVIER
SAUNDERS**

Radiol Clin N Am 43 (2005) 1119 – 1127

**RADIOLOGIC
CLINICS**
of North America

Angiographic Imaging of the Lower Extremities with Multidetector CT

Mark D. Hiatt, MD, Dominik Fleischmann, MD, Jeffrey C. Hellinger, MD, Geoffrey D. Rubin, MD*

Division of Cardiovascular Imaging, Department of Radiology, Stanford University Medical Center, Stanford, CA, USA

Multidetector CT (MDCT) has improved imaging of the arteries in the lower extremities. The main advantages of this novel technology are the exceptionally fast scan times, high spatial resolution, increased anatomic coverage, and capability to generate high-quality multiplanar reformations and three-dimensional (3-D) renderings from raw data that can be reprocessed easily and quickly. The applications of MDCT in imaging the lower extremities are multiple and varied. They include the evaluation of peripheral arterial occlusive and aneurysmal disease, the patency and integrity of bypass grafts, and arterial injury owing to trauma. This article describes the techniques of lower extremity MDCT angiography and its use in a few clinical applications.

Multidetector CT

Imaging of the arteries in the extremities was attempted with single detector row scanners in the past [1]. A revolution in peripheral CT angiography began when it became possible to image with four-channel MDCT the inflow and outflow vessels in the entire lower extremity at an adequate resolution with a single intravenous administration of contrast material in a single acquisition [2].

---

* Corresponding author. Division of Cardiovascular Imaging, Department of Radiology, Stanford University Medical Center, 300 Pasteur Drive, Room S-072, Stanford, CA 94305-5105.

E-mail address: grubin@stanford.edu (G.D. Rubin).

In evolving from axial single-slice helical CT to MDCT, the acquisition time has been diminished considerably. For example, 16-detector row CT, with its rotation time of 500 ms, can acquire thin slices from the diaphragm to the ankles in less than 25 seconds. Such a scan may yield a data set of around 2000 axial images that can be processed for efficient review and volumetric analysis (Fig. 1).

MDCT angiography has many advantages over other modalities commonly used to image the lower extremities, including ultrasonography and digital subtraction angiography (DSA). Unlike ultrasonography, CT angiography of the lower limb is relatively investigator independent and can be performed easily, even on patients with calcified native arteries or patients who have recently undergone bypass surgery (who are sutured and wrapped in surgical dressing).

When compared with conventional catheter angiography, CT angiography is less invasive, less expensive, and exposes the patient to less radiation [2]. CT angiography also assesses aspects external to the lumen of the vessel that DSA cannot, including mural thrombus, atheroma, inflammation, and periarterial tissues.

The diagnostic performance of MDCT in detecting arterial athero-occlusive disease relative to DSA is good, as reported in several studies (Table 1) [3–9]. Martin and colleagues [4] reported that MDCT angiography (using a four-detector scanner) had excellent specificity in revealing severe (>75%) stenoses and arterial occlusions (97% and 98%, respectively), with acceptable sensitivity (92% and 89%, respectively). Advances in MDCT with the release of 8-, 16-, and even 64-detector scanners should yield results that are even more promising.

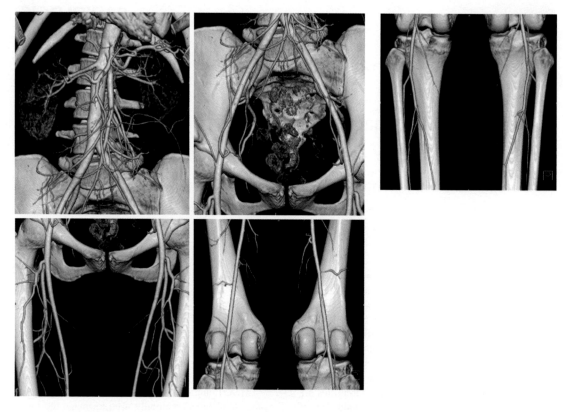

Fig. 1. CT angiography of normal lower extremities. Note the absence of any lesion or stenosis affecting the arteries.

MR angiography has contraindications and challenges that do not pose a similar restriction or problem when performing CT angiography. For example, patients who have undergone bypass surgery often have surgical clips or metallic stents, artifact from which interferes with the interpretation of MR angiography. Furthermore, patients with pacemakers or cardiac defibrillators cannot undergo MR angiography, yet many patients with these devices need to be evaluated for athero-occlusive disease because of their likelihood of additional cardiac disease (such as obstructive coronary arterial disease or cardiac arrhythmia) owing to frequent comorbid diabetes mellitus or long-term nicotine use. Another challenge of MR angiography is that tortuous arteries may appear occluded if they are not carefully included in the plane of imaging. MR angiography does not offer visualization of bony landmarks as well as CT for assisting surgeons in planning operations. On the other hand, MR angiography remains a preferred option for patients who should not receive iodinated contrast material because of renal dysfunction or allergy. MR angiography may also be more valuable in patients with extensive calcification of the crural arteries.

CT angiography is readily available as the first modality to image patients with an initial acute onset of symptoms. In particular, if a catheter-based intervention is not anticipated, noninvasive MDCT may be preferred to DSA. CT angiography may also be valuable as a 3-D guide to performing subsequent catheter-based interventions as well as for observing patients on whom procedures have been performed, such as the long-term surveillance of peripheral artery bypass grafts [10], endovascular aneurysm repair, and transluminal revascularization of the lower extremities [11].

Scanning technique

When performing angiographic imaging of the lower extremities from the diaphragm to the ankles, factors related to patient positioning, technical parameters, and contrast administration must be considered. The patient should lie supine on the table, feet first with the knees and ankles secured together in a neutral comfortable position to reduce artifact from motion during the scan and to minimize the

Table 1
Results of recent studies comparing multidetector CT with digital subtraction angiography

First author, year [Ref.]	No. of patients	MDCT rows	Section thickness (mm)	Images available for interpretation	Sensitivity (%)	Specificity (%)	Additional patent segments (%)
Willmann, 2005 [10]	39	16 × 0.75	0.75	VR, MIP, MPR, and transverse sections	96–97	96–97	NR
Edwards, 2005 [9]	44	4 × 2.5	3.2	VR and transverse sections only. No MPR, MIP, or CPR.	72–79	93	7.3
Romano, 2004 [8]	42	4 × 2.5	3.2	VR, MIP, MPR, and transverse sections	93	95	NR
Catalano, 2004 [7]	50	4 × 2.5	3.0	VR, MIP, MPR, and transverse sections	96	93	NR
Ota, 2004 [5]	24	4 × 2	2.0	VR, MIP, MPR, and transverse sections	99	99	2
Martin, 2003 [4]	41	4 × 5	5.0	VR, MIP, MPR, and transverse sections	92	97	9.3
Ofer, 2003 [3]	18	4 × 2.5	3.2	MIP following arterial wall calcium removal, CPR, and transverse sections	91	92	0

Summary of publications of MDCT angiography of lower extremity arterial occlusive disease with DSA as a reference standard. All sensitivities and specificities are reported for detection of ≥50% stenosis with the exception of [4], which is for ≥75% stenoses.
Abbreviation: NR, not reported.

display field of view. The legs should be as close to the isocenter of the scanner as possible to avoid off-center stair-step artifacts [12]. The feet should not be excessively plantar flexed to avoid artifactual stenosis or even occlusion of the dorsalis pedis artery.

The full study consists of a digital radiograph (the "scout" image), an optional unenhanced acquisition, a series for bolus testing or triggering, the angiographic acquisition, and an optional late-phase acquisition. A scout image, or topogram, should first be acquired to identify the area of coverage. Anatomic coverage usually extends from just cranial to the origins of the renal arteries through the feet, with an average scan length of around 120 cm. Next, unenhanced imaging may be helpful, particularly in evaluating traumatized patients to assess for foreign bodies and hemorrhage. Peripheral CT angiography can be performed with all current multiple-detector row scanners. Parameters that may be used for 4- and 16-slice CT of the lower extremities are presented in Table 2.

A few adjustments to the suggested protocol may be required. In obese patients, the x-ray tube current and potential voltage may need to be increased. If the distal vessels are not well opacified (eg, in cases of femoropopliteal aneurysm or slow circulation in the setting of cardiac failure), a second acquisition may be necessary. This optional late-phase scanning of the

popliteal and infrapopliteal vasculature should be initiated only on demand by the technologist upon seeing poor opacification on initial imaging.

The proper administration of nonionic contrast material is key to opacifying sufficiently the arteries of the lower extremities. The objective is to image these vessels while enhancing them homogenously without venous or tissue contamination. Factors related to the technology and to the patient need to be considered. First, the reduced scan time of MDCT requires a higher rate of injection to enhance the peripheral arteries sufficiently. Second, patients with

Table 2
Sample parameters for multidetector CT angiography of the lower extremities

Parameter	4-row	16-row
Anatomic region	Celiac axis to feet	Celiac axis to feet
Patient position	Supine	Supine
Slice collimation (mm)	4 × 2.5	16 × 1–1.5
Gantry rotation (ms)	500	500
Tube current (mA)	300–440	300–440
Tube voltage (kV)	120	120
Table feed (mm/s)	~15	~30
Slice thickness (mm)	1.5–3	1–1.5
Increment (mm)	1.5	0.8
Acquisition time (s)	35–40	17–20

peripheral artery disease may have widely varying times of transit of contrast material from the intravenous injection site to the peripheral arteries. Diminished cardiac output may lengthen the transit time. The contrast medium transit time, or t_{CMT}, must be determined by using a test bolus or automatic bolus triggering in the abdominal aorta [13]. The former method is generally more reliable than the latter. The optimal delay time corresponds to the peak arrival time of a test bolus in the abdominal aorta. Measuring the arrival time of the contrast material in the aorta, as opposed to more distally, may be preferred because of a potentially significant difference between the legs in their arterial inflow.

Once the t_{CTT} has been determined, the contrast material can be injected, generally via an upper arm peripheral venous access. Two parameters need to be calculated—how much contrast medium to use and how fast to inject it. The total volume of contrast material needed depends on the duration of the scan. With the feed of the CT table, the scan follows the contrast bolus distally to the ankles; therefore, the length of the injection may be 5 to 10 seconds shorter than the actual time of scanning [14]. In patients with peripheral artery disease, the scanning may actually outpace the bolus if the table feed exceeds 50 mm/s. A total volume of 120 to 160 mL of contrast material may be needed to opacify all of the arteries of the lower extremities sufficiently. In general, about 0.5 to 0.7 g of iodine per kilogram of body weight may be necessary.

Using an iodine concentration of 300 to 370 mg/mL and an injection rate of 3.5 to 5.0 mL/s sufficiently opacifies the abdominal aorta and peripheral arteries [2–4]. The total volume of contrast material may be reduced if a higher concentration of iodine (eg, 370 mg/mL) is used [13]. Monophasic injections during which contrast material is injected at a single rate yield a short-lived peak on curves that track arterial attenuation over time. Biphasic injections during which the rate is high initially, followed by a different lower rate, may enhance the arteries more consistently [15,16]. For example, 40 mL could be injected initially at 5 mL/s, immediately followed by 80 mL at 3.5 mL/s.

After the contrast medium has been injected, flushing with saline pushes the residual material from the venous system into arterial circulation. Typically, 30 to 50 mL of saline is administered via a dual-chamber injector device. If a dual-chamber injector is unavailable, the saline may be afterloaded in a single-chamber injector.

Post processing

MDCT is associated with several advantages but also challenges. Along with the benefits of exceptionally fast scan times, high spatial resolution, and increased volume coverage, MDCT presents the cumbersome task of dealing with an extremely large potentially unwieldy data set. Interpreting and reporting on 1000 images for a study on the lower extremity inflow and run-off, much less presenting this multitude of images in an explicable form to clinicians, can be challenging [17]. Relying on axial images alone is not practical for run-off examinations that typically comprise 1000 or even 2000 separate images. Fortunately, high-quality post-processed

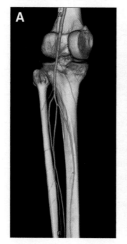 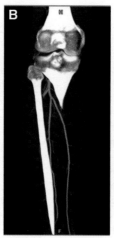 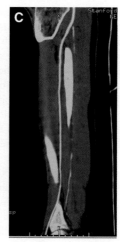

Fig. 2. CT angiography visualization techniques depicting the arteries of the lower leg. (*A*) VR. (*B*) MIP. (*C*) CPR.

imaging, such as multiplanar reconstruction (MPR), volume rendering (VR), maximum intensity projection (MIP), and curved planar reformation (CPR), can be generated easily and quickly to assist in interpretation and presentation [18]. Fig. 2 presents examples of the latter three techniques.

Understanding the basic principles behind the techniques of post processing helps one understand the limitations of these techniques. MPR allows rapid review of the acquired image data in sagittal, coronal, and oblique views, including information about adjacent parenchyma. Such multiplanar analysis may be

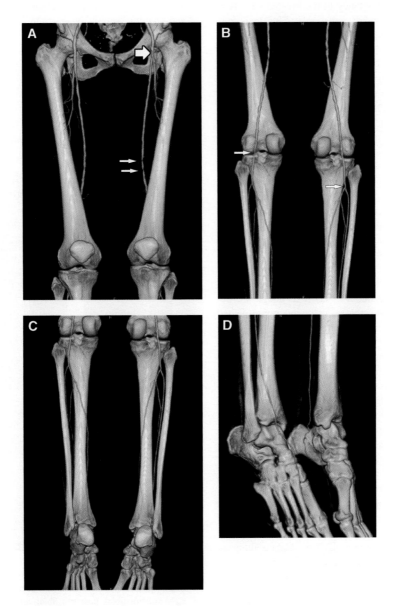

Fig. 3. CT angiography depicting the arteries of the lower extremities with moderate atherosclerotic disease and resulting multiple stenoses in a patient with left calf claudication. (*A*) Mild diffuse irregularity is present in the right superficial femoral artery. There is a focal approximately 50% stenosis at the distal aspect of the left common femoral artery just proximal to the takeoff of the profunda femoris (*wide arrow*) and two tandem stenoses of moderate-to-high grade of the distal left superficial femoral artery in the adductor canal (*narrow arrows*). (*B*) Mild diffuse atherosclerosis affects both popliteal arteries, resulting in focal moderate stenoses of these arteries (*arrows*) but no occlusion. (*C* and *D*) Both sides exhibit a normal trifurcation and three-vessel runoff, with both gradually tapering peroneal arteries no longer visible at the level of the ankle.

helpful in visualizing the artery wall that is otherwise obscured on MIP or VR imaging by calcified plaque, mural calcification, or an endoluminal stent. On the downside, the structure of interest must lie in one plane to be evaluated readily with this technique.

Three-dimensional VR provides a good overview of the anatomy and patency of the imaged vessels as well as the presence of collaterals. This technique renders the entire volume of data, rather than just its surfaces, revealing internal structures that may otherwise be hidden (Fig. 2A). The rendered volume of data can be analyzed interactively using various display algorithms to focus on tissues and relationships of interest. The resulting image can be cut and rotated in real time. The power of VR is the perspective it provides, particularly in depicting the course and integrity of vessels in patients with suspected embolic disease or vessel injury. Interactive rotation of a VR data set allows visualization of the full course of tortuous vessels all the way to the toes from different view angles, without the need to remove the bony structures, unlike the MIP technique.

The way MIPs are made renders this technique an excellent means for relaying results to referring physicians as well as for planning treatment in the operating room or angiography suite. The pixel values of a two-dimensional (2-D) MIP image are determined by the highest voxel value in a ray projected along the data set in a specified direction (Fig. 2B). MIPs consequently provide the images most similar to conventional angiography; however, this advantage is counterbalanced by at least three disadvantages or limitations. First, if another material of high density, such as calcification or an endoluminal stent, is along the ray through a vessel, the displayed pixel intensity will represent this denser material and contain no information about the intravascular contrast medium, possibly overestimating the degree of stenosis. Second, generating MIP images requires that bones be removed from the data set, which may be a time-consuming endeavor. Third, the inadvertent removal of vessels close to these bones may give rise to spurious lesions.

CPR displays a curved plane prescribed along an individual vessel contour, depicting the entire midline of the vessel on a single 2-D image. This technique is a single-voxel thick tomogram that is helpful in analyzing individual vessels, especially ones that are heavily calcified (Fig. 2C). Obscuration of the lumen of a vessel by extensive calcification, a major drawback of MIP and VR reconstructions, is not as much of a problem with CPR, which can allow evaluation of the lumen even in the presence of such calcification. A disadvantage of CPR is its limited spatial perception. Moreover, inaccurate centerline definition can lead to spurious stenoses and occlusions.

Despite all of their advantages, post-processed images alone are inadequate in performing a thorough assessment. The axial source images must be reviewed to assess extravascular pathology. Such review is also beneficial to obtain an overview of the vasculature. Source images can help distinguish between artifacts and true lesions when reformatted images suggest abnormalities.

Applications

The applications of MDCT for imaging the lower extremities are multiple and varied. With a single

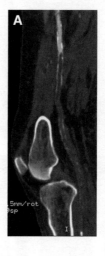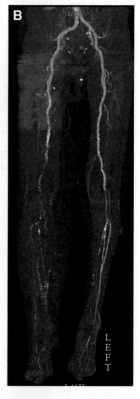

Fig. 4. CT angiography depicting acute clot occluding (*A*) the distal right superficial femoral and popliteal arteries and (*B*) right anterior tibial, posterior tibial, and peroneal arteries in the swollen right lower extremity of an 88-year-old woman. The arteries of both lower extremities manifest marked diffuse atherosclerotic disease. Although the left popliteal artery is patent, it contains multiple high-grade stenoses and short occlusions, most pronounced in its mid and distal portions. As on the right side, the left posterior and distal anterior tibial arteries are occluded without reconstitution.

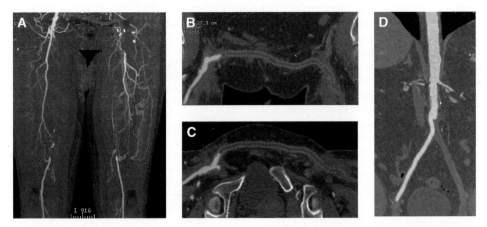

Fig. 5. A 74-year-old man with decreased pulses in the left foot had occlusions of both his femorofemoral bypass grafts (*A–C*) and the left iliac limb of an aortobifemoral bypass graft (*D*). The femorofemoral graft was completely occluded except for a 2-cm segment at its most proximal right aspect. In the right lower extremity, the proximal aspects of superficial femoral arteries was occluded, but the deep femoral artery reconstituted the distal superficial femoral artery. On the left side, the iliac system and the proximal aspects of the superficial and deep femoral arteries were occluded, but the deep femoral artery reconstituted from collaterals and, in turn, reconstituted the distal superficial femoral artery.

acquisition, vessels over a meter long can be imaged with a contrast resolution that distinguishes the lumen of the artery from opacified veins, calcification, plaque, and thrombus. Indications for this robust technology include evaluating peripheral vascular atherosclerotic steno-occlusive disease, embolic phenomena, congenital abnormalities, popliteal entrapment syndrome, traumatic and iatrogenic injuries, inflammatory conditions, and aneurysms, as well as assessing the patency and integrity of bypass grafts and preoperative free-flap vascular pedicle assessment. A few of these applications are discussed herein.

MDCT can be used in the evaluation of the spectrum of diseases comprising peripheral vascular occlusive conditions (Fig. 3) [2]. The goal of this imaging is to characterize the steno-occlusive disease of inflow, femoral, and run-off vessels in these patients, who typically present with critical limb ischemia or claudication, to triage them into appropriate treatment groups. This modality can characterize fully any lesions detected, including their number, lengths, diameters (and diameters of adjacent normal vasculature), and degree of calcification, assisting in pretreatment planning with respect to the route of access, selection of balloon, and expected patency after intervention. MDCT can also evaluate for the presence of related atheroembolism (Fig. 4).

MDCT is also helpful in assessing peripheral arterial bypass grafts. It is an accurate and reliable technique to assess these grafts and detect graft-related complications, including stenosis, occlusion, aneu-

rysm, arteriovenous fistulas, and infection (Fig. 5) [10]. Ultrasound may be the first choice for routine surveillance because of its reliability and ease of operation; however, CT angiography is particularly useful in the immediate postoperative period when wounds and bandages may limit sonographic access and at other times when ultrasound may be nondiagnostic.

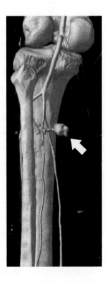

Fig. 6. CT angiography of a left peroneal artery disruption and resulting pseudoaneurysm (*arrow*) following a gunshot wound.

The increased acquisition speed of MDCT lends itself well to the rushed setting of the emergency department. Peripheral CT angiography can readily be performed within 15 minutes of total room time. The traumatized patient may have vascular injuries detected earlier, leading to more timely treatment and reduced morbidity and mortality [19]. Post-processed images provide helpful information for subsequent intervention (Fig. 6).

Limitations

Several factors limit the usefulness of CT angiography in evaluating vessels of the lower extremities. CT angiography may not even be attempted in patients with compromised renal function. Even if performed, it may not be executed optimally because of poor vascular opacification in obese patients or incorrect scan timing. Effective and efficient post processing may be time-consuming, although this limitation becomes less of a barrier with experience. The interpretation of CT angiography may be suboptimal owing to obscuration of vascular flow channels by calcification.

Summary

MDCT has improved imaging of the arteries in the lower extremities because of its fast scan times, high spatial resolution, and increased anatomic coverage, allowing cost-effective assessment of long vascular segments with higher spatial, contrast, and temporal resolution. To use this powerful tool to full advantage in evaluating diseases and injuries of vessels in the lower extremities, certain aspects of its use must be mastered, such as the timing of contrast administration and generation and the use of high-quality 3-D renderings and multiplanar reformations. CT angiography has become a routine means of evaluating a broad spectrum of arterial abnormalities in the lower extremities.

References

[1] Lawrence JA, Kim D, Kent KC, et al. Lower extremity spiral CT angiography versus catheter angiography. Radiology 1995;194(3):903–8.
[2] Rubin GD, Schmidt AJ, Logan LJ, et al. Multi-detector row CT angiography of lower extremity arterial inflow and runoff: initial experience. Radiology 2001;221(1):146–58.
[3] Ofer A, Nitecki SS, Linn S, et al. Multidetector CT angiography of peripheral vascular disease: a prospective comparison with intraarterial digital subtraction angiography. AJR Am J Roentgenol 2003;180(3):719–24.
[4] Martin ML, Tay KH, Flak B, et al. Multidetector CT angiography of the aortoiliac system and lower extremities: a prospective comparison with digital subtraction angiography. AJR Am J Roentgenol 2003;180(4):1085–91.
[5] Ota H, Takase K, Igarashi K, et al. MDCT compared with digital subtraction angiography for assessment of lower extremity arterial occlusive disease: importance of reviewing cross-sectional images. AJR Am J Roentgenol 2004;182(1):201–9.
[6] Romano M, Amato B, Markabaoui K, et al. Multidetector row computed tomographic angiography of the abdominal aorta and lower limbs arteries: a new diagnostic tool in patients with peripheral arterial occlusive disease. Minerva Cardioangiol 2004;52(1):9–17.
[7] Catalano C, Fraioli F, Laghi A, et al. Infrarenal aortic and lower-extremity arterial disease: diagnostic performance of multi-detector row CT angiography. Radiology 2004;231(2):555–63.
[8] Romano M, Mainenti PP, Imbriaco M, et al. Multidetector row CT angiography of the abdominal aorta and lower extremities in patients with peripheral arterial occlusive disease: diagnostic accuracy and interobserver agreement. Eur J Radiol 2004;50(3):303–8.
[9] Edwards AJ, Wells IP, Roobottom CA. Multidetector row CT angiography of the lower limb arteries: a prospective comparison of volume-rendered techniques and intra-arterial digital subtraction angiography. Clin Radiol 2005;60(1):85–95.
[10] Willmann JK, Mayer D, Banyai M, et al. Evaluation of peripheral arterial bypass grafts with multi-detector row CT angiography: comparison with duplex US and digital subtraction angiography. Radiology 2003;229(2):465–74.
[11] Lookstein RA. Impact of CT angiography on endovascular therapy. Mt Sinai J Med 2003;70(6):367–74.
[12] Fleischmann D, Rubin GD, Paik DS, et al. Stair-step artifacts with single versus multiple detector-row helical CT. Radiology 2000;216(1):185–96.
[13] Fleischmann D. Use of high concentration contrast media: principles and rationale—vascular district. Eur J Radiol 2003;45(Suppl 1):S88–93.
[14] Fleischmann D. Present and future trends in multiple detector-row CT applications: CT angiography. Eur Radiol 2002;12(Suppl 2):S11–5.
[15] Fleischmann D, Rubin GD, Bankier AA, et al. Improved uniformity of aortic enhancement with customized contrast medium injection protocols at CT angiography. Radiology 2000;214(2):363–71.
[16] Bae KT, Tran HQ, Heiken JP. Multiphasic injection

method for uniform prolonged vascular enhancement at CT angiography: pharmacokinetic analysis and experimental porcine model. Radiology 2000;216(3): 872–80.

[17] Rubin GD. Data explosion: the challenge of multidetector-row CT. Eur J Radiol 2000;36(2):74–80.

[18] Rubin GD. 3-D imaging with MDCT. Eur J Radiol 2003;45(Suppl 1):S37–41.

[19] Philipp MO, Kubin K, Mang T, et al. Three-dimensional volume rendering of multidetector-row CT data: applicable for emergency radiology. Eur J Radiol 2003;48(1):33–8.

ELSEVIER
SAUNDERS

Radiol Clin N Am 43 (2005) 1129–1162

RADIOLOGIC
CLINICS
of North America

Cumulative Index 2005

Note: Page numbers of article titles are in **boldface** type.

A

Abdomen, multidetector CT angiography of, **963–976**
  abdominal aorta, 965–968
    for endovascular therapy, 967–968
  gonadal veins, 973–974
  inferior vena cava, 974
  kidneys, 968–970
    before and after transplantation, 970
  liver, 973
  mesenteric vasculature, 970–971
  ovarian veins, 973
  pancreas, 971–973
    before and after transplantation, 972
  techniques for, 963–965
    maximum intensity projection, 964, 967
    multiplanar reconstruction, 964, 967
    volume rendering, 964–965

Abdominal aorta, multidetector CT angiography of, 965–968

Abdominal trauma, multidetector CT of, **1079–1095**
  bowel and mesenteric trauma, 1088–1090
    free intraperitoneal fluid, 1089–1090
    pneumoperitoneum, 1089
  gallbladder trauma, 1088
  hepatic trauma, 1084–1087
    and surgical management, 1087
    arteriovenous fistulas, 1087
    complications of, 1087
    contusions, 1085
    grading scales for, 1084–1085
    lacerations, 1085
    pseudoaneurysms, 1087
    retrohepatic vena cava injuries, 1085
    subcapsular hematomas, 1085, 1087
  renal trauma, 1090–1092
    grading scales for, 1090–1092

    hematomas, 1091
    infarctions, 1091
    lacerations, 1091
  splenic trauma, 1080–1084
    and surgical management, 1083–1084
    grading scales for, 1081
    infarctions, 1082
    vascular lesions and extravasation, 1082–1083
  techniques for, 1079–1080
    intraperitoneal fluid and
      hemoperitoneum, 1080
    isolated free intraperitoneal fluid, 1080
    total body scan, 1079–1080

Abdominal viscera, herniation of, in children, 278

Abduction external rotation position, in MR arthrography, of shoulders, 684, 685

Abscesses
  hepatic
    bacterial, multidetector CT of, 838
    fungal, multidetector CT of, 838
    MR imaging of, 868
  hepatic trauma and, multidetector CT of, 1087
  pancreatic, multidetector CT of, 1003
  pulmonary
    in children, 409
    in pneumonia, in immunocompetent children, 262–263
    infection patterns in, 499
  renal, multidetector CT of, 1037
  tubo-ovarian, multidetector CT of, 1102–1103
  with diabetic foot, MR imaging of, 750

Absence seizures, PET of, 87–88

Acetic acid injections, with radiofrequency ablation, of focal liver disease, 903

Achalasia, in children, 298

United States Postal Service
Statement of Ownership, Management, and Circulation

1. Publication Title	2. Publication Number	3. Filing Date
Radiologic Clinics of North America	0 0 3 3 - 8 3 8 9	9/15/05

4. Issue Frequency	5. Number of Issues Published Annually	6. Annual Subscription Price
Jan, Mar, May, Jul, Sep, Nov	6	$220.00

7. Complete Mailing Address of Known Office of Publication (Not printer) (Street, city, county, state, and ZIP+4)

Elsevier Inc.
6277 Sea Harbor Drive
Orlando, FL 32887-4800

Contact Person: Gwen C. Campbell
Telephone: 215-239-3685

8. Complete Mailing Address of Headquarters or General Business Office of Publisher (Not printer)

Elsevier Inc., 360 Park Avenue South, New York, NY 10010-1710

9. Full Names and Complete Mailing Addresses of Publisher, Editor, and Managing Editor (Do not leave blank)

Publisher (Name and complete mailing address)

Tim Griswold, Elsevier Inc., 1600 John F. Kennedy Blvd., Suite 1800, Philadelphia, PA 19103-2899

Editor (Name and complete mailing address)

Barton Dudlick, Elsevier Inc., 1600 John F. Kennedy Blvd., Suite 1800, Philadelphia, PA 19103-2899

Managing Editor (Name and complete mailing address)

Heather Cullen, Elsevier Inc., 1600 John F. Kennedy Blvd., Suite 1800, Philadelphia, PA 19103-2899

10. Owner (Do not leave blank. If the publication is owned by a corporation, give the name and address of the corporation immediately followed by the names and addresses of all stockholders owning or holding 1 percent or more of the total amount of stock. If not owned by a corporation, give the names and addresses of the individual owners. If owned by a partnership or other unincorporated firm, give its name and address as well as those of each individual owner. If the publication is published by a nonprofit organization, give its name and address.)

Full Name	Complete Mailing Address
Wholly owned subsidiary of	4520 East-West Highway
Reed/Elsevier, US Holdings	Bethesda, MD 20814

11. Known Bondholders, Mortgagees, and Other Security Holders Owning or Holding 1 Percent or More of Total Amount of Bonds, Mortgages, or Other Securities. If none, check box ☐ None

Full Name	Complete Mailing Address
N/A	

12. Tax Status (For completion by nonprofit organizations authorized to mail at nonprofit rates) (Check one)
The purpose, function, and nonprofit status of this organization and the exempt status for federal income tax purposes:
☐ Has Not Changed During Preceding 12 Months
☐ Has Changed During Preceding 12 Months (Publisher must submit explanation of change with this statement)

(See Instructions on Reverse)

PS Form 3526, October 1999

13. Publication Title	14. Issue Date for Circulation Data Below
Radiologic Clinics of North America	July 2005

15.			Extent and Nature of Circulation	Average No. Copies Each Issue During Preceding 12 Months	No. Copies of Single Issue Published Nearest to Filing Date
a.			Total Number of Copies (Net press run)	8417	7900
b.	Paid and/or Requested Circulation	(1)	Paid/Requested Outside-County Mail Subscriptions Stated on Form 3541. (Include advertiser's proof and exchange copies)	4507	4433
		(2)	Paid In-County Subscriptions Stated on Form 3541 (Include advertiser's proof and exchange copies)		
		(3)	Sales Through Dealers and Carriers, Street Vendors, Counter Sales, and Other Non-USPS Paid Distribution	1903	2039
		(4)	Other Classes Mailed Through the USPS		
c.			Total Paid and/or Requested Circulation [Sum of 15b. (1), (2), (3), and (4)]	6437	6472
d.	Free Distribution by Mail (Samples, complimentary, and other free)	(1)	Outside-County as Stated on Form 3541	137	139
		(2)	In-County as Stated on Form 3541		
		(3)	Other Classes Mailed Through the USPS		
e.			Free Distribution Outside the Mail (Carriers or other means)		
f.			Total Free Distribution (Sum of 15d. and 15e.)	137	139
g.			Total Distribution (Sum of 15c. and 15f.)	6574	6611
h.			Copies not Distributed	1843	1289
i.			Total (Sum of 15g. and h.)	8417	7900
j.			Percent Paid and/or Requested Circulation (15c. divided by 15g. times 100)	98%	98%

16. Publication of Statement of Ownership
☐ Publication required. Will be printed in the November 2005 issue of this publication.
☐ Publication not required

17. Signature and Title of Editor, Publisher, Business Manager, or Owner   Date

John Fanucci - Executive Director of Subscription Services   9/15/05

I certify that all information furnished on this form is true and complete. I understand that anyone who furnishes false or misleading information on this form or who omits material or information requested on the form may be subject to criminal sanctions (including fines and imprisonment) and/or civil sanctions (including civil penalties).

Instructions to Publishers

1. Complete and file one copy of this form with your postmaster annually on or before October 1. Keep a copy of the completed form for your records.
2. In cases where the stockholder or security holder is a trustee, include in items 10 and 11 the name of the person or corporation for whom the trustee is acting. Also include the names and addresses of individuals who are stockholders who own or hold 1 percent or more of the total amount of bonds, mortgages, or other securities of the publishing corporation. In item 11, if none, check the box. Use blank sheets if more space is required.
3. Be sure to furnish all circulation information called for in item 15. Free circulation must be shown in items 15d, e, and f.
4. Item 15h., Copies not Distributed, must include (1) newsstand copies originally stated on Form 3541, and returned to the publisher, (2) estimated returns from news agents, and (3), copies for office use, leftovers, spoiled, and all other copies not distributed.
5. If the publication had Periodicals authorization as a general or requester publication, this Statement of Ownership, Management, and Circulation must be published; it must be printed in any issue in October or, if the publication is not published during October, the first issue printed after October.
6. In item 16, indicate the date of the issue in which this Statement of Ownership will be published.
7. Item 17 must be signed.
Failure to file or publish a statement of ownership may lead to suspension of Periodicals authorization.

PS Form 3526, October 1999 (Reverse)

Changing Your Address?

Make sure your subscription changes too! When you notify us of your new address, you can help make our job easier by including an exact copy of your Clinics label number with your old address (see illustration below.) This number identifies you to our computer system and will speed the processing of your address change. Please be sure this label number accompanies your old address and your corrected address—you can send an old Clinics label with your number on it or just copy it exactly and send it to the address listed below.

We appreciate your help in our attempt to give you continuous coverage. Thank you.

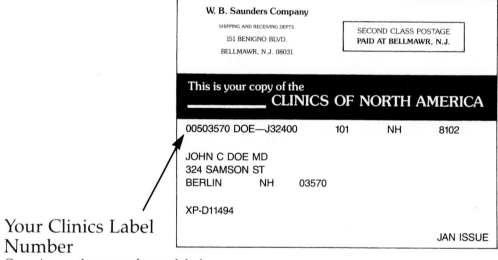

Your Clinics Label Number

Copy it exactly or send your label
along with your address to:
W.B. Saunders Company, Customer Service
Orlando, FL 32887-4800
Call Toll Free 1-800-654-2452

Please allow four to six weeks for delivery of new subscriptions and for processing address changes.